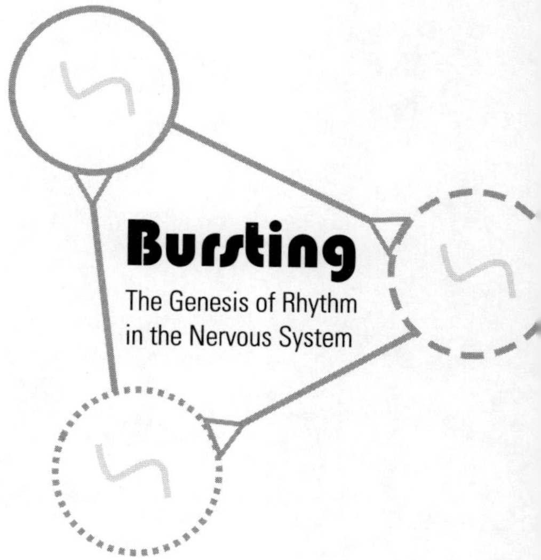

Bursting

The Genesis of Rhythm in the Nervous System

Bursting

The Genesis of Rhythm in the Nervous System

editors

Stephen Coombes
The University of Nottingham, UK

Paul C. Bressloff
University of Utah, USA

World Scientific

NEW JERSEY • LONDON • SINGAPORE • BEIJING • SHANGHAI • HONG KONG • TAIPEI • CHENNAI

Published by

World Scientific Publishing Co. Pte. Ltd.

5 Toh Tuck Link, Singapore 596224

USA office: 27 Warren Street, Suite 401-402, Hackensack, NJ 07601

UK office: 57 Shelton Street, Covent Garden, London WC2H 9HE

Library of Congress Cataloging-in-Publication Data

Bursting: the genesis of rhythm in the nervous system / edited by Stephen Coombes, Paul C. Bressloff.

p. cm.

Includes bibliographical references and index.

ISBN 981-256-506-X

1. Neural transmission. 2. Sensory neurons. I. Coombes, Stephen. II. Bressloff, Paul C.

QP364.5.B57 2005

612.8'1--dc22

2005051845

British Library Cataloguing-in-Publication Data

A catalogue record for this book is available from the British Library.

Printed in Singapore by World Scientific Printers (S) Pte Ltd

PREFACE

Neurons in the brain communicate with each other by transmitting sequences of electrical spikes or action potentials. One of the major challenges in neuroscience is to understand the basic physiological mechanisms underlying the complex spatiotemporal patterns of spiking activity observed during normal brain functioning, and to determine the origins of pathological dynamical states such as epileptic seizures and Parkinsonian tremors. A second major challenge is to understand how the patterns of spiking activity provide a substrate for the encoding and transmission of information, that is, how do neurons compute with spikes? It is likely that an important element of both the dynamical and computational properties of neurons is that they can exhibit bursting.

Bursting is a relatively slow rhythmic alternation between an active phase of rapid spiking and a quiescent phase without spiking. It is exhibited by a wide range of nerve and endocrine cells, including pancreatic β-cells, respiratory pacemaker neurons in the pre-Bötzinger complex, dopaminergic neurons of the mammalian midbrain, thalamic relay cells, and pyramidal neurons in the neocortex. Following the seminal work of John Rinzel and collaborators, a general framework for understanding the biophysical origins of bursting has been developed using mathematical and computational modeling. The fundamental idea is to dissect the full dynamics of a neuron into a fast subsystem coupled to a slowly varying subsystem. Typically, the fast subsystem has a time-scale of milliseconds and models the membrane potential and spike generation process, whereas the slow subsystem operates on a time-scale of seconds and models slow trans-membrane ionic currents. For many types of bursting, as exemplified by square wave bursting in pancreatic β-cells, the fast subsystem exhibits bistability between a quiescent fixed point and an active oscillatory state. At least one slow variable is then required to alternate back and forth through the region of bistability such that the neuron periodically jumps between the active and quiescent phases along a hysteresis loop. It is also possible to generate bursting without bistability in the fast subsystem, provided that there are at least two variables in the slow subsystem that periodically sweep the fast subsystem through a sequence of bifurcations. This is exemplified by parabolic bursting in the abdominal ganglion neuron of Aplysia.

In recent years, several classification schemes of the various forms of bursting behavior have been developed by investigating the detailed bifurcation structure of the fast and slow subsystems. From a mathematical perspective, these classifications characterize the bursting behavior in terms of the topologies of the invariant sets (fixed points, periodic orbits etc.) that the solutions visit, and the various transitions between these sets. From a phenomenological perspective, they describe various properties of bursting such as the amplitude and shape of spikes, the evolution of the spiking frequency during the active phase, and the duration of the quiescent phase. These phenomena can also be measured experimentally and used to classify biological bursters. Although most studies of bursting mechanisms have been based on isopotential point neuron models, it is also possible for bursting to arise through interactions between different parts of the cell, namely the soma and dendrites, or through interactions between cells. In the latter case individual cells may themselves not be intrinsic bursters.

This book provides a detailed overview of the current state-of-the-art in the mathematical and computational modeling of bursting, with contributions from many of the leading researchers in the field. It is a natural complement to the more pedagogical work of Eugene M. Izhikevich (Dynamical Systems in Neuroscience: The Geometry of Excitability and Bursting, The MIT Press, to appear), and is divided into two parts. Part I (chapters 1–6) covers bursting at the single cell level and Part II (chapters 7–14) covers bursting at the network level. The first few chapters describe some specific examples of conductance-based models of bursting: the Hindmarsh-Rose model of a bursting neuron (chapter 1), the Chay-Keizer model of insulin secreting pancreatic cells (chapter 2), and a recent model of bursting in endocrine cells of the hypothalamus (chapter 3). This is followed by a bifurcation analysis of a reduced bursting model that highlights some important features regarding the decomposition into fast/slow subsystems (chapter 4). The final two chapters of Part I concern bursting in two-compartment models, consisting of a soma electrically coupled to an active dendritic compartment. The first shows how geometric methods can be used to study the well known Pinsky-Rinzel model of a hippocampal CA3 pyramidal neuron (chapter 5), and the second reviews a recent model of "ghostbursting", which is a novel type of bursting observed in sensory processing neurons of weakly electric fish (chapter 6). In the latter case, some possible computational advantages of bursting are discussed. Part II begins with an analysis of phase-locking in small networks of coupled bursting neurons using phase resetting curves (chapter 7). This is followed by an analysis of bursting in two-cell systems using symmetric bifurcation theory (chapter 8), which illustrates how local singularity theory rather than global geometric methods can also be used to classify different bursting mechanisms. The next four chapters consider the effects of coupling on bursting at the network level. First, a computationally efficient method for studying networks of cells is described, based on coupled bursting maps (chapter 9). This is followed by an analysis of diffusively coupled square-wave bursters (chapter 10). Two examples of bursting in excitatory networks are then considered. The first concerns a mean field model of spontaneous episodic activity in developing spinal cord networks, in which the individual cells are not themselves intrinsic bursters and the slow process arises from synaptic depression (chapter 11). The second involves a model of oscillatory bursting in an excitatory network of synaptically coupled respiratory neurons of the pre-Bötzinger complex (chapter 12). The last two chapters of Part II consider wave propagation in bursting networks: a geometric analysis of traveling waves in models of thalamic networks (chapter 13) and the effects of depolarization block on wave propagation in a model of disinhibited cortical slices (chapter 14).

S. Coombes
School of Mathematical Sciences
University of Nottingham, UK.

P. C. Bressloff
Department of Mathematics
University of Utah, USA.

June, 2005.

CONTENTS

PART II: BURSTING AT THE NETWORK LEVEL

PART I:
BURSTING AT THE SINGLE CELL LEVEL

CHAPTER 1

THE DEVELOPMENT OF THE HINDMARSH-ROSE MODEL FOR BURSTING

Jim Hindmarsh
Philip Cornelius
Cardiff School of Mathematics, Cardiff University, Senghenydd Road, Cardiff CF24 4AG, Wales UK
e-mail: hindmarsh@cardiff.ac.uk; philip.cornelius@croftvillas.com

We review the development of the Hindmarsh-Rose equations of 1982 and 1984. After a brief description of bifurcations in a model for subthreshold oscillations, that can generate bursting, we show that similar bifurcations will not be found in the Hindmarsh-Rose nor in other similar equations.

1.1. Introduction

The collaboration that led to the Hindmarsh-Rose model began in 1979 shortly after Malcolm Rose joined Cardiff University. The particular project was to model the synchronization of firing of two snail neurons in a relatively simple way that did not use the full Hodgkin-Huxley equations [6]. A natural choice at the time was to use equations of the FitzHugh [2] type

$$\dot{x} = a(y - f(x) + I(t)) \,, \tag{1}$$

$$\dot{y} = b(g(x) - y) \,, \tag{2}$$

where x represents the membrane potential and y an internal, or recovery, variable. The function f is cubic, the function g is linear, a, b are time constants, and $I(t)$ is the external, applied, or clamping current at time t.

A problem with this choice was that these equations do not provide a very realistic description of the rapid firing of the neuron compared to the relatively long interval between firing. Attempts were made to achieve a more realistic description by making the time constants a, b voltage dependent. In particular so the rates of change of x and y were much smaller in the subthreshold or recovery phase. These were not convincing and it was not until Malcolm raised the question about whether the FitzHugh equations could account for "tail current reversal" that progress was made[a].

The modification of the FitzHugh equations to account for tail current reversal was crucial for the development of the Hindmarsh-Rose model.

1.2. Tail Current Reversal

This effect is described by the following numerical experiment on the Hodgkin-Huxley equations. Suppose the Hodgkin-Huxley equations are voltage clamped to an initial potential of -40mv (where the resting potential is -60mv). This means that a suitable external, or clamping, current is applied so that the membrane potential is held constant at -40mv. If the potential to which the equations are voltage clamped is now instantaneously changed to -50mv the clamping current will change over a period of time until equilibrium is reached. The behaviour in time of this clamping current has two stages, an initial response followed by a long 'tail' current. The initial response is a steep increase and the tail current is a slow decrease. If instead of instantaneously clamping the equations from -40mv to -50mv they are clamped from -40mv to -80mv then the tail current is increasing. The reason for this reversal of direction is that the behaviour of these tail currents in this situation is dominated by the Potassium current $I_K = g_K n^4(V_c - V_K)$ which changes sign as the clamping potential V_c goes below V_K = -72mv.

To see what the FitzHugh model has to say about this, assume that the model described by equations (1) and (2) is voltage clamped to some initial potential x_i. This means, from equation (2), that $y(t)$ changes to its equilibrium value $g(x_i)$. Now, at time $t = 0$, clamp the cell to a new potential $x_c < x_i$. The applied current at times $t \geq 0$ is given from equation (1), with $\dot{x} = 0$ (because we have clamped the voltage) and $x = x_c$, by

$$I(t) = f(x_c) - y(t)\,, \tag{3}$$

where y satisfies

$$\dot{y} = b(g(x_c) - y)\,, \quad y(0) = g(x_i)$$

whose solution is

$$y(t) = g(x_c) - \big(g(x_c) - g(x_i)\big)e^{-bt}\,. \tag{4}$$

[a]When asked about this many years afterwards Malcolm could not recall what had prompted him to ask this question.

From equations (3), and (4) we see that

$$I(t) = f(x_c) - g(x_c) + \big(g(x_c) - g(x_i)\big)e^{-bt}\,. \tag{5}$$

The tail current $I(t)$, given by equation (5), is decreasing if $g(x_c)-g(x_i) > 0$ and increasing if $g(x_c)-g(x_i) < 0$. It follows that if the model is to describe tail current reversal then $g(x_c) - g(x_i)$ must change sign as x_c is lowered. This cannot happen if g is a linear function of x. Clearly the y-nullcline, whose equation is

$$y = g(x)\,, \tag{6}$$

has to be modified. In keeping with the qualitative nature of the FitzHugh model, the simplest change to the y-nullcline that would allow a change in sign for $g(x_c) - g(x_i)$, would be to make g a quadratic function. This was overlooked at the time because the analysis of tail current reversal using the FitzHugh model suggested the experimental approach described in the next section.

1.3. The 1982 Model

The equations for the 1982 model [4] came from voltage clamp data obtained from pond snails[b]. The experiment performed was as follows.

(i) Adjust the applied current so that the cell is in equilibrium just below the firing threshold and recalibrate the applied current so that $I = 0$ for this equilibrium.

(ii) Assume the cell may be described by equations (1) and (2), and that this equilibrium is at $x = 0$ and $y = 0$. This means the y-nullcline, equation (6), passes through $(0,0)$ so

$$0 = g(0)\,, \tag{7}$$

and that our initial clamping potential $x_i = 0$.

(iii) Voltage clamp to potential x_c and record the applied current $I(t)$, in particular $I(0)$ and $I(\infty)$.

From equation (5), and using (7), we see

$$I(0) = f(x_c) - g(0) = f(x_c)\,,$$
$$I(\infty) = f(x_c) - g(x_c)\,,$$

[b] Malcolm had found a good supply of these in a canal in the Taff valley of South Wales. They had unusually large neurons which made the experimental work easier.

from which

$$f(x_c) = I(0)\,,$$
$$g(x_c) = I(0) - I(\infty)\,.$$

By measuring $I(0)$ and $I(\infty)$ for different x_c information was obtained about f and g. This suggested that $f - g$ could be described by an exponential function and f by a cubic function. The case for a cubic function for f was not convincing. It was possible to perform the above experiment for clamping potentials only just into the subthreshold region. The results were not inconsistent with a cubic, FitzHugh had used a cubic, and so a cubic was chosen. If the same experiment had been performed numerically with the Hodgkin Huxley equations then a cubic would almost certainly have been rejected and it is unlikely that any useful modification of the FitzHugh equations would have been found.

The time constant a was estimated by applying a constant current to the cell at equilibrium. Because this equilibrium is assumed to correspond to the equilibrium point at $(0,0)$ in the model, the initial rate of change of potential, using equation (1) with $x = 0, y = 0, f(0) = 0, t = 0$, is given by

$$\dot{x}(0) = aI\,.$$

Measuring $\dot{x}(0)$ and I gives a. The time constant b was obtained from recordings of $I(t)$ using equation (5). For more details of the above procedure see the 1982 model [4].

This provided all the information necessary to integrate the equations[c]. The first results showed, in the same way as the FitzHugh equations, these equations modelled the transition from a stable equilibrium to stable repetitive firing. There was was also the additional result that the potential showed a long period of slow change followed by a short period of rapid change. In other words a long interval between rapid firing.

This was completely unexpected because all that had been attempted was to modify the y-nullcline, in order to account for tail current reversal. It was however quickly explained by looking at the nullcline diagram shown qualitatively in Fig. 1.1.

When the limit cycle crosses the x-nullcline at C it is trapped in a "narrow channel" between the nullclines and cannot leave until near the top at A. Whilst the state is in this channel it is close to both nullclines

[c]This was done by giving a bundle of punched cards to a main frame computer and returning a few hours later to receive pages of printed output.

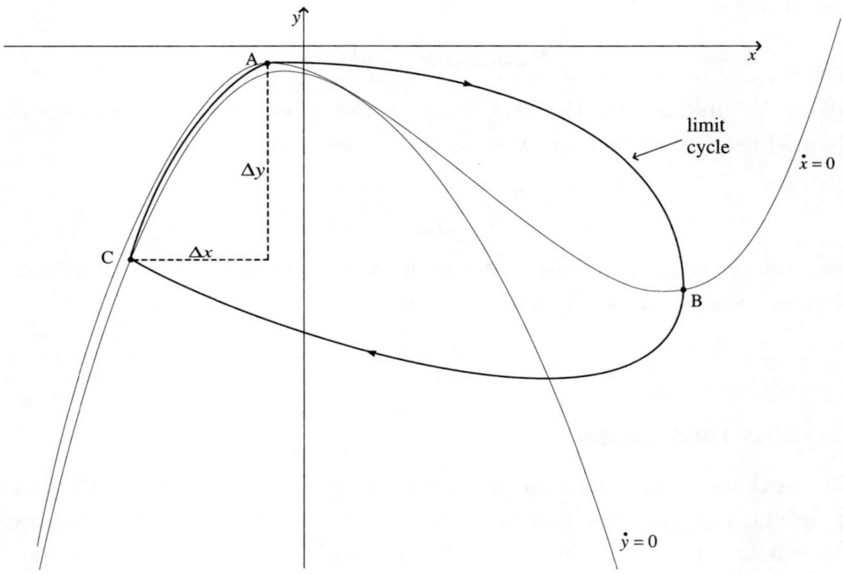

Fig. 1.1. Nullclines and firing limit cycle for the 1982 model. The limit cycle is the closed path A, B, C, A. The changes in x and y as the state changes up the narrow channel between the nullclines from C to A are Δx and Δy.

and so both $\dot{x}$ and $\dot{y}$ are small. This means the state changes slowly giving the long interspike interval.

The model also provided an explanation for the approximately linear relation between applied external current and the frequency of firing. This comes about as follows. Taking a linear combination of equations (1) and (2) we obtain

$$b\dot{x} + a\dot{y} = ab\big(g(x) - f(x)\big) + abI\,. \tag{8}$$

The interspike interval τ is approximately the time spent in the narrow channel because the firing spike is of comparatively short duration. Integrate both sides of equation (8) from time $t = 0$ when the state enters the channel to the time $t = \tau$ when it leaves the channel. Ignore the term $ab\big(g(x) - f(x)\big)$ because between C and A $g(x) \approx f(x)$ and over the range of applied current I considered

$$|\big(g(x) - f(x)\big)| \ll I\,.$$

The result is

$$b\Delta x + a\Delta y \approx abI\tau\,,$$

where Δx and Δy are the changes in x and y as the state moves up the channel from C to A. From this the frequency f is given by

$$f \propto \frac{1}{\tau} \approx \frac{abI}{b\Delta x + a\Delta y}\,.$$

Because Δx and Δy change very little with I we see that the frequency increases linearly with the applied current

$$f \propto I\,.$$

1.4. The 1984 Model

The next step was to create a model for neurons that exhibit triggered firing. This means they can be switched from a subthreshold stable resting state to a stable firing state by the application of a positive applied current pulse of short duration. The model required more than one equilibrium point. One inside the limit cycle corresponding to firing and one for the subthreshold stable resting state at a potential below the firing cycle. Because the nullclines were so close in the subthreshold region only a small deformation to the shape of the nullclines was required to make them intersect and create the extra equilibrium points.

At this point it seemed more attractive to abandon the quantitative models in favour of a qualitative model. The equations chosen were

$$\dot{x} = y - x^3 + 3x^2 + I\,, \tag{9}$$

$$\dot{y} = 1 - 5x^2 - y\,. \tag{10}$$

Whose nullclines are shown qualitatively in Fig. 1.2. This nullcline diagram shows how the model explains triggered repetitive firing. If the state of the system is initially in the stable resting state, and a positive current pulse of short duration is applied, the effect is to lower the x-nullcline so the middle equilibrium point B and the left hand equilibrium point C meet and vanish. This allows the state to rise up the narrow channel and enter a stable limit cycle. Termination of the positive current pulse does not force the state away from this limit cycle but application of a suitable negative current pulse does.

In order to terminate the firing an adaptation variable was added to the model. This variable, z, represented a slowly varying current that changed

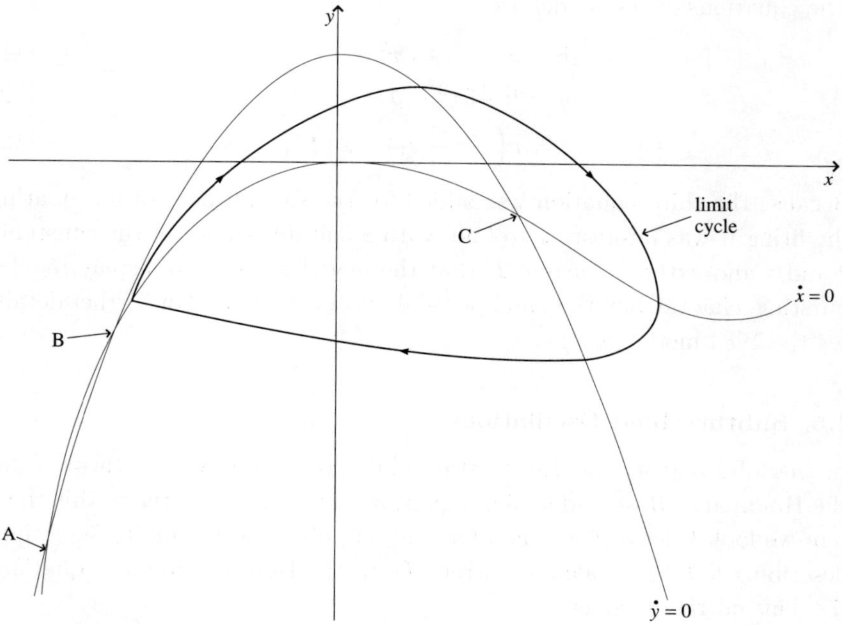

Fig. 1.2. Nullclines for the 1984 model when $I = 0$. The x-nullcline is above the y-nullcline between the stable equilibrium point A and the saddle equilibrium point B. The third equilibrium point C is unstable.

the applied current I to an effective applied current $I - z$. A differential equation was required that would raise the value of z when the model is firing and so lower the effective applied current leading to the termination of firing. The equation chosen was

$$\dot{z} = r\Big(s(x - x_1) - z\Big),$$

where x_1 is the x-coordinate of the stable subthreshold equilibrium point of the two dimensional system of equations (9) and (10) in the case $I = 0$[d].

[d]The x-coordinates of the three equilibrium points are $-\phi$, -1, and $\phi - 1$, where ϕ is the Golden Number $\frac{\sqrt{5}+1}{2}$. This fact appears to have no relevance whatsoever.

The equations of the model are

$$\dot{x} = y - x^3 + 3x^2 + I - z\,, \tag{11}$$

$$\dot{y} = 1 - 5x^2 - y\,, \tag{12}$$

$$\dot{z} = r\Big(s(x - x_1) - z\Big)\,, \tag{13}$$

Because the third equation was added for the sole purpose of terminating the firing it was interesting to find, with a suitable choice of the constants r and s and external current I, that the model would also display regular bursting, chaotic bursting, and post-inhibitory rebound. For further details see the 1984 model [5].

1.5. Subthreshold Oscillations

In the following section 1.6 we state and prove a bifurcation theorem for the Hindmarsh-Rose and similar equations. In order to motivate this theorem we look briefly at a model for bursting obtained by adding equations describing a T-type calcium current I_T to the Hodgkin Huxley equations [7]. This current is given by

$$I_T = g_T\, m_T^3\, h_T\, (V - V_{Ca})\ ,$$

where the activation variable m_T changes sufficiently rapidly that

$$m_T = m_{T_\infty}(V) = \frac{1}{1 + e^{-\gamma_{m_T}\left(V - \theta_{m_T}\right)}}\,,$$

whereas h_T changes according to

$$\frac{dh_T}{dt} = \tau_{h_T}^{-1}\,(h_{T_\infty}(V) - h_T)\ ,$$

where

$$h_{T_\infty}(V) = \frac{1}{1 + e^{\gamma_{h_T}\left(V - \theta_{h_T}\right)}}\,,$$

and θ_{m_T}, θ_{h_T}, γ_{m_T}, γ_{h_T} and τ_{h_T} are constants.

Adding the I_T current can generate subthreshold oscillations which in turn can generate bursting behavior. To see how this happens we look at the system in the case where the currents responsible for the firing cycle are absent. In other words we look at the subsystem

$$\dot{V} = C^{-1}\,(I - I_L - I_T)\ , \tag{14}$$

$$\dot{h}_T = \tau_{h_T}^{-1}\,(h_{T\infty}(V) - h_T)\ , \tag{15}$$

where

$$I_L = g_L(V - V_L)\,,$$

is a leakage current. To simplify the appearance of equations (14) and (15) we define the functions f and k by

$$\begin{aligned} f &: V \mapsto f(V) = g_L(V - V_L)\,, \\ k &: V \mapsto k(V) = m_{T_\infty}(V)(V - V_{Ca})\,, \end{aligned}$$

omit the sub-fix T_∞ from h_{T_∞}, and h_T from $\tau_{h_T}^{-1}$, put $C = 1$, and rename the variables V and h_T by x and y. Equations (14) and (15) become

$$\begin{aligned} \dot{x} &= f(x) - g_T k(x) y + I\,, \\ \dot{y} &= \tau^{-1}(h(x) - y)\,. \end{aligned}$$

We will look at current-voltage bifurcation diagrams for these equations where the external current I is the bifurcation parameter. As I varies so does the equilibrium point. Suppose there is an equilibrium point at (x_E, y_E) then this is completely specified by x_E because

$$y_E = h(x_E)\,.$$

For this equilibrium point the external current is given as a function of x_E by

$$I = I(x_E) = -f(x_E) + g_T k(x_E) y_E = -f(x_E) + g_T k(x_E) h(x_E)\,.$$

The stability of this equilibrium point is obtained from the linear approximation matrix

$$A = \begin{bmatrix} f'(x) - g_T k'(x) y & -g_T k(x) \\ \tau^{-1} h'(x) & -\tau^{-1} \end{bmatrix}.$$

Evaluating these matrix elements at the equilibrium point (x_E, y_E), and using $y_E = h(x_E)$, we obtain the matrix

$$A(x_E) = \begin{bmatrix} f'(x_E) - g_T k'(x_E) h(x_E) & -g_T k(x_E) \\ \tau^{-1} h'(x_E) & -\tau^{-1} \end{bmatrix}.$$

The stability is determined by the trace and determinant of $A(x_E)$ which are

$$\begin{aligned} \mathrm{Tr}\,(A(x_E)) &= f'(x_E) - g_T k'(x_E) h(x_E) - \tau^{-1}\,, \\ \mathrm{Det}\,(A(x_E)) &= -\tau^{-1} f'(x_E) + \tau^{-1} g_T k'(x_E) h(x_E) + \tau^{-1} g_T k(x_E) h'(x_E) \\ &= \tau^{-1}\left(-f'(x_E) + g_T\,(kh)'\,(x_E)\right). \end{aligned}$$

We will be interested in equilibrium points where

$$\text{Det}\,(A(x_E)) > 0\,.$$

For such equilibrium points we have

$$I'(x_E) = -f'(x_E) + g_T\,(kh)'\,(x_E) = \tau\text{Det}\,A(x_E) > 0$$

and so I is strictly increasing with x_E. This means we may use x_E as the bifurcation parameter instead of I.

As x_E varies the values of Tr $(A(x_E))$ and Det$(A(x_E))$ determine a point on a path in the trace-determinant stability diagram. We call such a path

$$\gamma : x_E \mapsto \gamma(x_E) = \big(\text{Tr}\,A(x_E), \text{Det}\,A(x_E)\big)$$

the stability path. Figure 1.3 shows three stability paths obtained for different values of the constants θ_{m_T}, θ_{h_T}, γ_{m_T}, γ_{h_T} and τ_{h_T}. The innermost (a) lies wholly inside the top left quadrant so all its equilibrium points are stable, the next one (b) touches the positive Det-axis and the third (c) crosses into the top right quadrant and so has unstable equilibrium points. For each stability path there is a corresponding current voltage diagram showing the position of equilibrium points and upper and lower points on the limit cycles for each value of current. These are shown in Fig. 1.4.

In Fig. 1.4(a) there is a path of stable equilibrium points and there are also stable and unstable limit cycles corresponding to the two closed curves. The stable limit cycle is outermost. In Fig. 1.4(b) there is a figure of eight bifurcation diagram corresponding to the stability path that touches the positive Det-axis. In Fig. 1.4(c) there are two subcritical Hopf Bifurcations where the branching small amplitude limit cycles are unstable. What is happening, as one or more parameters change, is the stability path approaches, touches and crosses the positive Det-axis. When it touches the positive Det-axis, and we have the figure of eight current-voltage bifurcation diagram, the small amplitude limit cycles are unstable just as they are for the subcritical Hopf bifurcations that appear once the stability path has crossed the positive Det-axis.

Suppose a stability path touches the positive Det-axis at the point

$$\gamma(x_B) = \big(\text{Tr}\,A(x_B), \text{Det}\,A(x_B)\big)\,.$$

At this point in the stability diagram, which corresponds to the equilibrium

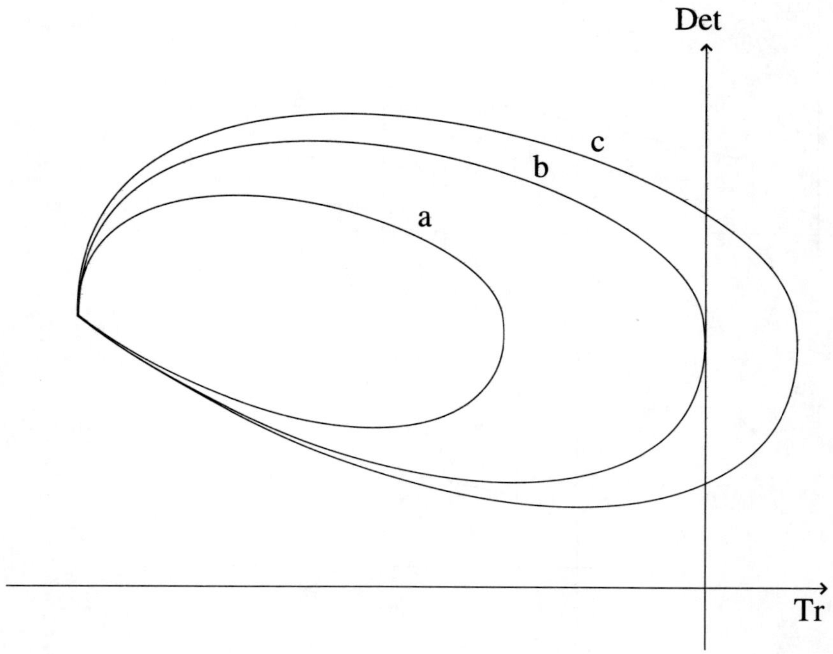

Fig. 1.3. Stability paths for equations (14) and (15) obtained for different values of the constants θ_{m_T}, θ_{h_T}, γ_{m_T}, γ_{h_T} and τ_{h_T}. Each point on a path corresponds to an equilibrium point of these equations which is stable if the path point lies in the top left quadrant.

point (x_B, y_B), we have

$$\begin{aligned} \operatorname{Tr} A(x_B) &= 0\,, \\ (\operatorname{Tr} A)'(x_B) &= 0\,, \\ (\operatorname{Tr} A)''(x_B) &< 0\,, \\ \operatorname{Det} A(x_B) &> 0\,. \end{aligned}$$

The values of θ_{m_T}, θ_{h_T}, γ_{m_T}, γ_{h_T} and τ_{h_T} required to obtain the stability paths of Fig. 1.3 and the current voltage diagrams of Fig. 1.4 have to be chosen with care. This was done analytically using the conditions above together with the condition that the Hopf bifurcations create small amplitude limit cycles which are unstable [1].

The reason for our interest in this situation is that for systems having

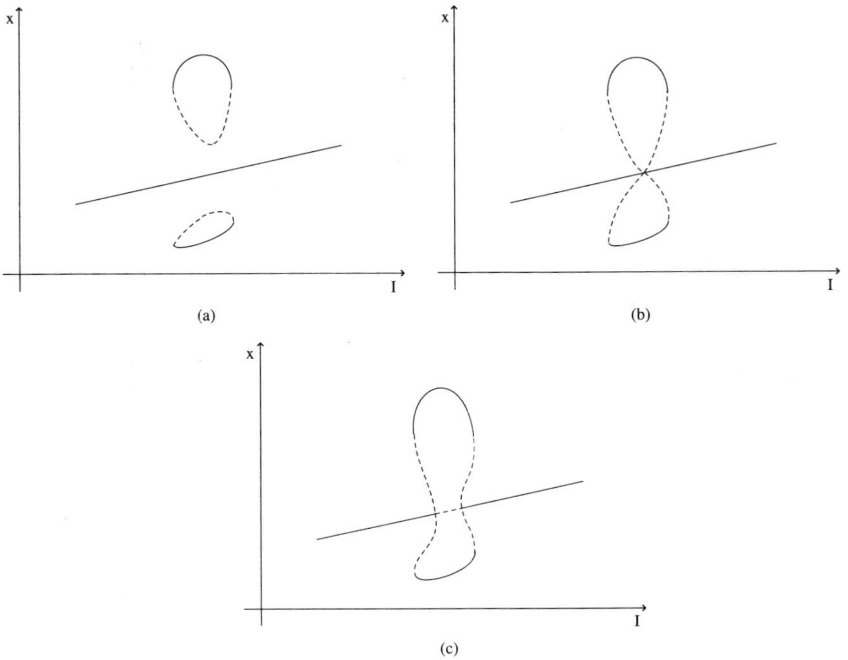

Fig. 1.4. Current-voltage (I-x) diagrams for each of the three stability paths shown in Fig. 1.3.

bifurcation diagrams like the one shown in Fig. 1.4(a) slow changes in the current I through the range shown will keep the system in a stable equilibrium point. This would not happen in the case shown in Fig. 1.4(c) where the equilibrium point becomes unstable when I reaches a Hopf bifurcation value. In the case of Fig. 1.4(a) suppose the system is at a stable equilibrium point for an I value in the range where the system also has a stable limit cycle. If the current I is subject to a rapid change, for example a current pulse, the state of the system may be displaced to the limit cycle. Alternatively the limit cycle could be reached by resonance induced by periodic stimulation. These effects may provide a mechanism for information processing.

In order to examine this possibility in the simpler context of qualitative models an attempt was made to modify the Hindmarsh-Rose equations so that they had a figure of eight current-voltage bifurcation diagram. This was unsuccessful for reasons explained in the next section.

1.6. A Bifurcation Theorem

We will show that models such as those of Hindmarsh-Rose, Fitzhugh-Nagumo and Morris-Lecar whose equations may, after scaling if necessary, be written in the form

$$\dot{x} = y - f(x) + \alpha\, x\, y + I\,,$$
$$\dot{y} = g(x) - y\,,$$

where α is a constant, cannot have a figure of eight bifurcation diagram as found in section 1.5.

Theorem 1: Suppose the equations

$$\dot{x} = y - f(x) + \alpha\, x\, y + I \tag{16}$$
$$\dot{y} = g(x) - y \tag{17}$$

have a stability path which contains an equilibrium point (x_B, y_B) for which

$$\mathrm{Tr}\, A(x_B) = 0\,, \tag{18}$$
$$(\mathrm{Tr}\, A)'(x_B) = 0\,, \tag{19}$$
$$(\mathrm{Tr}\, A)''(x_B) < 0\,, \tag{20}$$
$$\mathrm{Det}\, A(x_B) > 0\,, \tag{21}$$

then the nonlinear normal form at this equilibrium point is

$$\dot{r} = Lr^3 + O(r^5) + \ldots$$
$$\dot{\theta} = \omega + O(r^2) + \ldots\,,$$

where

$$L = \frac{1}{16}(\mathrm{Tr}\, A)''(x_B) < 0$$
$$\omega^2 = \mathrm{Det}\, A(x_B)\,.$$

Proof: The linear approximation matrix for the system described by equations (16) and (17) at equilibrium point (x_B, y_B) is

$$A(x_B) = \begin{bmatrix} -f'(x_B) + a\, y_0 & 1 + a\, x_B \\ g'(x_B) & -1 \end{bmatrix}.$$

The trace of which is

$$\mathrm{Tr}\, A(x_B) = -f'(x_B) + a\, g(x_B) - 1\,,$$

which, using conditions (18) and (19) gives us,

$$\operatorname{Tr} A(x_B) = -f'(x_B) + \alpha y_B - 1 = -f'(x_B) + \alpha g(x_B) - 1 = 0\,, \qquad (22)$$

$$(\operatorname{Tr} A)'(x_B) = -f''(x_B) + \alpha g'(x_B) = 0\,. \qquad (23)$$

We define

$$\omega^2 = \operatorname{Det} A(x_B) = f'(x_B) - \alpha\, g(x_B) - g'(x_B)(1 + \alpha\, x_B)\,. \qquad (24)$$

From equations (22), (23), and (24) we have

$$-f'(x_B) + \alpha g(x_B) = 1\,, \qquad (25)$$

$$g'(x_B) = \frac{f''(x_B)}{\alpha}\,, \qquad (26)$$

$$1 + \alpha\, x_B = \frac{\alpha(\omega^2 + 1)}{f''(x_B)}\,. \qquad (27)$$

Now expand equations (16) and (17) as Taylor series about (x_B, y_B) and use new coordinates $X = x - x_B, Y = y - y_B$. The equations for X and Y are

$$\begin{aligned}\dot{X} &= (-f'(x_B) + \alpha\, y_B)X + (1 + \alpha y_B)Y + \alpha XY \\ &\quad - \frac{f''(x_B)}{2}X^2 - \frac{f'''(x_B)}{6}X^3 \ldots\,, \\ \dot{Y} &= g'(x_B)X - Y + \frac{g''(x_B)}{2}X^2 + \frac{g'''(x_B)}{6}X^3 \ldots\,.\end{aligned}$$

Using (25), (26), and (27) the above equations become

$$\begin{aligned}\dot{X} &= X + \frac{\alpha(\omega^2 + 1)}{f''(x_B)}Y + \alpha XY \\ &\quad - \frac{f''(x_B)}{2}X^2 - \frac{f'''(x_B)}{6}X^3 \ldots\,, \qquad (28) \\ \dot{Y} &= \frac{f''(x_B)}{\alpha}X - Y + \frac{g''(x_B)}{2}X^2 + \frac{g'''(x_B)}{6}X^3 \ldots\,. \qquad (29)\end{aligned}$$

Finally we make the transformation

$$\begin{aligned}X &= v\,, \\ Y &= \frac{f''(x_B)}{\alpha(\omega^2 + 1)}(-\omega u + v)\,,\end{aligned}$$

which transforms equations (28) and (29) into

$$\dot{u} = -\omega\, v - \frac{f''(x_B)}{\omega^2+1}\, uv - \left(\frac{f''(x_B)(\omega^2-1)}{\omega\,(\omega^2+1)} + \frac{\alpha\,(\omega^2+1)\, g''(x_B)}{\omega f''(x_B)}\right)\frac{v^2}{2}$$
$$- \left(\frac{f'''(x_B)}{\omega} + \frac{\alpha\,(\omega^2+1)\, g'''(x_B)}{\omega f''(x_B)}\right)\frac{v^3}{6} + \dots, \tag{30}$$
$$\dot{v} = \omega\, u - \frac{\omega f''(x_B)}{\omega^2+1}\, uv - f''(x_B)\left(\frac{\omega^2-1}{\omega^2+1}\right)\frac{v^2}{2} - f'''(x_B)\,\frac{v^3}{6} + \dots. \tag{31}$$

Our equations are now of the form

$$\dot{u} = P(u,v),$$
$$\dot{v} = Q(u,v)$$

with an equilibrium point whose linear approximation matrix is

$$\begin{bmatrix} 0 & -\omega \\ \omega & 0 \end{bmatrix}$$

where $\omega \neq 0$.

These equations can now be transformed into the higher order normal form

$$\dot{r} = Lr^3 + O(r^5) + \dots,$$
$$\dot{\theta} = \omega + O(r^2) + \dots,$$

where L is given [3] in terms of partial derivatives of P and Q by

$$L = \frac{1}{16}\left(P_{uuu} + Q_{uuv} + P_{uvv} + Q_{vvv}\right)$$
$$+ \frac{1}{16\omega}\left(P_{uv}\left(P_{uu} + P_{vv}\right) - Q_{uv}\left(Q_{uu} + Q_{vv}\right) - P_{uu}\, Q_{uu} + P_{vv}\, Q_{vv}\right).$$

The partial derivatives may be obtained from equations (30) and (31). It seems remarkable that L simplifies to

$$L = \frac{1}{16}\Big(\alpha\, g''(x_B) - f'''(x_B)\Big)$$
$$= \frac{1}{16}\mathrm{Tr}\, A''(x_B)$$

so that $L < 0$ because, from (19), $\mathrm{Tr}\, A''(x_B) < 0$. □

Assuming L depends continuously on the parameters of the system we have $L < 0$ for sufficiently small parameter changes. So for the small parameter changes necessary to create a pair of Hopf bifurcations, as in Fig. 1.4(c), we get supercritical Hopf bifurcations where the branching small amplitude limit cycles are stable. This means equations of the form (16) and (17) cannot have a figure of eight bifurcation diagram as was found in section 1.5.

Acknowledgments

The first author is grateful to Stephen Coombes for allowing him one last chance to talk about equations that are now over twenty years old. Both authors are grateful to Mark Weston for help with the preparation of this paper.

References

[1] P. Cornelius, *Bifurcation Theory Applied to Neuron Models*, PhD Thesis, University of Wales, (2001).

[2] R. FitzHugh, Impulses and physiological states in theoretic models of nerve membrane. *Biophys. J.* **1**, 445–466, (1961).

[3] P. Glendinning, *Stability, Instability and Chaos*, Cambridge University Press, p. 227, (1994),

[4] J. L. Hindmarsh and R. M. Rose, A model of the nerve impulse using two first-order differential equations. *Nature, Lond.* **296**, 162–164, (1982).

[5] J. L. Hindmarsh and R. M. Rose, A model of neuronal bursting using three coupled first-order differential equations. *Proc. Roy. Soc. Lond.* **B 221**, 87–102, (1984).

[6] A. L. Hodgkin and A. F. Huxley, A quantitative description of membrane current and its application to conductance and excitation in nerve. *J. Physiol. Lond.* **117**, 500–544, (1952).

[7] X. J. Wang, Multiple dynamic modes of thalamic relay neurons: rhythmic bursting and intermittent phase-locking. *Neuroscience* **59**, 21–31, (1994).

CHAPTER 2

NEGATIVE CALCIUM FEEDBACK: THE ROAD FROM CHAY-KEIZER

Richard Bertram
Department of Mathematics and Institute of Molecular Biophysics
Florida State University
Tallahassee, FL 32306, USA
e-mail: bertram@math.fsu.edu

Arthur Sherman
Laboratory of Biological Modeling, NIDDK
National Institutes of Health
Bethesda, MD 20892, USA
e-mail: asherman@nih.gov

We trace the development of negative feedback by Ca^{2+} as a driving mechanism for bursting in the Chay-Keizer model for insulin-secreting pancreatic β-cells and successor models. We focus on the role of the endoplasmic reticulum in providing the slow kinetic components needed to obtain bursting that lasts more than a few seconds. The fast/slow analysis applied by Rinzel to Chay-Keizer is generalized to elucidate the properties of bursting when there are two slow, negative feedback variables. Citations are provided to the current literature on further ramifications to Chay-Keizer that can be dissected by similar techniques.

2.1. Introduction

One of the earliest bursting models was developed by Chay and Keizer [15] as a description of the insulin-secreting pancreatic β-cell. This cell type is of great interest because defects in insulin secretion are important for the pathogenesis of Type 2 Diabetes Mellitus (T2DM). In fact, in recent years data has accumulated implicating electrical properties of β-cells, specifically channel polymorphisms, in T2DM [3].

Here, however, our focus will be on two other aspects of the Chay-Keizer (CK) model. One is the underlying bifurcation structure of the model, which is described as square-wave [33] or fold-homoclinic [26] or Type I bursting [6]. This easy-to-understand pattern has provided a template for models describing a wide variety of cells and systems, such as neuroendocrine pituitary melanotropes [17], thalamic neurons [24], respiratory pacemaker neurons in the pre-Bötzinger complex [11], and episodic network activity in embryonic spinal cord [41]; the last three are reviewed in chapters 1, 12, and 11 respectively.

A second aspect of general interest is the paradigm of slow negative feedback by cytosolic Ca^{2+}, which in CK targets a Ca^{2+}-activated K^+ channel. This was a natural choice following the success of the early Plant model for the R-15 neuron of *Aplysia* [32]. However, this seductive hypothesis has traveled a hard road, falling into disfavor before the age of 10 and making a comeback before the age of 20. The Ca^{2+}-feedback hypothesis has emerged from these trials altered, but still recognizable, and strengthened by insights into new areas of cellular Ca^{2+} handling, including sequestration and release by the endoplasmic reticulum (ER), and exotic effects on metabolism, including mitochondrial respiration and glycolytic oscillations.

In addition, we have found that the simplest square-wave burster models, with a single slow variable, are not adequate to account for the complexity of β-cell activity patterns. Adding a second or third slow variable, while mathematically redundant, greatly enhances the robustness and dynamic range and can lead to qualitative changes in some properties, such as phase resetting.

In this chapter we will trace out a pedagogically streamlined history of the twin ideas of square-wave bursting and calcium feedback, focusing in detail on the properties of the ER.

2.2. Before the Beginning

The square-wave bursting typical of β-cells is dynamically similar to a relaxation oscillation. The prototypical relaxation oscillator was developed by van der Pol and van der Mark as a description of an oscillatory cardiac pacemaker [44]. Later, FitzHugh and Nagumo developed simple neural models, recognizing that an action potential or electrical impulse could be described as a relaxation oscillation [19]. The key features of what came to be called the FitzHugh-Nagumo model are (1) a cubic voltage nullcline, and (2) a separation of time scales of the two variables, so that one changes much more rapidly than the other. The Morris-Lecar model for a barnacle muscle fiber, developed two decades later, also possesses these features, although the voltage nullcline is only approximately cubic in this case [31]. Because Morris-Lecar includes expressions for ionic currents, it is more suitable for describing biophysical phenomena, such as the effects of channel blockers.

We use a modification of the Morris-Lecar model to describe impulses in the β-cell:

$$C_m \frac{dV}{dt} = -[I_{Ca} + I_K + I_{K(Ca)} + I_{K(ATP)}] \tag{1}$$

$$\frac{dn}{dt} = \lambda(n_\infty(V) - n)/\tau_n \ , \tag{2}$$

where C_m is the membrane capacitance of the cell, V is membrane potential or voltage, I_{Ca} is an inward Ca^{2+} current, I_K is an outward K^+ current of the delayed rectifier type, $I_{K(Ca)}$ is a Ca^{2+}-activated K^+ current and $I_{K(ATP)}$ is an ATP-sensitive K^+ current (ATP=adenosine triphosphate). The latter two currents, $I_{K(Ca)}$ and $I_{K(ATP)}$, were not included in the Morris-Lecar model, but have been added here because they play important roles in β-cells. Additional variables and parameters in the model are n, the activation variable for I_K, its equilibrium function $n_\infty(V)$, and its activation time constant, τ_n. The parameter λ is used as a convenient means to speed up or slow down the time scale of the variable n. Additional equations are:

$$I_{Ca} = g_{Ca} m_\infty(V)(V - V_{Ca}) \tag{3}$$

$$I_K = g_K n(V - V_K) \tag{4}$$

$$I_{K(Ca)} = g_{K(Ca)} \left(\frac{c^3}{c^3 + K_d^3} \right) (V - V_K) \tag{5}$$

$$I_{K(ATP)} = g_{K(ATP)}(V - V_K) \tag{6}$$

$$m_\infty(V) = [1 + \exp((v_m - V)/s_m)]^{-1} \tag{7}$$

$$n_\infty(V) = [1 + \exp((v_n - V)/s_n)]^{-1} \ . \tag{8}$$

With the parameter values listed in Table 1 the system is oscillatory, producing a continuous train of impulses. One impulse is shown in Fig. 2.1(A). This is characterized by a rapid upstroke (due to the inward current I_{Ca}) and a rapid downstroke (due to the outward current I_K), with slow changes between impulses. Figure 2.1(B) illustrates the impulse trajectory (oriented curve) in the n-V-phase plane. The scaling parameter λ is small in this simulation ($\lambda = 0.01$), so the activation variable n changes much more slowly than V. As a result, the trajectory is attracted to the V-nullcline and moves along either the top or bottom branch of the cubic until the branch switches back. The trajectory moves slowly to the left (since $dn/dt < 0$) along the bottom branch between impulses. When the branch ends the trajectory moves rapidly to the top branch and travels rightward (since $dn/dt > 0$) until this branch ends, after which the trajectory moves rapidly to the lower branch. Motion along the upper branch and the rapid transitions between branches constitute the impulse. The full orbit is a classic relaxation oscillation. It is important that the nullclines intersect only along the middle branch of the V-nullcline. Otherwise, the intersection point, a steady state of the system, would be stable, and periodic motion would not occur.

Table 1: Parameter Values for the Morris-Lecar Model

Parameter	Value	Parameter	Value
g_{Ca}	1000 pS	g_K	2700 pS
$g_{K(Ca)}$	400 pS	$g_{K(ATP)}$	180 pS
V_{Ca}	25 mV	V_K	−75 mV
C_m	5300 fF	λ	1
τ_n	20 msec	K_D	0.4 μM
v_n	−16 mV	s_n	5 mV
v_m	−20 mV	s_m	12 mV

In most β-cell models the time scale separation is not as extreme as in this example. Thus, rather than $\lambda = 0.01$ a value closer to $\lambda = 1$ is used. With the n dynamics now 100 times faster, the trajectory no longer rides along the branches of the V-nullcline, but instead travels along an elliptical path between the upper and lower branches of the nullcline. The resulting impulse is of lower amplitude, with peak value less than −10 mV (Fig. 2.2(A)). For more detailed phase-plane analysis see Sherman [36] and corresponding exercises at http://mrb.niddk.nih.gov/sherman, where the XPP source files used here may also be found. Smaller impulses like these are characteristic of impulses recorded in β-cells [45], and henceforth we use $\lambda = 1$.

Calcium-activated K^+currents, $I_{K(Ca)}$, are found in many neurons [23]. In β-cells, Ca^{2+}-activated and voltage-independent K(Ca) channels were proposed to be responsible for packaging impulses into bursts [4], which led to the Chay-Keizer model described in the next section. For now we treat the cytosolic Ca^{2+} concentration, c, as a parameter. Increasing this parameter increases the outward K(Ca) current (Eq. (5)), which has a hy-

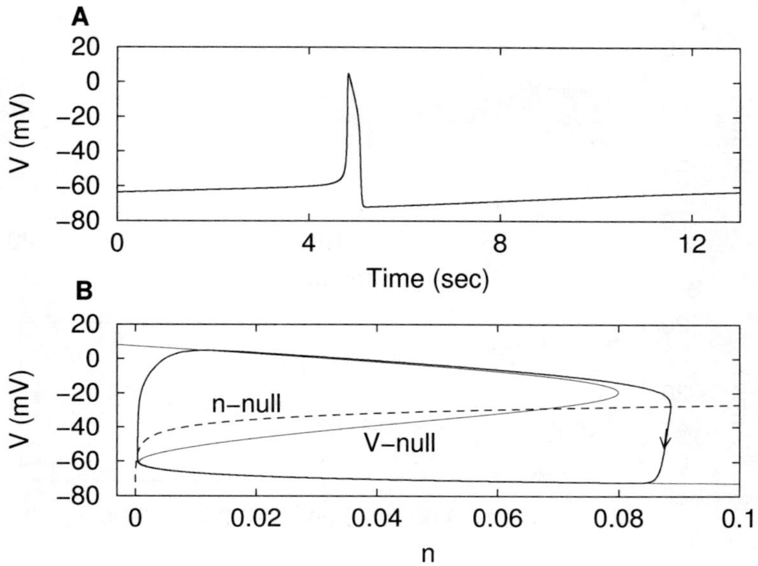

Fig. 2.1. (**A**) A single impulse from a train of impulses generated by the Morris-Lecar-like model. (**B**) Phase plane view of an impulse. The trajectory (oriented curve) moves along the top and bottom branches of the V-nullcline, and is a typical relaxation oscillation. The time scale parameter is small, $\lambda = 0.01$, accentuating the separation in time scales of the V and n variables. Cytosolic calcium, c, is fixed at 0.1 μM.

perpolarizing effect on the cell. In terms of the phase plane, increasing c translates the V-nullcline leftward (Fig. 2.2(B)). This may result in an intersection of the two nullclines on the lower branch of the V-nullcline, creating a hyperpolarized stable steady state (indicated by a circle). When this occurs the system moves from a state of continuous spiking to a resting state at a low voltage (Fig. 2.2(A)). Thus, the dynamics of the system depend critically on the cytosolic Ca^{2+} concentration.

The scenarios described in Fig. 2.2 reflect two extreme cases, where the system has either a globally attracting periodic solution or a globally attracting steady state. An important intermediate case occurs for $0.12 < c < 0.165$. Here, a stable periodic solution coexists with a stable steady-state (Fig. 2.3). There are three steady state solutions. The solution with the highest voltage (open circle) is an unstable spiral, which is surrounded by a stable limit cycle. The middle steady-state solution (open triangle) is a saddle point, whose stable manifold (dot-dashed curve) forms the separatrix

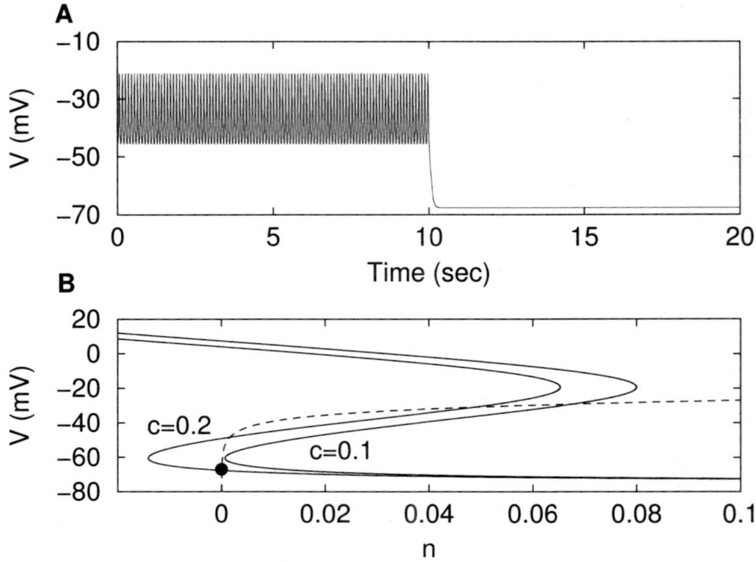

Fig. 2.2. (**A**) A train of β-cell-like impulses is terminated when the cytosolic Ca^{2+} concentration is increased from $c = 0.1$ to $c = 0.2$. (**B**) Increasing c from 0.1 to 0.2 shifts the V-nullcline leftward. The filled circle represents a stable steady-state solution.

between the basins of attraction of the stable limit cycle and the stable steady state (filled circle). In this bistable system the ultimate fate of a trajectory is determined by its starting location. If the trajectory starts between the two branches of the stable manifold, then it is attracted to the limit cycle. If it starts below this region, then the trajectory is attracted to the stable steady state. We shall see below that bistability between a steady state and a periodic solution is a key ingredient for square-wave bursting.

2.3. The Beginning

All current models for β-cell electrical activity are descendants of the Chay-Keizer model [15]. Even though this model did not contain all of the features subsequently shown to be important in β-cell electrical activity, it successfully identified the key elements of square-wave bursting and provided a scaffold onto which additional elements could be added. The appealing simplicity accounts for its impact on bursting models in general. Chay-Keizer was based on the earlier hypothesis of Atwater and Rojas that bursting is due to the slow rise and fall of the cytosolic Ca^{2+} concentration, acting on

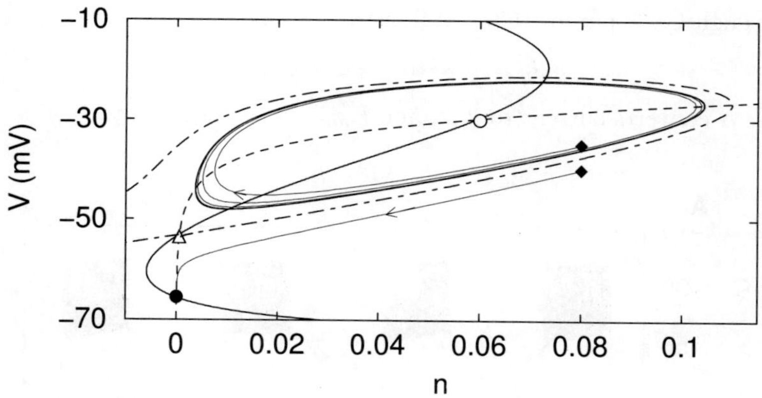

Fig. 2.3. For intermediate values of the parameter c (here $c = 0.15$) the system is bistable. A stable limit cycle coexists with a stable hyperpolarized steady state (filled circle). Trajectories starting within the two branches of the saddle point's stable manifold (dot-dashed curve) are attracted to the limit cycle. Those starting below this region are attracted to the stable steady state.

K(Ca) channels [4].

Historically, however, Chay-Keizer was preceded by a less well-known model developed by Matthews and O'Connor [30]. It anticipated many features of Chay-Keizer, such as a central role for K(Ca) channels, as well as features not introduced until much later, such as metabolic oscillations. However, the Matthews-O'Connor model was much more complex than Chay-Keizer because special currents were assigned roles in producing the plateau and pacemaker functions, features that arose organically from a much simpler set of currents in Chay-Keizer. This perhaps accounts for why it left no apparent progeny.

Chay and Keizer used modified squid axon Hodgkin-Huxley equations [25] to describe action potentials. We use the simpler Morris-Lecar model, supplemented by a differential equation for the cytosolic Ca^{2+} concentration:

$$\frac{dc}{dt} = f_{cyt} J_{mem} \quad , \tag{9}$$

where c is the cytosolic Ca^{2+} concentration, f_{cyt} is the fraction of cytosolic Ca^{2+} that is not bound to buffers, and J_{mem} is the Ca^{2+} flux across the plasma membrane. The Ca^{2+} influx is through Ca^{2+} channels and the efflux is through Ca^{2+} pumps (Ca^{2+} ATPases):

$$J_{mem} = -(\alpha I_{Ca} + k_{pmca} c) \ , \tag{10}$$

where α converts current to flux, and k_{pmca} is the pump rate.

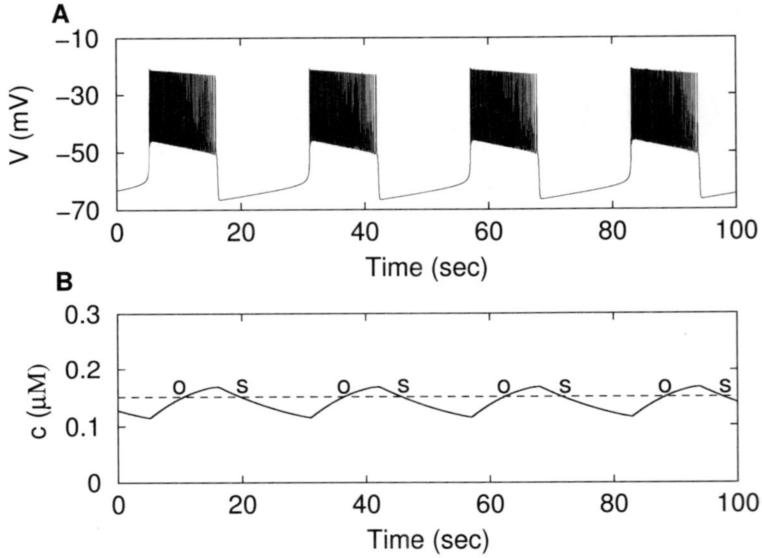

Fig. 2.4. (**A**) Bursting produced by the Chay-Keizer model. (**B**) Bursting is driven by slow activity-dependent oscillations in the cytosolic Ca^{2+} concentration. The Ca^{2+} concentration rises during the active phase and falls during the silent phase of bursting. The horizontal dashed line is used to illustrate that the fast subsystem is bistable: for the same value of c the fast subsystem may be oscillatory ("O") or stationary ("S"). Fraction of free Ca^{2+} is $f_{cyt} = 0.00025$.

This three-variable model is able to reproduce the square-wave bursting that characterizes β-cells (Fig. 2.4(A)). During the oscillatory or active phase, Ca^{2+} channels are mostly open, so that Ca^{2+} accumulates in the cell. Thus, c rises during the active phase ("O" in Fig. 2.4(B)). This rise is slow, since the effective time scale for c is large. (The time scale can be easily adjusted using the parameter f_{cyt}, which is currently set to a very small value, $f_{cyt} = 0.00025$.) The rise in c activates K(Ca) current, translating the V-nullcline leftward (Fig. 2.2). Eventually c rises to a large enough value that the limit cycle oscillation disappears, terminating the active phase of spiking. Now that the system has entered the silent phase and V is in a low rest state the Ca^{2+} channels close. This results in a slow decline in c ("S" in Fig. 2.4(B)). As a result, hyperpolarizing K(Ca) current is shut off and the V-nullcline is translated rightward. Eventually, the stable intersection of the V- and n-nullclines is lost and the system re-enters the oscillatory active phase. Note that the burst period is tens of seconds (here about 22 sec). This is typical of most *in vitro* electrical recordings from β-cells within intact islets, but is very slow compared with bursting produced by most neurons.

A standard way to analyze bursting oscillations is to separate the variables into slow and fast subsystems, and then to treat the slow variable as a parameter of the fast subsystem. This "fast/slow analysis" was pioneered by Rinzel, building on concepts developed by Fitzhugh [19] in his phase-plane analysis of the Hodgkin-Huxley model, and used to analyze several types of bursting oscillations, including the square-wave bursting characteristic of β-cells [35]. In our case, the fast subsystem consists of Eqs. (1)–(2), with fast variables V and n. The calcium concentration c is the single slow variable. For large values of c, now treated as a parameter of the fast subsystem, the V nullcline is shifted far to the left (see Fig. 2.2) and the model cell is silent at a hyperpolarized voltage. As c is reduced the V nullcline is translated rightward, so the intersection with the n-nullcline occurs at higher voltages. For sufficiently small values of c the lower knee of the V-nullcline is to the right of the n-nullcline. That is, a saddle-node bifurcation (SN) has occurred. This is illustrated in the bifurcation diagram of Fig. 2.5. The lower branch of this diagram corresponds to the lower, stable, steady state of the fast subsystem. The middle, unstable, branch corresponds to steady states on the middle branch of the V-nullcline, and is a branch of saddle points. This saddle point branch begins at the SN bifurcation with the stable steady state branch, and ends at a second SN bifurcation with a branch of unstable equilibria. The SN bifurcations are marked by triangles in Fig. 2.5.

The branch of upper unstable equilibria continues for lower values of c, and eventually goes through a supercritical Hopf bifurcation (circle). Beyond this the branch is stable. A branch of stable periodic solutions emerges from the Hopf bifurcation. Each of these periodic solutions represents a continuous train of action potentials (as in the left portion of Fig. 2.2(A)). The periodic branch terminates at a homoclinic bifurcation, where the limit cycle connects with a saddle point, forming an infinite-period homoclinic orbit. The bistability illustrated in Fig. 2.3 occurs for all values of c between the left SN (triangle) and the homoclinic bifurcation (square).

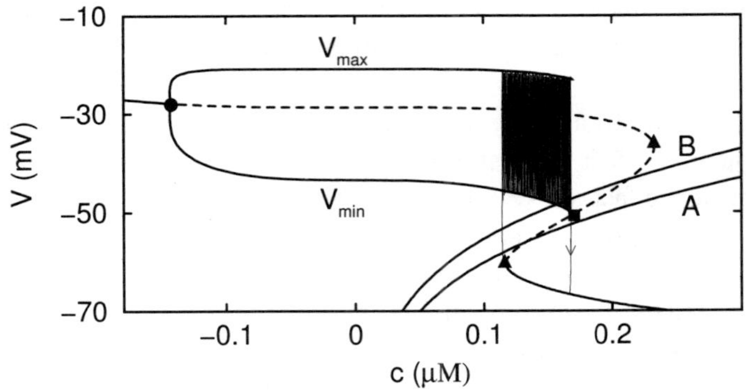

Fig. 2.5. Fast/slow analysis of bursting. The burst trajectory and c-nullcline (A or B) are superimposed on a bifurcation diagram (z-curve) of the fast subsystem. On the z-curve, solid curves represent stable solutions and dashed curves represent unstable solutions. There are two saddle-node bifurcations (triangles), a supercritical Hopf bifurcation (circle), and a homoclinic bifurcation (square). The periodic branch is represented using the minimum (V_{min}) and maximum (V_{max}) voltage of the oscillations. A: $k_{pmca} = 0.13$, B: $k_{pmca} = 0.18$.

The z-shaped fast-subsystem bifurcation diagram, called the "slow manifold" or "z-curve", is defined as the curve on which V and n are at steady state and can be constructed numerically using XPPAUT [18] by treating c as a parameter. The z-curve can also be calculated analytically by defining the fraction of activated K(Ca) channels,

$$\omega = \frac{c^3}{c^3 + K_d^3}, \tag{11}$$

setting $\frac{dV}{dt} = 0$ in Eq. (1) and solving for ω,

$$\omega = -\frac{g_{Ca} m_\infty(V)(V - V_{Ca}) + g_K n(V - V_K)}{g_{K(Ca)}(V - V_K)} + \frac{g_{K(ATP)}}{g_{K(Ca)}}, \tag{12}$$

and solving Eq. (11) for c.

We now add in the slow dynamics of c, and view Fig. 2.5 as a c-V phase plane. The c-nullcline, obtained from Eq. (9), is superimposed (curve A or B). Below the nullcline $dc/dt < 0$, while above the nullcline $dc/dt > 0$. Finally, we superimpose the burst trajectory. This moves along the z-curve since the fast subsystem dynamics are much faster than the slow subsystem dynamics. This relaxation-like oscillation is similar to the relaxation oscillation shown in Fig. 2.1. The burst trajectory rides along the bottom branch of the z-curve during the silent phase, traveling to the left since it is below the c-nullcline. When the trajectory reaches the SN bifurcation it moves to the periodic branch, since the limit cycle is now the only remaining attractor. At this point the trajectory travels rightward since it is above the c-nullcline. The active phase of bursting ends when the trajectory reaches the homoclinic bifurcation. This completes one cycle of bursting.

The bistability of the fast subsystem is a crucial feature of square-wave bursting. Without bistability there would be no bursting. Also, bursting does not occur if the c-nullcline intersects the lower branch of the z-curve, since in this case the intersection is a stable equilibrium of the full system of equations. Likewise, if the nullcline crosses deep into the periodic branch the system will spike continuously. Thus, for bursting to occur, the c-nullcline must cross the z-curve either between the lower SN and the homoclinic bifurcation, or slightly above the homoclinic bifurcation. If the slow variable were infinitely slow then bursting would occur only if the crossing occurred between the saddle node and the homoclinic bifurcation [42].

The similarity between the fast/slow analysis of bursting and the dynamics of a relaxation oscillation is emphasized in Fig. 2.6. Here the periodic branch is represented not only by the maximum and minimum voltage curves, but also by a curve showing the average voltage (V_{avg}). The average voltage of the burst trajectory then travels along the V_{avg} branch during the active phase, and the lower branch of the z-curve during the silent phase (Fig. 2.6, heavy curve). (We note that the equivalent V curve, V_{eqv}, defined in Bertram *et al.*[6] would be more representative of the periodic branch than the average V curve. However, V_{avg} is much easier to compute, and in this case a sufficiently good approximation of V_{eqv}.) The union of the z-curve with the V_{avg} curve is then analogous to the V-nullcline in the relaxation oscillator of Fig. 2.1.

In addition to exhibiting bursting, Chay-Keizer was able to reproduce the effects on membrane potential of increasing the glucose concentration. This is physiologically important because β-cells adjust their output (insulin secretion) according to the glucose level in the blood. The insulin

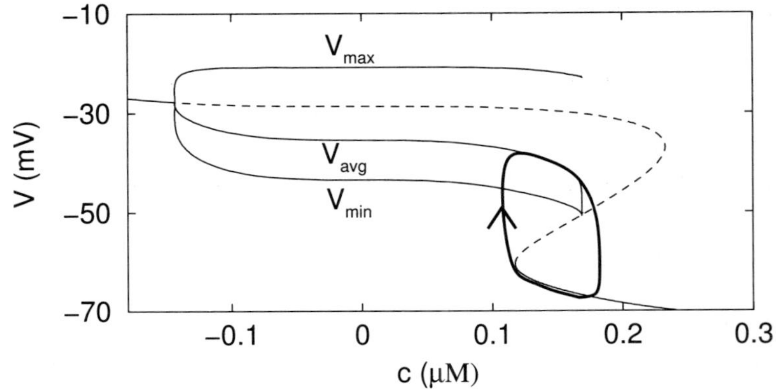

Fig. 2.6. The z-curve is similar in shape to the cubic V-nullcline of the Morris-Lecar relaxation oscillator when the periodic branch is represented by the average voltage curve.

secretion rate is roughly proportional to the *plateau fraction*, the ratio of the active phase duration to the total burst period. At low glucose levels the cell is silent, so the plateau fraction is 0 and the rate of insulin secretion is low. With glucose concentrations just beyond about 5 mM the β-cells burst, but the plateau fraction is relatively low, less than 0.5. As the glucose concentration is increased, the plateau fraction increases, raising the mean rate of insulin secretion. At very high glucose concentrations, ≈ 20 mM, the cell spikes continuously and the plateau fraction reaches a value of 1 [5].

Chay and Keizer simulated the effect of glucose by increasing the Ca^{2+} pump rate k_{pmca}. This is biophysically reasonable, since Ca^{2+} pumps are powered by ATP, and the ATP level in the β-cell increases when the glucose level is increased. Figure 2.7 shows that the mechanism used by Chay and Keizer to simulate an increase in the glucose level is able to reproduce the glucose effect on the β-cell's electrical activity. In this figure, k_{pmca} is increased from 0.1, to 0.13, 0.22, and 0.25. With each step increase in k_{pmca} the duration of the silent phase decreases while the duration of the active phase increases, until the cell finally enters a continuous spiking state. In terms of the fast/slow analysis, the c-nullcline is translated upward when k_{pmca} is increased (Fig. 2.5, from A to B). This increases the distance between the nullcline and the bottom branch of the z-curve, so the trajectory traverses this branch more quickly and the silent phase duration

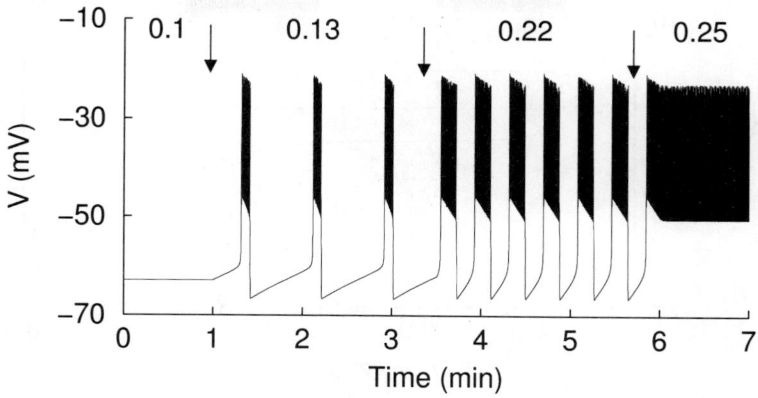

Fig. 2.7. Simulation of a gradual increase in the glucose concentration. The parameter k_{pmca} is increased from 0.1 to 0.13, then 0.22, and finally 0.25 (at arrows). The response of the model is similar to what has been observed in islets (Beigelman *et al.*, 1977). Fraction of free Ca^{2+} is $f_{cyt} = 0.00025$.

is reduced. At the same time, the distance between the nullcline and the periodic branch (or V_{avg} curve) is decreased, so that the trajectory moves more slowly along this branch, increasing the duration of the active phase. With k_{pmca} small the nullcline intersects the bottom branch of the z-curve and the model cell is at rest. With k_{pmca} large the nullcline intersects deep into the periodic branch and the cell spikes continuously.

It is now believed that a factor more important than Ca^{2+} pumps is the inhibitory effect that glucose has on ATP-sensitive K^+ channels [2]. When these channels were discovered after the Chay-Keizer model was published, it was easy to demonstrate that reduction of $g_{K(ATP)}$ could also increase plateau fraction [34]. Geometrically, increasing k_{pmca} moves the c nullcline to the left (Eqs. (9), (10)), whereas reducing $g_{K(ATP)}$ moves the z-curve to the right (Eq. (12)), both of which prolong the active phase at the expense of the silent phase.

Another feature of islet behavior captured by the Chay-Keizer model is the ability to reset. That is, the model predicts that it should be possible to reset the system from the silent phase to the active phase, and vice versa, by giving a brief voltage perturbation. This is due to the bistability of the fast subsystem (Fig. 2.8). Furthermore, when the system is reset from the silent phase to the active phase, the active phase should be shorter than usual. This is because the distance that the trajectory must travel along

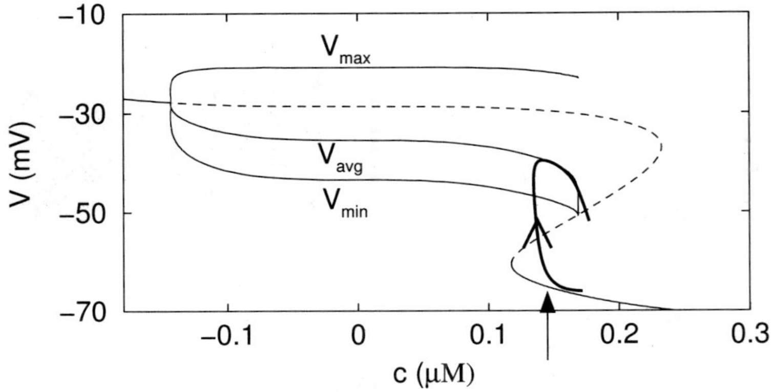

Fig. 2.8. The Chay-Keizer model predicts that it should be possible to reset from the silent phase to the active phase (at arrow). The active phase is shorter than usual. Resetting should also be possible from the active phase to the silent phase.

the periodic branch is less than during a typical active phase. The same can be said for resetting from active to silent phase. Thus, the model predicts that resetting is phase-dependent.

Resetting experiments were performed on islets by Cook *et al.* [16]. They found that it was possible to reset an islet from one phase of bursting to the other, consistent with the model. However, this resetting was phase-independent, contrary to the Chay-Keizer model. That is, when the islet was reset from the silent phase to the active phase (or active to silent), the active phase duration was similar to that of a typical active phase. A later modeling study showed that phase-independent resetting could be obtained in a model with two negative-feedback variables, one slow during the active phase and one slow during the silent phase [39]. Although the Chay-Keizer model failed in this respect, it still established the important principle that bursting oscillations based on bistability are resettable. This is in contrast to bursting oscillations driven by an endogenous oscillatory process, such as the glycolytic oscillations mentioned later in this chapter.

2.4. The Demise of K(Ca)

The most obvious prediction of the Chay-Keizer model is that the cytosolic Ca^{2+} concentration rises slowly during the active phase and declines slowly during the silent phase (Fig. 2.4(B)). When Ca^{2+} was first measured some years after publication of the model, it was indeed found to oscillate [43], but not with the sawtooth shape predicted by the model. Instead, the concentration often shows two time scales, a rapid rise to a plateau followed by a slowly rising plateau, and a similar pattern in the silent phase (Fig 2.9(A)). Even worse, some records showed Ca^{2+} declining before the end of the active phase (Fig. 2.9(B)). These measurements seemed to be incompatible with a burst mechanism driven by Ca^{2+} acting on K(Ca) channels.

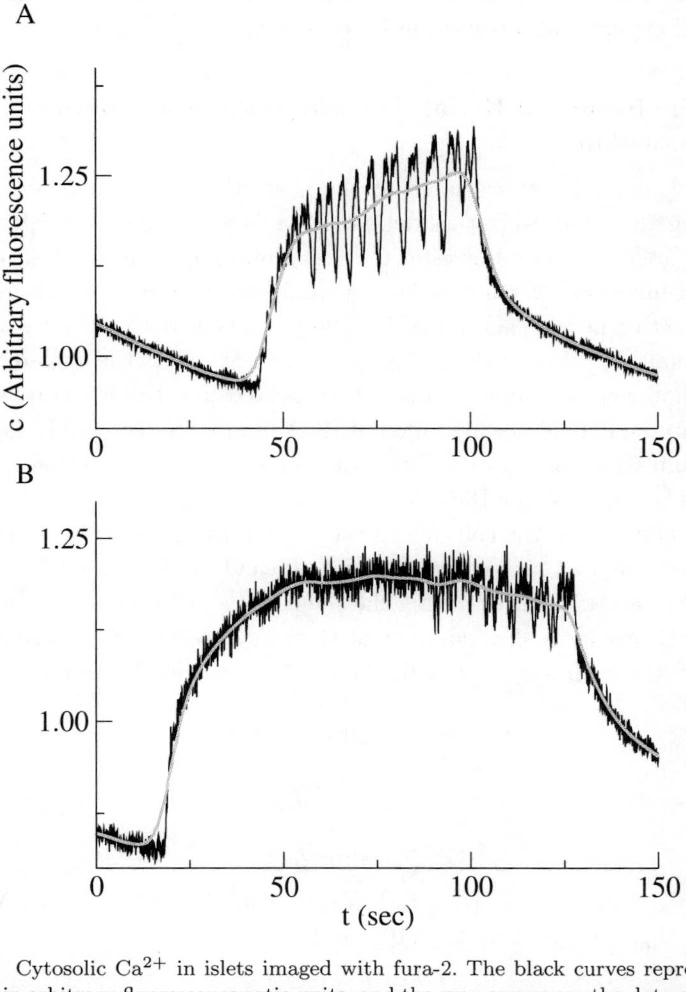

Fig. 2.9. Cytosolic Ca^{2+} in islets imaged with fura-2. The black curves represent the raw data in arbitrary fluorescence ratio units, and the grey curves are the data smoothed to highlight the trends. Data courtesy of Craig Nunemaker and Les Satin, Virginia Commonwealth University.

With cytosolic Ca^{2+} out of favor as a slow variable to drive bursting, a succession of other models with different slow variables was proposed. These included slow inactivation of a voltage-dependent Ca^{2+} current [14, 28]; slow changes in the ratio of ATP to ADP, acting on K(ATP) channels [27, 38]; and the effects of the endoplasmic reticulum (ER) acting either indirectly on cytosolic Ca^{2+} or directly through Store-Operated-Current [12, 13]. The mathematical template established by the Chay-Keizer model made it relatively easy to devise new models, but in the end none of these survived experimental testing in its pure form.

2.5. The Return of K(Ca): Help from the Endoplasmic Reticulum

Although not fully appreciated at the time, the most important advance following the Chay-Keizer model was Chay's addition of the ER [12, 13]. This organelle is a storehouse for Ca^{2+}, maintaining a free Ca^{2+} level on the order of hundreds of micromolar (by comparison, the cytosolic free Ca^{2+} concentration never reaches 1 μM.) The ER acts as both a Ca^{2+} source and a Ca^{2+} sink [10]. When the cell is spiking, Ca^{2+} enters the cytosol through Ca^{2+} channels and some of this is transported into the ER through Ca^{2+} pumps in the ER membrane called SERCA pumps (Sarco- and Endoplasmic Reticulum Calcium pumps). Thus, the ER acts as a sink during the active phase of bursting. When the cell is silent, Ca^{2+} channels are closed and there is a net efflux from the cell due to the plasma membrane Ca^{2+} pumps. At the same time, Ca^{2+} is released back into the cytosol from the ER. Thus, the ER acts as a Ca^{2+} source during the silent phase of bursting. These actions of the ER provide a slow component to the cytosolic Ca^{2+} concentration.

With the addition of the ER, the Ca^{2+} subsystem becomes

$$\frac{dc}{dt} = f_{cyt}(J_{mem} - J_{er}) \tag{13}$$

$$\frac{dc_{er}}{dt} = f_{er}\frac{\nu_{cyt}}{\nu_{er}}J_{er} \tag{14}$$

$$= f_{cyt}\sigma_{er}J_{er} \ , \tag{15}$$

where $\sigma_{er} = (\nu_{cyt}/f_{cyt})/(\nu_{er}/f_{er})$ is the ratio of effective cytosolic to ER volume, J_{mem} is given by Eq. (10), and

$$J_{er} = J_{serca} - J_{leak} \tag{16}$$

where $J_{serca} = k_{serca}c$ is the flux into the ER through SERCA pumps and $J_{leak} = p_{leak}(c_{er} - c)$ is the leak out of the ER into the cytosol. Although it

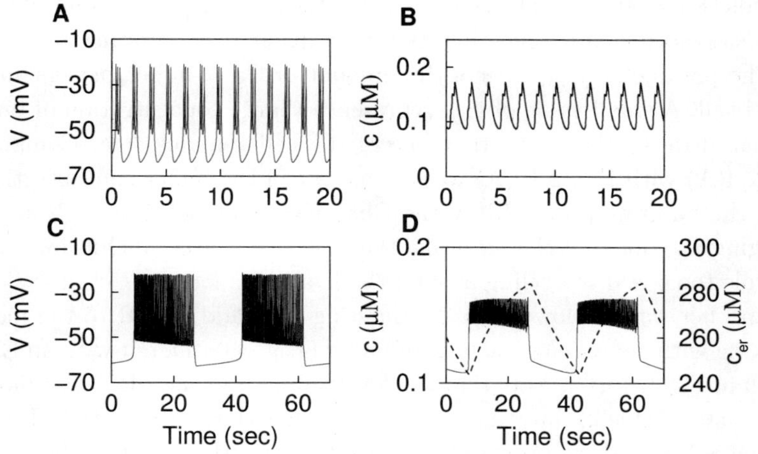

Fig. 2.10. (**A**) The Chay-Keizer model with the fraction of free cytosolic Ca^{2+} increased by a factor of 40 produces fast bursting ($f_{cyt} = 0.01$, $g_{K(Ca)} = 500$ pS, $g_{K(ATP)} = 185$ pS). (**B**) The cytosolic Ca^{2+} concentration has a sawtooth shape. (**C**) When an ER compartment is added to the model the bursting slows down dramatically. (**D**) Cytosolic Ca^{2+} now has a square shape with a slow decline, similar to experimental measurements. The model predicts that the ER Ca^{2+} concentration (dashed) has a sawtooth shape.

would be more correct to model the flux terms with non-linear Hill functions (as in Li *et al.*, [29]), the properties of the ER described here do not depend on non-linearity, and the linear formulas simplify the analysis.

Table 2: Additional Parameter Values for the Chay-Keizer Model with ER

Parameter	Value	Parameter	Value
f_{cyt}	0.01	k_{pmca}	$0.18\ \text{msec}^{-1}$
α	$4.5 \times 10^{-6}\ \text{fA}^{-1}\ \mu\text{M msec}^{-1}$	f_{er}	0.01
k_{SERCA}	$0.4\ \text{msec}^{-1}$	p_{leak}	$0.0002\ \text{msec}^{-1}$
ν_{cyt}	$10\ \mu\text{m}^3$	ν_{er}	$0.3\ \mu\text{m}^3$

Figure 2.10 illustrates the bursting and Ca^{2+} oscillations produced by the Chay-Keizer model without (panels (A) and (B)) and with (panels (C) and (D)) an ER. The fraction of Ca^{2+} in the cytosol that is free (f_{cyt}) has been increased from 0.00025 to a more physiological value of 0.01. The effect of this change is to speed up changes in c by a factor of 40. Thus, with this change the Chay-Keizer model bursts with a short period of a few

seconds (Fig. 2.10(A)). The time course of the cytosolic Ca^{2+} concentration has a sawtooth shape, reflecting its role in driving the bursting.

The parameter f_{cyt} reflects the amount of Ca^{2+} buffer present in the model cell. A small value of f_{cyt} represents a large concentration of buffer, so that little of the Ca^{2+} that enters the cell remains free. Comparing Fig. 2.4(A) with Fig. 2.10(A) we see that when the buffer concentration is high, the bursting produced by the Chay-Keizer model is slow. Note that changing f_{cyt} does not change either the z-curve or the c-nullcline but rather controls the speed of cycling around the hysteresis loop.

Another way to slow down the bursting is to add an ER to the model. Bursting with a physiological level of buffer ($f_{cyt} = 0.01$), but with an ER, is shown in Fig. 2.10(C). Note that the level of buffer in the ER is also modest ($f_{er} = 0.01$, Table 2), but that c_{er} is nonetheless slow because the ER Ca^{2+} concentration is three orders of magnitude larger than that of the cytosol (Fig. 2.10(D), dashed). The burst period, ≈ 35 sec, is much longer than that produced by the model with no ER (Fig. 2.10(A)). In addition, the cytosolic Ca^{2+} concentration no longer has a sawtooth shape (Fig. 2.10(D)), but instead has fast and slow components, in better agreement with experiment (Fig. 2.9).

Thus, while one often speaks casually of the ER acting to buffer Ca^{2+}, the model shows that the kinetic effect is quite different: Because buffering is rapid compared to the intrinsic timescale of c, it produces a uniform slowing of the c time course (compare Figs. 2.10(B), 2.4(B)), whereas c_{er} is much slower than c and introduces a second slow kinetic component (Fig. 2.10(D)).

The new quantity in the model, c_{er}, has a sawtooth appearance, and is largely responsible for driving the bursting (Fig. 2.10(D)). This model prediction has not yet been tested experimentally, due to the technical difficulty of measuring the Ca^{2+} concentration in the ER, separate from the cytosolic Ca^{2+}, in an intact islet. Thus, a variable that we believe to be important for bursting in β-cells, the ER Ca^{2+}, is practically invisible to current experimental measurements, and can only be observed indirectly through its effects on the cytosolic Ca^{2+}.

The most robust feature in experiments is the biphasic decline of cytosolic Ca^{2+} during the silent phase (Fig. 2.9). The initial rapid decline reflects the abrupt cessation of Ca^{2+} entry, while the much slower decline that follows reflects the slow reduction of release from the ER as Ca^{2+} that was taken up by the ER during the active phase slowly drains out. This interpretation is supported by the observation that the slow component disappears when SERCA pumps are blocked pharmacologically or genetically [1].

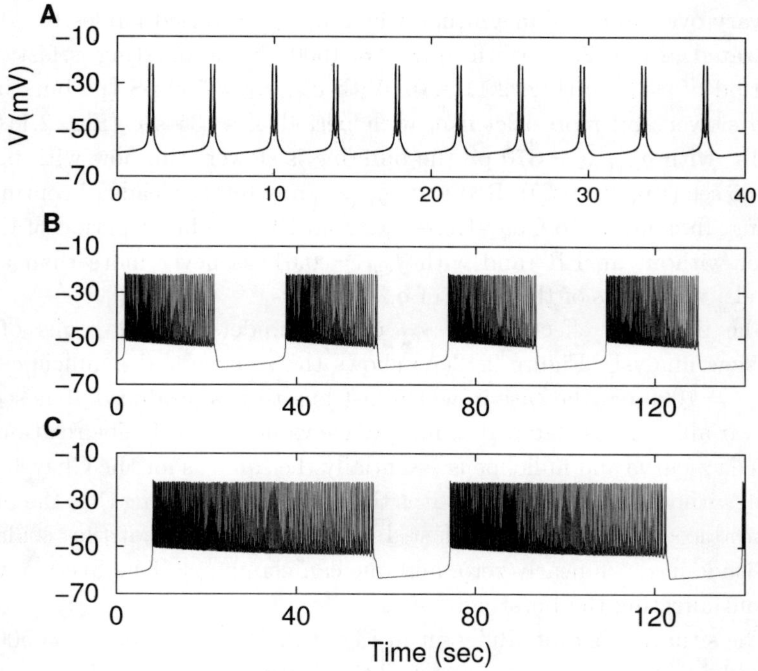

Fig. 2.11. The Chay-Keizer model with an ER can generate bursting with a wide range of periods. (**A**) Fast bursting is produced when $g_{K(Ca)} = 1000$ pS. (**B**) Slower bursting is produced when $g_{K(Ca)}$ is reduced to 500 pS. (**C**) Bursting becomes slower yet when $g_{K(Ca)}$ is reduced to 370 pS. The range of burst periods obtained by varying $g_{K(Ca)}$ is much smaller without an ER.

The addition of an ER compartment to the model also adds a great deal of flexibility to the system dynamics. That is, the period of bursting now ranges from a few seconds to more than a minute, and changes in period can be achieved by varying a single parameter, $g_{K(Ca)}$ (below we show that other parameters can also be varied to achieve a similar range of periods). From a biophysical perspective, if $g_{K(Ca)}$ is decreased it will take more Ca^{2+} to terminate the spiking since more K(Ca) channels must be activated, so the active phase duration will increase. Since the extra Ca^{2+} that accumulated during the active phase must be removed when the cell is hyperpolarized, the silent phase duration also increases. Thus, we expect the burst period to increase when $g_{K(Ca)}$ is reduced. While this would be true even without an ER, the role of the ER as a Ca^{2+} sink and source accentuates the effect of reducing $g_{K(Ca)}$, so that now the burst period can vary over orders of magnitude when $g_{K(Ca)}$ is varied modestly. This is illustrated in Fig. 2.11. With $g_{K(Ca)} = 1000$ pS the bursting is fast, with a period of ≈ 3 sec (Fig. 2.11(A)). With $g_{K(Ca)} = 500$ pS the bursting is much slower and more islet-like, with period of ≈ 35 sec (Fig. 2.11(B)). Finally, with $g_{K(Ca)} = 370$ pS the bursting is slower still, now with period of ≈ 65 sec (Fig. 2.11(C)). Reducing $g_{K(Ca)}$ any further leads to continuous spiking. In contrast to Chay-Keizer with an ER, the burst period of Chay-Keizer without an ER (and with $f_{cyt} = 0.01$) is never more than a few seconds, regardless of the value of $g_{K(Ca)}$.

The dramatic effect of $g_{K(Ca)}$ can be understood in terms of the fast/slow analysis. Figure 2.12(A) shows the z-curve and c-nullcline with $g_{K(Ca)} = 1000$ pS, the case in which fast bursting is produced. The second slow variable, c_{er}, is clamped at its average value, 181 μM. The relationship between z-curve and nullcline is essentially the same as for the Chay-Keizer model without an ER (Fig. 2.5). It is therefore not surprising that the bursting produced by this system is fast. Indeed, it is so fast that the oscillation amplitude in c_{er} is nearly zero, and one can clamp c_{er} at its average value without affecting the bursting.

The situation is quite different in Fig. 2.12(B), where $g_{K(Ca)} = 500$ pS. The reduction in $g_{K(Ca)}$ has stretched the z-curve, moving the knees farther apart, and moving the homoclinic bifurcation farther to the right. (This can also be seen from Eqs. (11), (12).) As a result, the c-nullcline now intersects both the bottom branch and the periodic branch. Thus, during the silent phase the trajectory moves along the bottom branch until it reaches the intersection with the nullcline. At this point the trajectory stalls, and in the absence of an ER would remain at this point. However, c_{er} influences the c-nullcline: when c_{er} declines (as it would during the silent phase) the nullcline moves leftward. This can be seen by setting the right-hand-side of Eq. (13) to 0, viewing c_{er} as a parameter, to get

$$c = \frac{-\alpha I_{Ca} + p_{leak} c_{er}}{k_{pmca} + k_{serca} + p_{leak}} \tag{17}$$

on the c-nullcline. Eventually, the nullcline moves past the lower knee of the z-curve, and the trajectory escapes the silent phase and enters the active phase. Once again, though, the trajectory stalls, this time on the periodic branch during the active phase. However, as the cell spikes, Ca^{2+} accumulates in the ER, shifting the c-nullcline to the right. Eventually, the nullcline moves past the homoclinic bifurcation and the trajectory escapes the periodic branch to re-enter the silent phase.

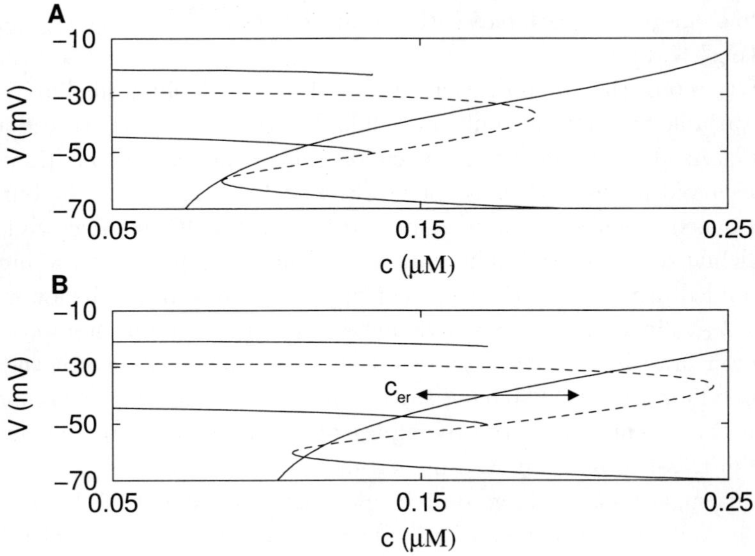

Fig. 2.12. The z-curve and c-nullcline for two different values of $g_{K(Ca)}$ and with c_{er} clamped. (**A**) With $g_{K(Ca)} = 1000$ pS the dynamics are similar to those of the Chay-Keizer model without an ER. Here, $c_{er} = 181$ μM. (**B**) Decreasing $g_{K(Ca)}$ to 500 pS stretches the z-curve, so that the knees are farther apart and the homoclinic bifurcation is further to the right. Now the trajectory stalls at intersections with the nullcline, awaiting slow changes in c_{er} to shift the nullcline to the right or the left (the nullcline moves to the right when c_{er} increases). Unlike the case above, if c_{er} is clamped bursting will not occur. To make this diagram, c_{er} is set at 267 μM.

Unlike the "classical" bursting of the Chay-Keizer model, where the period was set by the time scale of c, the period of the bursting produced by the model with an ER is determined by the time scales of both c and c_{er}. The c time scale determines the time required for the trajectory to move along the z-curve until it reaches an intersection with the c-nullcline. The c_{er} time scale determines the time required for the nullcline to move past the knee during the silent phase and past the homoclinic bifurcation during the active phase. Since c_{er} changes more slowly than c, the burst period is dominated by the c_{er} time scale. Another factor in setting the burst period is the distance that the nullcline must travel for the trajectory to escape the silent or active phase. This is determined by how much the z-curve has been stretched, and thus by the value of $g_{K(Ca)}$. It is for this reason that such a large range of burst periods is achieved by varying this parameter. This scenario, in which the bursting is driven by activity-dependent oscillations in two or more slow variables with disparate time scale, is called "phantom bursting" [7, 9].

It is interesting to note that the mechanism of phantom bursting, a slow variable translating a nullcline while the other "nullcline" (the z-curve) remains fixed, is similar to the mechanism for Chay-Keizer bursting itself when viewed in the n-V phase plane (Figs. 2.2 and 2.3). That is, bursting is produced when slow changes in c translate the V-nullcline while the n-nullcline remains fixed. The duration of the silent phase of the burst is determined primarily by the length of time required to move the lower knee of the V-nullcline past the n-nullcline, so that there is no intersection on the lower branch. The active phase duration is also determined by the time required for changes in c to move the V-nullcline, this time past a homoclinic bifurcation point. Thus, the dynamics of phantom bursting recapitulate those of classical bursting at a higher level.

This suggests that we go on to view c as a component of the fast subsystem and consider a stack of c-V phase-planes for different values of c_{er}. That is, we construct the bifurcation diagram of the V-n-c subsystem with respect to c_{er}. The z-curve for V with respect to c_{er} is then the curve on which V, n, and c are at steady state. It can be computed analytically by inverting Eq. (17) to get c_{er} in terms of c, and using Eqs. (11), (12) to express c in terms of V. Although the algebra is the same as before, when we viewed Eq. (17) as the equation for the c-nullcline and c as a slow variable, the point of view has changed. We now view c as a fast variable in equilibrium with V. The results are shown in Fig. 2.13 for the default parameters (A) and for increased ER leak (B). The oscillations become faster (see insets) because the the z-curve is squashed when the ER leak is greater, decreasing the amplitude of c_{er}. This is the case that was considered by Chay [12, 13], in an early unappreciated example of phantom bursting. The increase in frequency is physiologically relevant for β-cells, representing part of the effect of acetylcholine to increase burst frequency and insulin secretion. Eqs. (11), (12), (17) also predict an increase in frequency when stores are depleted by reducing k_{serca}, another phenomenon seen in β-cells. See Bertram and Sherman [9] for details.

Varying k_{serca} and p_{leak} in proportion changes the rate of ER Ca^{2+} turnover without depleting or overfilling the ER. This also affects burst kinetics, with reduced turnover reducing burst period and also attenuating the slow tail in cytosolic Ca^{2+} (not shown). Thus, the ratio of ER flux to plasma membrane flux is an important parameter for adjusting β-cell models to produce realistic Ca^{2+} timecourses.

It may seem paradoxical that c_{er} is now the slow, negative-feedback variable because it does not affect the plasma membrane ion channels directly. The resolution of the paradox is contained in Eq. (17), which can be rewritten in the following form:

$$\begin{aligned} c &= \frac{-\alpha I_{Ca}(V)}{k_{pmca} + k_{serca} + p_{leak}} + \frac{p_{leak} c_{er}}{k_{pmca} + k_{serca} + p_{leak}} \\ &= c_{fast} + c_{slow} \ . \end{aligned} \tag{18}$$

Thus, c can be decomposed into a fast component, which is in equilibrium with V and a slow component, which is in equilibrium with c_{er}. The slow rise and fall of c_{er} is communicated to $g_{K(Ca)}$ through the latter component. From this point of view, the increase in burst frequency as p_{leak} is increased reflects the increased efficiency with which the ER can influence $g_{K(Ca)}$. This "subtle inhibitory effect" of the ER was noted by Shorten and Wall [37] in a model for pituitary corticotrophs exhibiting a range of non-square-wave bursting patterns. We point out that the ER does not play solely an inhibitory role: during the early part of the active phase, it blunts the rise of c and hence the activation of $g_{K(Ca)}$. This stimulatory effect prolongs the active phase, setting the stage for the delayed inhibitory effect that ultimately terminates the active phase.

2.6. Further Modifications to the Model

The model presented here is in reasonable agreement with the data in Fig. 2.9(A), in which cytosolic Ca^{2+} rises throughout the active phase, but not with Fig. 2.9(B), in which cytosolic Ca^{2+} declines towards the end of the active phase. Here we point to several modifications to the model in the current literature where this issue is addressed in different but complementary ways.

One way is to incorporate a hidden Ca^{2+} compartment that communicates with $g_{K(Ca)}$ in which $[Ca^{2+}]$ rises throughout the active phase [21]. Such a compartment was postulated in order to account for data showing that block of SERCA pumps eliminated $I_{K(Ca)}$.

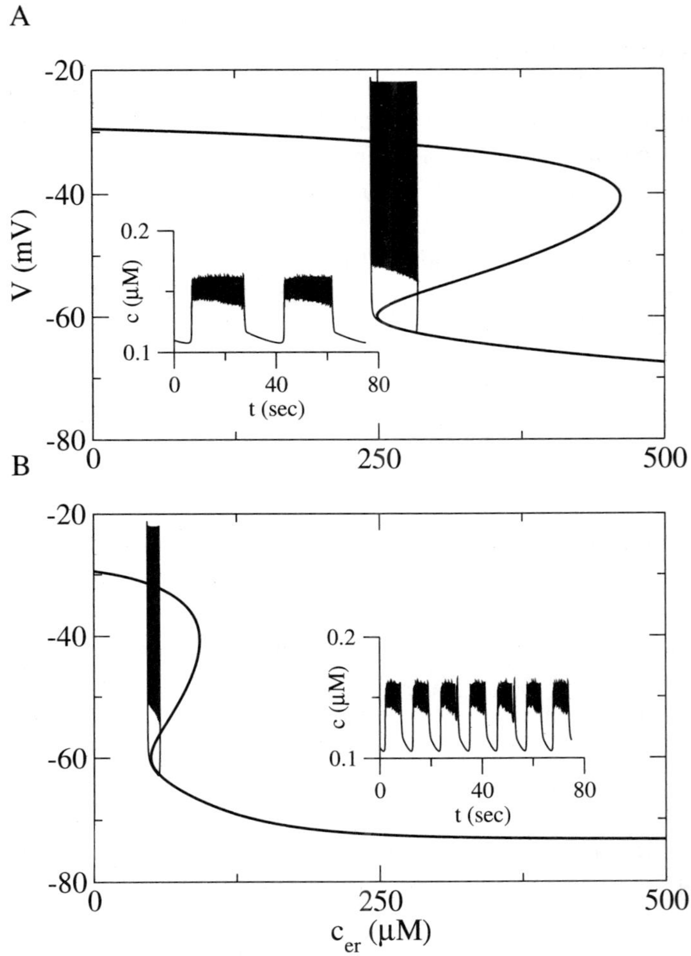

Fig. 2.13. Increasing ER efflux reduces c_{er} amplitude and increases burst frequency. BDs with respect to c_{er}. (**A**) $p_{leak} = 0.0002$, (**B**) $p_{leak} = 0.001$ (insets, c vs. t).

A second way is to incorporate a slow negative feedback process that is triggered by a rise in c but outlasts the rise in c. The hypothesis of Keizer and Magnus [27] that the rise in c inhibits mitochondrial ATP production and hence reopens K(ATP) channels fits this description, and complements the effects of c_{er} in phantom-type models by sliding the V-c z-curve horizontally. (See Eqs. (11), (12) and Bertram and Sherman [9]).

A third proposal is that c is not the primary ionic negative feedback process, but rather Na^+, which enters through the Na^+-Ca^{2+} exchanger and activates the Na^+-K^+ pump [20].

Finally, data on compound oscillations ("bursts of bursts") in membrane potential, cytosolic Ca^{2+}, and metabolic variables, such as oxygen, glucose, and mitochondrial membrane potential, have led to models in which glycolytic oscillations interact with electrical oscillations [8]. These oscillations of metabolism would again slide the V-c z-curve, but, because they are independent of or only weakly dependent on cytosolic Ca^{2+}, the trajectory can be dragged outside the region of bistability. One consequence is that the oscillation may no longer be resettable by brief perturbations of membrane potential.

This is an area in which rapid development is in progress, but the dynamic foundation described here should continue to be useful in analyzing new models as they appear.

2.7. Discussion

We have traced the development of ideas on negative feedback by cytosolic Ca^{2+} via K(Ca) channels in β-cell models, starting with the Chay-Keizer model [15]. That model was successful in a number of ways, but its prediction of the kinetics of Ca^{2+} oscillations appeared to be fatally in disagreement with experiments showing both fast and slow components in c. Here we showed how adding a slow ER to Chay-Keizer could account for much of the discrepancy. The essential idea is that cytosolic Ca^{2+} is not very slow (viewed on the timescale of tens of seconds to minutes as found in β-cell bursting electrical activity), but that the ER can impart an effective slow component.

More generally, one can speak of bi-directional communication between the plasma membrane and the ER. Oscillations of membrane potential cause oscillations of cytosolic Ca^{2+}, which are propagated into the ER. In turn, oscillations of ER Ca^{2+} modulate the kinetics of cytosolic Ca^{2+} and can thus affect membrane potential through cytosolic Ca^{2+}-dependent ion channels. This idea was used by Li *et al.* [29] to explain how the ER promotes its own refilling after being emptied by agonists: when the ER is refilling, it takes up Ca^{2+} from the cytosol, deactivating K(Ca) channels and thus increasing action potential frequency and Ca^{2+} entry through the plasma membrane.

With regard to the β-cell, we caution that it has only been shown that K(Ca) channels can, with assistance from the ER, function as a slow negative feedback mechanism. While this hypothesis has also received some support from the identification for the first time of an appropriate non-voltage dependent K(Ca) channel in β-cells [21, 22], it remains to be established experimentally that these K(Ca) channels play the role we have attributed to them.

We know that K(Ca) channels can not be solely responsible for bursting, because slow cytosolic Ca^{2+} oscillations persist in mice in which the low-affinity SERCA3 pump has been knocked-out [1]. In this case, the cytosolic oscillations lack the slow tail seen normally (Fig. 2.9), which likely means that ER Ca^{2+} is flat. Thus, one can have oscillations of c without oscillations in c_{er}, raising the question of what role the latter serves. One intriguing possibility is that oscillations in the ER are at least as important for other functions of the cell, such as protein trafficking and gene expression, as for regulating cytosolic Ca^{2+} and membrane potential. This would be parallel to cytosolic Ca^{2+}, which serves both signaling and rhythmogenic roles.

Even if ER Ca^{2+} uptake is intact, the ER may fail to oscillate if it is too slow (eg. if σ_{er} is very small in Eq. (15)). In the model decribed here, the ER only has an effect when it is sourcing or sinking Ca^{2+}. However, it is believed that β-cells, like many other cells, also possess store-operated channels (SOC) that carry an inward current directly activated by the level of c_{er}. SOC was previously proposed by us to mediate the response to acetylcholine-dependent store dumping [36] in a model with a very slow ER. Alternatively, when the ER is fast enough to oscillate in response to bursting, SOC can provide a gross depolarization that complements the increased frequency we showed here when ER efflux is activated (Fig. 2.13; Bertram and Sherman [9]). It has also been suggested that SOC itself can drive bursting, since influx would be attenuated by ER filling during the active phase and would recover during the silent phase [13, 20]. A different proposal is that Ca^{2+} influx triggers Ca^{2+} release from the ER by calcium-induced calcium release (CICR) and thus activates SOC to help sustain the active phase. This scenario seems unlikely, however, because disabling SERCA pumps increases, rather than decreases, the amplitude of c [10].

The dynamical consequences of having two negative feedback variables (here, cytosolic and ER Ca^{2+}) in a square-wave bursting model obviously generalize well beyond the β-cell. We have illustrated the concept of phantom bursting by means of bifurcation diagrams in the V-c plane, with c_{er} used as a parameter, and in the V-c_{er} plane, with c treated as a fast variable. The reader may wish to consider yet another point of view, the two-slow-variable plane (here, c vs. c_{er}), as described by Smolen *et al.* [40]. Another interesting case to consider is the model of Cornelisse *et al.* [17] for pituitary melanotropes, which lacks an ER but has two slow variables because the K(Ca) channels are assumed to respond slowly to Ca^{2+}.

Acknowledgements

R. B. was supported by NSF DMS-0311856.

References

[1] A. Arredouani, Y. Guiot, J. C. Jonas, L. H. Liu, M. Nenquin, J. A. Pertusa, J. Rahier, J. F. Rolland, G. E. Shull, M. Stevens, F. Wuytack, J. C. Henquin, and P. Gilon, SERCA3 ablation does not impair insulin secretion but suggests distinct roles of different sarcoendoplasmic reticulum Ca^{2+} pumps for Ca^{2+} homeostasis in pancreatic β-cells, *Diabetes.* **51**, 3245–3253, (2002).

[2] F. M. Ashcroft, D. E. Harrison, and S. J. H. Ashcroft, Glucose induces closure of single potassium channels in isolated rat pancreatic β-cells, *Nature.* **312**, 446–448, (1984).

[3] F. M. Ashcroft and P. Rorsman, Type 2 diabetes mellitus: not quite exciting enough?, *Human Mol. Gen.* **13**, R21–R31, (2004).

[4] I. Atwater, C. M. Dawson, A. Scott, G. Eddlestone, and E. Rojas. The nature of the oscillatory behavior in electrical activity for pancreatic β-cell, *Horm. Metab. Res. Suppl.* **10**, 100–7, (1980).

[5] P. M. Beigelman, B. Ribalet, and I. Atwater, Electrical activity of mouse pancreatic beta–cells: II. Effects of glucose and arginine, *J. Physiol. (Paris).* **73**, 201–217, (1977).

[6] R. Bertram, M. J. Butte, T. Kiemel, and A. Sherman, Topological and phenomenological classification of bursting oscillations, *Bull. Math. Biol.* **57**, 413–439, (1995).

[7] R. Bertram, J. Previte, A. Sherman, T. A. Kinard, and L. S. Satin, The phantom burster model for pancreatic β-cells, *Biophys. J.* **79**, 2880–2892, (2000).

[8] R. Bertram, L. Satin, M. Zhang, P. Smolen, and A. Sherman, Calcium and glycolysis mediate multiple bursting modes in pancreatic islets, *Biophys. J.* **87**, 3074–3087, (2004).

[9] R. Bertram and A. Sherman, A calcium-based phantom bursting model for pancreatic islets, *Bull. Math. Biol.* **66**, 1313–1344, (2004).

[10] R. Bertram and A. Sherman, Filtering of calcium transients by the en-

doplasmic reticulum in pancreatic β-cells, *Biophys. J.* **87**, 3775–3785, (2004).

[11] R. J. Butera Jr., J. Rinzel, and J. C. Smith, Models of respiratory rhythm generation in the pre-Bötzinger complex. I. Bursting pacemaker neurons, *J. Neurophysiol.* **81**, 382–397, (1999).

[12] T. R. Chay, Electrical bursting and luminal calcium oscillation in excitable cell models, *Biol. Cybern.* **75**, 419–431, (1996).

[13] T. R. Chay, Effects of extracellular calcium on electrical bursting and intracellular and luminal calcium oscillations in insulin secreting pancreatic β-cells, *Biophys. J.* **73**, 1673–1688, (1997).

[14] T. R. Chay and D. L. Cook, Endogenous bursting patterns in excitable cells, *Math. Biosci.* **90**, 139–153, (1988).

[15] T. R. Chay and J. Keizer, Minimal model for membrane oscillations in the pancreatic β-cell, *Biophys. J.* **42**, 181–190, (1983).

[16] D. L. Cook, W. E. Crill, and D. Porte, Jr., Plateau potentials in pancreatic islet cells are voltage-dependent action potentials, *Nature.* **286**, 404–406, (1980).

[17] L. N. Cornelisse, W. J. J. M. Scheenen, W. J. H. Koopman, E. W. Roubos, and S. C. A. M. Gielen, Minimal model for intracellular calcium oscillations and electrical bursting in melanotrope cells of *Xenopus Laevis*, *Neural Comput.* **13**, 113–137, (2000).

[18] G. B. Ermentrout, *Simulating, analyzing, and animating dynamical systems: A guide to XPPAUT for researchers and students.* (SIAM Books, Philadelphia, 2002).

[19] R. FitzHugh, Impulses and physiological states in theoretical models of nerve membrane, *Biophys. J.* **1**, 445–466, (1961).

[20] L. E. Fridlyand, N. Tamarina, and L. H. Philipson, Modeling of Ca^{2+} flux in pancreatic β-cells: role of the plasma membrane and intracellular stores, *Am. J. Physiol. (Endocrinol. Metab.).* **285**, E138–E154, (2003).

[21] P. B. Goforth, R. Bertram, F. A. Khan, M. Zhang, A. Sherman, and L. S. Satin, Calcium-activated K^+ channels of mouse pancreatic β-cells are controlled by both store and cytoplasmic Ca^{2+}: Experimental and theoretical studies, *J. Gen. Physiol.* **120**, 307–322, (2002).

[22] S. O. Göpel, T. Kanno, S. Barg, L. Eliasson, J. Galvanovskis, E. Renström, and P. Rorsman, Activation of Ca^{2+}-dependent K^+ channels contributes to rhythmic firing of action potentials in mouse pancreatic β cells, *J. Gen. Physiol.* **114**, 759–769, (1999).

[23] B. Hille, *Ionic channels of excitable membranes.* (Sinauer Associates,

Sunderland, MA, 2001).

[24] J. L. Hindmarsh and R. M. Rose, A model of neuronal bursting using three coupled first order differential equations, *Proc. R. Soc. Lond. B.* **221**, 87–102, (1984).

[25] A. L. Hodgkin and A. F. Huxley, A quantitative description of membrane current and its application to conduction and excitation in nerve, *J. Physiol. (Lond.).* **117**, 500–544, (1952).

[26] E. M. Izhikevich, Neural excitability, spiking, and bursting, *Int. J. Bifur. Chaos.* **10**, 1171–1266, (2000).

[27] J. Keizer and G. Magnus, ATP-sensitive potassium channel and bursting in the pancreatic β cell, *Biophys. J.* **56**, 229–242, (1989).

[28] J. Keizer and P. Smolen, Bursting electrical activity in pancreatic β cells caused by Ca^{2+}- and voltage-inactivated Ca^{2+} channels, *Proc. Natl. Acad. Sci. USA.* **88**, 3897–3901, (1991).

[29] Y.-X. Li, S. S. Stojilkovic, J. Keizer, and J. Rinzel, Sensing and refilling calcium stores in an excitable cell, *Biophys. J.* **72**, 1080–1091, (1997).

[30] E. K. Matthews and M. D. L. O'Connor, Dynamic oscillations in the membrane potential of pancreatic islet cells, *J. Exp. Biol.* **81**, 75–91, (1979).

[31] C. Morris and H. Lecar, Voltage oscillations in the barnacle giant muscle fiber, *Biophys. J.* **35**, 193–213, (1981).

[32] R. E. Plant, The effects of Ca^{2+} on bursting neurons, *Biophys. J.* **21**, 217–237, (1978).

[33] J. Rinzel. A formal classification of bursting mechanisms in excitable systems. In eds. E. Teramoto and M. Yamaguti, *Mathematical Topics in Population Biology, Morphogenesis and Neurosciences*, vol. 71, *Lecture Notes in Biomathematics*, pp. 267–281, Berlin, (1987). Springer–Verlag.

[34] J. Rinzel, T. R. Chay, D. Himmel, and I. Atwater. Prediction of the glucose-induced changes in membrane ionic permeability and cytosolic Ca^{2+} by mathematical modeling. In eds. I. Atwater, E. Rojas, and B. Soria, *Biophysics of the Pancreatic β-Cell*, pp. 247–263. Plenum Publishing Co., New York and London, (1986).

[35] J. Rinzel and Y. S. Lee. On different mechanisms for membrane potential bursting. In ed. H. G. Othmer, *Nonlinear oscillations in biology and chemistry*, vol. 66, *Lecture Notes in Biomathematics*, pp. 19–33, Berlin, (1985). Springer–Verlag.

[36] A. Sherman. Calcium and membrane potential oscillations in pancreatic β-cells. In eds. H. G. Othmer, F. R. Adler, M. A. Lewis, and J. C.

Dallon, *Case Studies in Mathematical Modeling—Ecology, Physiology, and Cell Biology*, pp. 199–217. Prentice-Hall, New Jersey, (1997).

[37] P. R. Shorten and D. J. N. Wall, A Hodgkin-Huxley model exhibiting bursting oscillations, *Bull. Math. Biol.* **62**, 695–715, (2000).

[38] P. Smolen and J. Keizer, Slow voltage inactivation of Ca^{2+} currents and bursting mechanisms for the mouse pancreatic β–cell, *J. Membrane Biol.* **127**, 9–19, (1992).

[39] P. Smolen and A. Sherman, Phase independent resetting in relaxation and bursting oscillators, *J. Theor. Biol.* **169**, 339–348, (1994).

[40] P. Smolen, D. Terman, and J. Rinzel, Properties of a bursting model with two slow inhibitory variables, *SIAM J. Appl. Math.* **53**, 861–892, (1993).

[41] J. Tabak, J. Rinzel, and M. J. O'Donovan, The role of activity-dependent network depression in the expression and self-regulation of spontaneous activity in the developing spinal cord, *J. Neurosci.* **21**, 8966–8978, (2001).

[42] D. Terman, The transition from bursting to continuous spiking in excitable membrane models, *J. Nonlinear Sci.* **2**, 135–182, (1992).

[43] M. Valdeolmillos, R. M. Santos, D. Contreras, B. Soria, and L. M. Rosario, Glucose-induced oscillations of intracellular Ca^{2+} concentration resembling bursting electrical activity in single mouse islets of Langerhans, *FEBS Lett.* **259**, 19–23, (1989).

[44] B. van der Pol and J. van der Mark, The heartbeat considered as a relaxation oscillation, and an electrical model of the heart, *Phil. Mag.* **6**, 763–775, (1928).

[45] M. Zhang, P. Goforth, R. Bertram, A. Sherman, and L. Satin, The Ca^{2+} dynamics of isolated mouse β-cells and islets: Implications for mathematical models, *Biophys. J.* **84**, 2852–2870, (2003).

CHAPTER 3

AUTOREGULATION OF BURSTING OF AVP NEURONS OF THE RAT HYPOTHALAMUS

Peter Roper

Laboratory of Biological Modelling, NIDDK,
12A South Drive, National Institutes of Health, Bethesda, MD 20892, USA
e-mail: proper@helix.nih.gov

Colin H. Brown

Centre for Neuroendocrinology and Department of Physiology, School of Medical Sciences, University of Otago, P.O. Box 913, Dunedin, New Zealand
e-mail: colin.brown@stonebow.otago.ac.nz

Charles W. Bourque

Centre for Research in Neuroscience, Montréal General Hospital, Montréal, Canada
e-mail: charles.bourque@mcgill.ca

William E. Armstrong

Department of Anatomy and Neurobiology, University of Tennessee College of Medicine, Memphis, TN, USA
e-mail: warmstrong@utmem.edu

3.1. Introduction

Arginine vasopressin (AVP) is the hormone that controls both blood osmolality and pressure, and it is secreted directly into the blood by certain neurones of the neuroendocrine system. In contrast to most other CNS neurones these cells do not release neurotransmitter[a] from their terminals at a synapse, but rather secrete AVP into the blood system, *via* exocytosis, in response to invasion of the nerve terminal by incident action potentials (spikes). In the absence of appropriate physiological stimuli, such as dehydration or a sudden drop in blood pressure, the basal secretion is low but is sufficient to maintain homeostasis. To effect this level of release the neurones emit a slow (<1.5Hz), Poisson distributed spike train. However the autonomic nervous system defends aggressively homeostasis of both blood pressure and osmolality, and a swift increase in secretion of the hormone occurs during dehydration, during haemorrhage and during carotid occlusion. Under such stimuli the cells start to fire lengthy (>20s), repeating bursts of action potentials which are separated by equally lengthy silent periods [63]. Mean firing rates during bursts can attain ~10Hz which significantly elevates the secretion rate, while the long periods of quiescence presumably allow the cells to recover and rebuild their readily-releasable stores of the peptide. In fact these protracted bursts and silences are the most efficient mode of firing for release from AVP nerve terminals [8]. There are more than 6000 AVP cells in the brain and since the entire population fires asynchronously, the total amount of peptide secreted into the blood increases smoothly with increasing stress. Phasic activity persists in *in vitro* preparations, as shown in Fig. 3.1, although there do appear to be subtle differences between *in vivo* and *in vitro* activity [54]. *In vitro* bursting can be evoked by either varying the osmolality of the perfusing media, or by direct depolarization [1, 40].

AVP is not the sole peptide released from these cells, but it is both copackaged and co-released with several other substances in the secretory vesicles, the most notable of which is the opioid peptide dynorphin. When released into the pituitary gland, dynorphin diffuses and acts on κ-opioid receptors on the terminals of neighbouring oxytocin (OT) cells to inhibit the secretion of their hormone [9, 60] by blocking calcium influx into the terminal [53], as shown in Fig. 3.2. Thus dynorphin is thought to act in the neurohypophysis as a paracrine neuromodulating agent.

Release of both AVP and dynorphin occurs also within the hypothalamus *via* dense-core granule (DCG) exocytosis from the somato-dendritic region of AVP cells. However here both the range of action and the modulatory roles of both peptides differ from their counterparts in the neuro-

[a]In fact, as in common with most neuropeptides, AVP has a dual role and can also act as a neurotransmitter, but this will not be discussed here.

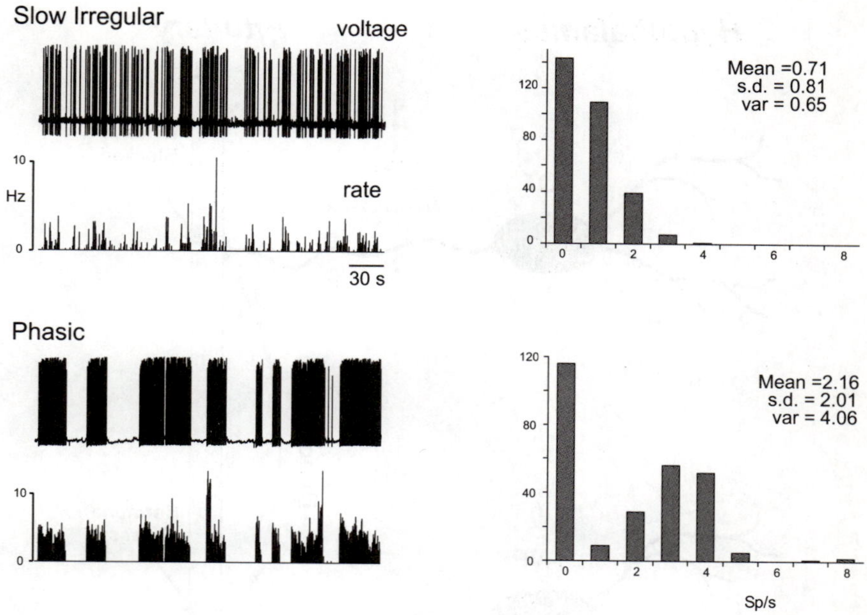

Fig. 3.1. Slow-irregular and phasic discharge *in vitro* in a hypothalamic slice preparation, *cf.* Fig. 1 of [44]. See [50, 51] for a description of experimental protocols. Mean firing rates are computed by averaging over a 300 second spike train divided into consecutive 1 second epochs. Slow irregular activity is the discharge pattern seen *in vivo* under basal conditions and is characterized by a Poissonian (variance/mean $\simeq 1$) distribution of firing rates with a skewed distribution. Phasic bursting occurs in AVP cells *in vivo* during times of stress, such as dehydration or haemorrhage, and is associated with a bimodal distribution of firing rates with a high (typically ~ 2.5) variance-to-mean ratio [44].

hypophysis. AVP cells express both V_{1a} and V_{1b} AVP autoreceptors, and these both increase calcium influx through voltage gated channels [21] when activated, and furthermore V_1 receptor activation also reduces the amplitude of incident excitatory synaptic potentials [36]. AVP diffuses widely within the nuclei before enzymatic degradation and so its release can affect both the secreting cell and also its neighbours. In contrast the diffusion of dynorphin is strongly constrained by the action of endopeptidases and so its influence is restricted to a small region around the site of secretion. Thus in the hypothalamus, AVP can be both an autocrine and a paracrine agent whilst dynorphin tends to act preferentially as an autocrine modulator. A further level of autoregulatory complexity is that the secretory vesicles also contain dynorphin sensitive κ-opioid receptors which are inserted into the cell membrane during exocytosis and thus can amplify the effects of the

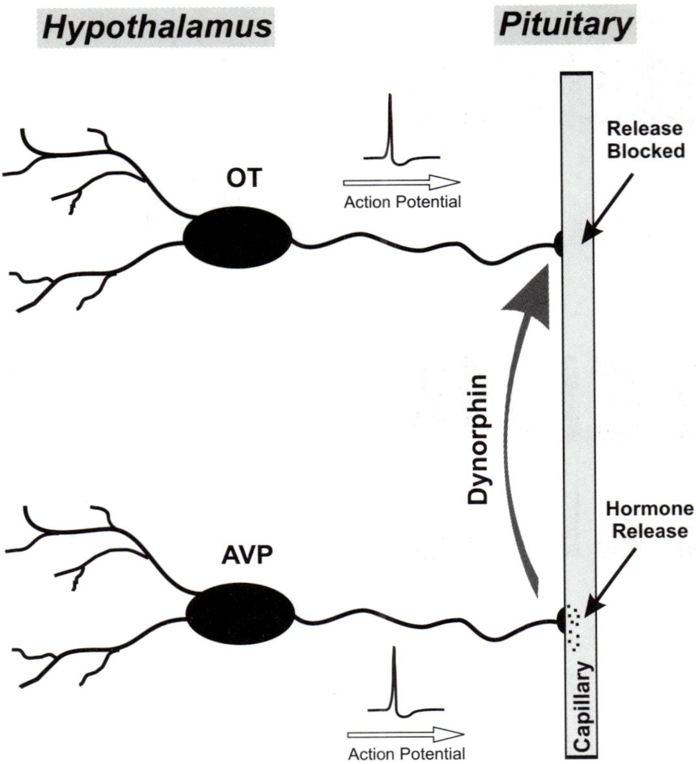

Fig. 3.2. Paracrine actions of dynorphin in the pituitary gland. The opioid peptide dynorphin is secreted from terminals of AVP cells in the neurohypophysis. It can diffuse and act *via* κ-opioid receptors on terminals of neighbouring oxytocin-secreting neurones to block calcium influx and so inhibit release of OT.

secreted opioid in a stimulus dependent manner [55].

In this chapter we will concentrate specifically on the autocrine action of dynorphin in the supraoptic nucleus, and show how it is a key modulator of phasic bursting. Our mathematical model is based solely on *in vitro* data, but we discuss how our findings may extrapolate to *in vivo* preparations. A complete elucidation of the mathematical model can be found in [50, 51], and our experimental protocols are discussed fully in [15, 50, 51].

3.2. Electrical Properties of AVP Cells

AVP cells *in vitro* have a resting potential close to -65mV and fire action potentials that typically reach $+40$mV and have a half-width of $\sim$1.2ms

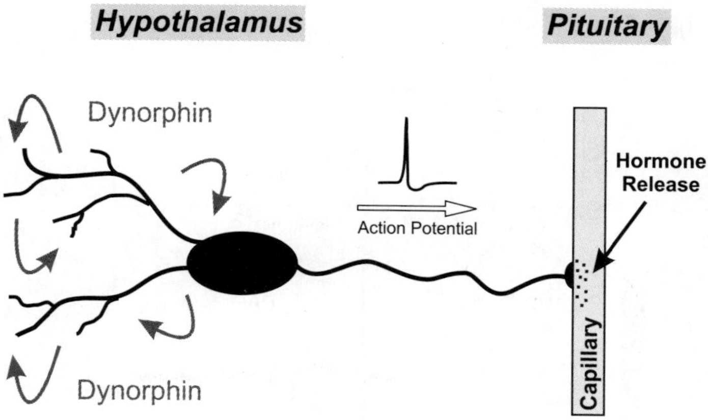

Fig. 3.3. Autocrine actions of dynorphin in the hypothalamus. Dynorphin is released by dense-core granule exocytosis from the somato-dendritic region of AVP neurones in the hypothalamus. It acts on κ-autoreceptors on the secreting cell to modulate the cell's own electrical activity. Its diffusion is restricted by the action of endo-peptidases, and so it tends to act in an autocrine rather than a paracrine fashion.

[6]. Spike repolarization transiently overshoots rest and merges into a brief hyperpolarization, the hyperpolarizing afterpotential (HAP), which decays mono-exponentially with τ_{HAP} ~17.5ms and hyperpolarizes the cell by ~7.4mV [13]. A single spike briefly elevates intracellular calcium, probably *via* influx through high-voltage gated calcium channels, and the transient subsequently decays slowly. Calcium clearance after short trains of spikes follows a single exponential with time constant τ_{Ca} = 2.33s and decays toward a rest state of $C_r \equiv [\mathrm{Ca}^{2+}]_{rest} \sim 113\mathrm{nM}$ [51].

Single, isolated, spikes *in vitro* are succeeded by a small, lengthy transient depolarization of the membrane potential, known as the depolarizing after-potential (DAP) and shown in Fig. 3.4(i)(c). The DAP is both calcium- and voltage-dependent, lasts for up to 6 seconds, raises the membrane potential by ~3mV and its decay tracks that of $[\mathrm{Ca}^{2+}]_i$, as shown in Fig. 3.4(ii). It is thought to be caused by the temporary, calcium-mediated inhibition of a persistent potassium channel, $I_{K,leak}$, that otherwise contributes to maintenance of the resting potential (but see also [27]). The DAPs that follow two or more closely spaced spikes sum to a much larger afterpotential and the resulting depolarization can take the cell above spike threshold.

Trains of evoked spikes also activate a long-lasting hyperpolarization of the membrane potential, the AHP shown in Fig. 3.4(b) [3, 5, 13, 35]. The

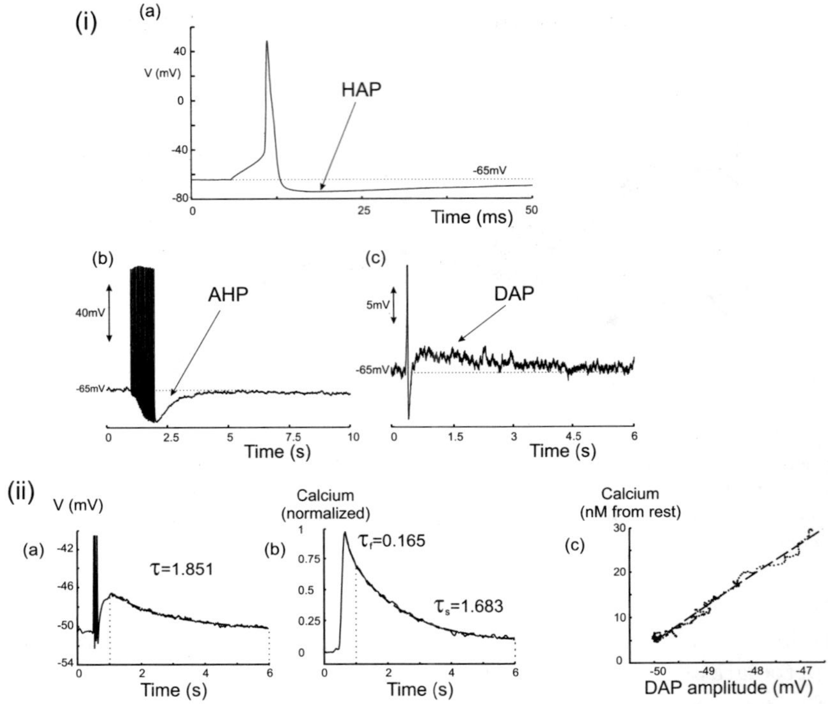

Fig. 3.4. (i) Spike after-potentials in AVP MNCs: (a) The hyperpolarizing after-potential (HAP) follows each spike and typically hyperpolarizes the cell by $\sim$ 7.5mV and lasts for 25–125ms. (b) An after-hyperpolarizing potential (AHP) follows each spike train. It decays mono-exponentially with $\tau \sim 500$ ms and has a maximum amplitude $\sim$12.5mV. (c) The depolarizing after-potential (DAP) succeeds the HAP. DAPs can last for several seconds and a single DAP can depolarize the cell by $\sim$3mV. Note that the spike has been truncated for clarity. The traces are taken from whole cell (a, b) and sharp electrode (c) recordings in the slice and explant respectively. (ii) The dependency of the DAP on intracellular calcium: (a) An average of 15 DAPs from different neurones evoked with 3 spikes at 20 Hz. The baseline membrane potential was offset to be near -50mV for all cells to reduce DAP amplitude variability and obtain a smooth decay. The decay was fit to a single exponential of 1.851, as shown by the dashed line. (b): The average somatic calcium response for the 15 DAPs. Each response was normalized to its peak. This curve was fit with a double exponential with a fast time constant of 0.165s and a slow time constant of 1.683s, the latter is shown by the dashed line. The vertical lines show the region of this curve (*i.e.* $1 \leq t \leq 6$s) matching the DAP decay shown in the left panel. (c): The decay of the averaged DAP is plotted against the average Ca^{2+} decay. For calcium, values were converted to nM using the average peak value (41 nM) in order to appreciate the relationship between elevations in bulk calcium and the activation of the DAP. The linear fit to these responses is shown by the dashed line. Figures modified from [51].

AHP decays with a single time constant (400–500ms) [5, 61], is abolished by removal of calcium, and is markedly abbreviated by apamin [5, 11, 34, 35], although it is not entirely abolished [28]. During a train of spikes the AHP becomes manifest as a progressive increase in the inter-spike interval, and this is termed spike frequency adaptation (SFA). The AHP and the DAP overlap in time, but since the former activates more quickly than does the latter, it can overwhelm the DAP and cause an initial net hyperpolarization of the membrane. However since the AHP then decays more quickly, the more protracted DAP can appear when the AHP is attenuated.

3.3. Mathematical Model

We have developed a mathematical model for the electrical activity of AVP neurones *in vitro* that is based on a set of Hodgkin-Huxley equations, and whose parameters are derived from experimental data. The full model and parameter set can be found in [51], but briefly it comprises a set of five currents that give rise to individual action potentials ($I_{spike} \equiv I_{Na} + I_{Ca} + I_K + I_A + I_c$), a calcium-dependent potassium AHP current I_{AHP}, and a leak current $I_{leak} = G_{leak}(V - E_{leak})$ that sets both the resting potential and the membrane time constant

$$\frac{\mathrm{d}V}{\mathrm{d}t} = -\frac{1}{\mathcal{C}}(I_{Na} + I_{Ca} + I_K + I_A + I_c + I_{AHP} + I_{leak} + I_{app}) \quad (1)$$

$$\equiv -\frac{1}{\mathcal{C}}(I_{spike} + I_{AHP} + I_{leak} + I_{app}) \quad (2)$$

The specific capacitance is $\mathcal{C} = 1\mu\mathrm{F\ cm}^{-2}$, and I_{app} denotes the effects of any external applied current.

The active currents, (I_{spike} and I_{AHP}) have the usual Hodgkin-Huxley form (for inactivating and non-inactivating currents respectively):

$$I_\gamma = g_\gamma m^\alpha h^\beta (V - E_\gamma) \quad \text{or} \quad I_\gamma = g_\gamma m^\alpha (V - E_\gamma) \quad (3)$$

and their corresponding activation (*e.g.* $m(t)$) or inactivation ($h(t)$) function $x(t)$ evolves to its equilibrium state x_∞ with time constant τ_x, according to

$$\frac{\mathrm{d}}{\mathrm{d}t}x(t) = \frac{x_\infty - x(t)}{\tau_x} \quad (4)$$

Full discussion of the spiking currents can be found in [51] and their specifics will not be considered in detail here. If the leak current has a constant conductance ($G_{leak} = \text{const}$), then Equation (2) has a steady state when the applied current, I_{app}, is zero, but passes through a saddle-node bifurcation to repetitive spiking when I_{app} is increased beyond some threshold, I_{thresh} [52]. For $I_{app} < I_{thresh}$ the stable rest-state is excitable, and single action potentials can be elicited by transient supra-threshold stimulation. The bifurcation is characterized by a switch to repetitive firing with a frequency, ν, that increases with distance above threshold.

Equation (2) does not exhibit bistability (*cf.* the Morris-Lecar model presented in [47]) and if the bifurcation is approached from above, by reducing I_{app} below I_{thresh}, then the system reverts again to its steady state.

The neurone is considered to be isopotential and is treated as a single point, and since bulk calcium is well mixed throughout the cell it is described by a single scalar variable, $C_i \equiv [\mathrm{Ca}^{2+}]_i$, which obeys

$$\frac{\mathrm{d}}{\mathrm{d}t} C_i = -\alpha I_{Ca} - \frac{1}{\tau_{Ca}} (C_i - C_r) \tag{5}$$

In addition the two calcium sensitive K^+-currents, I_c and I_{AHP} are each activated by distinct calcium microdomains, $[\mathrm{Ca}^{2+}]_i^c$ and $[\mathrm{Ca}^{2+}]_i^{AHP}$ respectively, which again are scalar variables and evolve independently of $[\mathrm{Ca}^{2+}]_i$, but for simplicity their dynamics will not be considered here.

We model the current that gives rise to the apamin-sensitive AHP as a non-inactivating K^+-current which depends solely on the calcium concentration ($C_{SK} \equiv [\mathrm{Ca}^{2+}]_i^{AHP}$) in a small domain around the mouth of the channel

$$I_{AHP} = G_{AHP} q_\infty^2 (V - E_K) \tag{6}$$

where the activation, $q_\infty(C_{SK})$, is given by the Boltzman function [51]

$$q_\infty(C_{SK}) = \left(1 + \exp\left[-1.120 - 2.508 \log\left(\frac{C_{SK} - C_r}{1000}\right)\right]\right)^{-1} \tag{7}$$

We assume that the current activates instantaneously since calcium dynamics are already slow, and so the AHP decays sharply once activity has ceased, typically within 30ms of cessation of the spike train [29]. More recent evidence [28] has shown that the AHP has a second, slower, apamin-insensitive component, termed the sAHP. This afterpotential is also mediated by a K^+ current, but needs many more spikes to fully activate. We have not yet incorporated this current into our model.

The DAP is modelled by dividing the leak current into separate sodium and potassium components ($I_{leak} = I_{Na,leak} + I_{K,leak}$), and while the sodium leak current is constant,

$$I_{Na,leak} = G_{Na,leak}(V - E_{Na}) \tag{8}$$

we let the conductance of $I_{K,leak}$ depend on both $[\text{Ca}^{2+}]_i$ and voltage according to

$$I_{K,leak} = G_{K,leak}(1 - R)(V - E_K) \tag{9}$$

where $G_{K,leak}$ is the maximum conductance of the current and $E_K = -90\text{mV}$ is the K^+ reversal potential.

Although $(1 - R)$ describes the modulation of a K^+-leak conductance, it is simpler to think of R as being an activation function for the DAP. It is made up of a calcium- $(a(C_i))$ and a voltage-sensitive $(b_\infty(V))$ component

$$R(C_i, V) = \lambda - \Gamma a(C_i) b_\infty(V) \tag{10}$$

where λ and Γ are constants to account for the possibility that $I_{K,leak}$ can only be partially inhibited. b_∞ activates instantaneously, while a decays exponentially, with time-constant $\tau_a = 75\text{ms}$, according to Equation (4). a_∞ and b_∞ are given by

$$a_\infty(C_i) = \tanh\left(\frac{C_i - C_r}{k_a}\right) \quad \text{and} \quad b_\infty(V) = \left[1 + \exp\left(-\frac{V + V_b}{k_b}\right)\right]^{-1} \tag{11}$$

and the steady state R_∞ is shown in Fig. 3.5.

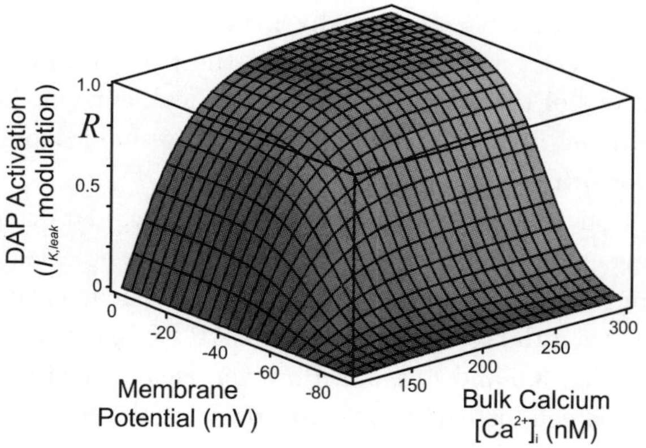

Fig. 3.5. Putative steady-state voltage- and calcium-dependent modulation of the potassium leak current, $I_{K,leak}$, or equivalently the fractional activation of the depolarizing afterpotential. See Equations (10) and (11) (reproduced from [51]).

Thus the calcium that enters the cell during an action potential increases R which partially inactivates $I_{K,leak}$ and so momentarily depolarizes the cell. After the spike, calcium starts to clear, R slowly resets and

$I_{K,leak}$ returns to its rest state. This sequence of events is manifest as a transient depolarization of the membrane, and underlies the depolarizing after-potential.

Note that a_∞, and hence so too R_∞, can go negative if $[\mathrm{Ca}^{2+}]_i$ is brought below rest ($C_i < C_r$), and so $I_{K,leak}$ can be both up- and down-regulated by intracellular calcium.

3.4. Firing Patterns

During the basal (ν <1.5Hz) firing pattern, and in the absence of stimulation, *in vitro* cells lie subthreshold for spiking and single action potentials may be evoked when spike threshold is crossed by transient synaptic input. The cells depolarize during stimulation and this progressively increases their firing rate. If the mean firing rate exceeds ~1.5Hz, then the DAPs that follow two or more closely spaced spikes can sum to a much larger afterpotential and the resulting depolarization can take the cell above spike threshold (but see also [18]), as shown in Fig. 3.6(i), and this bootstrapping also occurs in the model Fig. 3.6(ii). The consequent action potential then brings in more calcium, this in turn elicits another DAP which keeps the cell above threshold and the process then repeats. This spike-dependent, positive-feedback appears as a sustained plateau potential which supports repetitive spiking, and which typically persists for ~20s before abruptly collapsing [1]. In the model, the DAP and the plateau potential are thus both incarnations of the inhibition of the K^+ -leak current, however to be consistent with the literature we refer to sub-threshold depolarizations as DAPs and supra-threshold potentials as plateaus.

The transition from Poisson distributed, slow-irregular firing to repeated phasic bursting can be replicated *in vitro* by direct depolarization. Furthermore, if two or three action potentials are evoked concurrently during slow-irregular firing then the resulting summed DAP can elicit a single burst, as shown in both Fig. 3.6 and Fig. 3.9. However such evoked bursts tend not to repeat and the cell instead returns to slow-irregular firing once the burst has ended.

3.5. Burst Structure

To elucidate the mechanism that drives phasic activity we first consider the progression of a single, evoked burst in a cell that is otherwise not firing phasically. Such bursts can be triggered, both *in vivo* and *in vitro*, by antidromic stimulation; by brief spike trains triggered by short depolar-

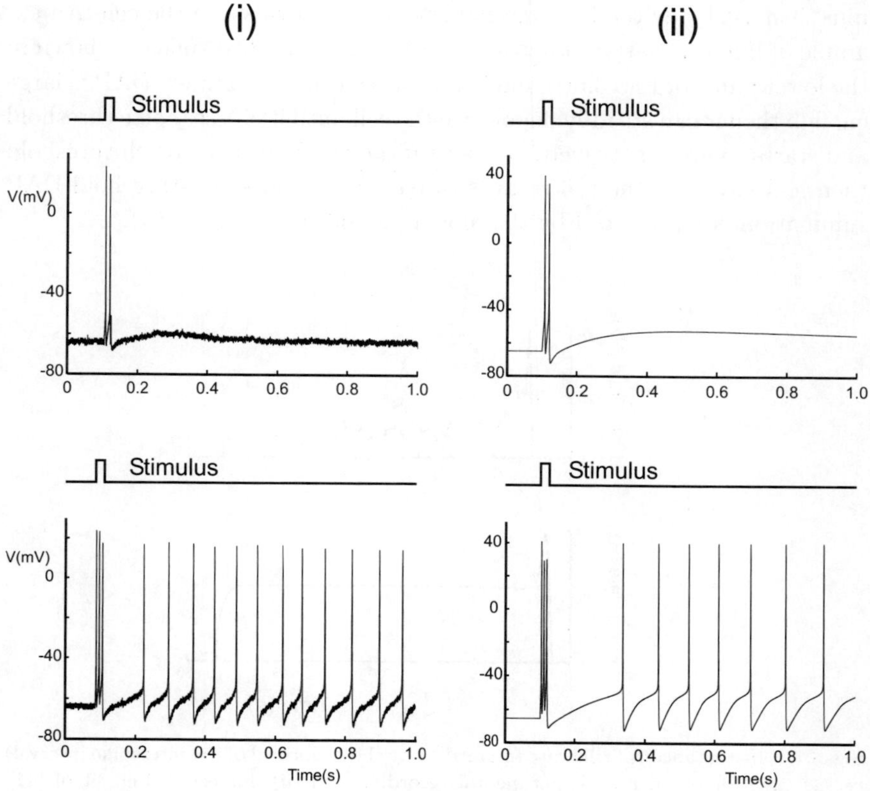

Fig. 3.6. (i) Experimental and (ii) model sub- and supra-threshold depolarizing afterpotentials (DAPs). Data taken from a whole cell recording from the SON of a hypothalamic slice, spikes evoked with a 5ms depolarizing pulse and have been truncated for clarity. Upper panels: two spikes are followed by a DAP that is sub-threshold for firing. The decay of the DAP tracks that of intracellular calcium and returns to rest with a time constant of $\tau \sim 1.85\text{s}^{-1}$ (recall Fig. 3.4(i) and see [51]). Lower panels: DAP summation and the initiation of phasic activity: the stimulation protocol elicits three spikes and the resulting summed DAP crosses spike threshold. The consequent action potentials further raise intracellular calcium, which in turn maintains the suppression of $I_{K,leak}$ and so supports a regenerative plateau potential. This plateau then persists, and continues to support repetitive spiking, until it is inactivated by dynorphin, as discussed in section 3.7.

izing pulses; and also by clusters of excitatory synaptic events. Although the present model includes neither synaptic input nor a mechanism for antidromic activation, current pulses can be injected by choosing a suitable protocol for the applied current, I_{app}.

Since the burst continues for many seconds beyond the end of the stimulus, it must be driven by a mechanism that is intrinsic to the cell. An example of burst initiation *in vitro* by consecutively evoked spikes is shown in the lower panel of Fig. 3.6(i) and it is clear that if the summed DAP is large enough then it can steadily depolarize the cell until it crosses spike threshold and starts to fire repetitively. However if the DAP does not reach threshold then it decays and the cell returns to rest. Sub- and supra-threshold DAP summation is reproduced by the model, as shown in Fig. 3.6(ii).

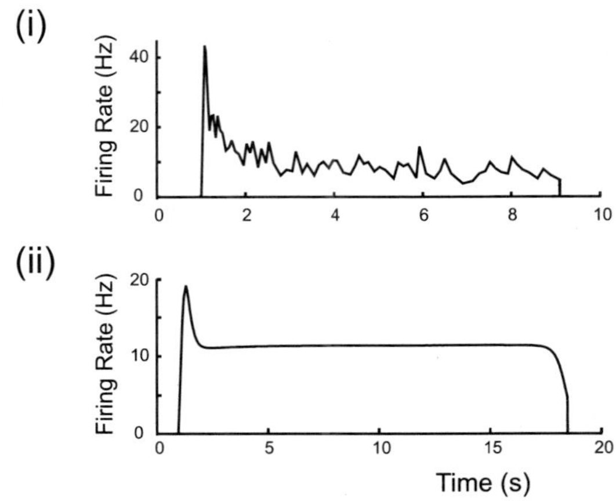

Fig. 3.7. Instantaneous firing rate (quantified by the reciprocal of the interspike interval) *versus* time for (i) *in vitro* experimental recording and (ii) model, *cf.* Fig. 11 of [44]. Note that the rate first rises rapidly to a peak, and then slowly adapts to ∼10Hz as the apamin sensitive AHP becomes slowly activated. Firing then remains steady until the burst abruptly terminates. Figure modified from [50].

The firing rate within a burst, both *in vivo* and *in vitro*, shows strong spike frequency adaptation (SFA) [35, 44], and following an initial rapid acceleration to ∼30Hz the firing gradually slows over the first couple of seconds to ∼10Hz [2] and then remains steady until the end of the burst (but see section 3.7), as shown in Fig. 3.7(i). The firing rate does decrease further during the final few spikes of the burst (see Fig. 3.8), but termination is otherwise abrupt [24] and is not correlated with any further adaptation.

The initial spike-frequency adaptation can be abolished by application of 50–300nM apamin [11, 35] so that the firing frequency remains high (∼30Hz) throughout the burst, and thus SFA is due to the progressive activation of the apamin sensitive AHP current (I_{AHP}) [3, 11]. Such a scenario for spike frequency adaptation also occurs in the model, as shown in the lower panel of Fig. 3.7(ii). However, in contrast to the Plant model for *Aplysia* R15 [43], apamin block *in vitro* decreases, rather than increases, the burst length [35]. Furthermore the time-course of spike frequency adaptation indicates I_{AHP} is strongly activated early, rather than late, in the burst. Thus since $[Ca^{2+}]_i$ also attains its plateau early (see section 3.6 and Fig. 3.9) and does not precipitously rise during the latter stages of the burst, the primary role of I_{AHP} is likely to be the control of the firing rate within the burst and it is unlikely to contribute to burst termination.

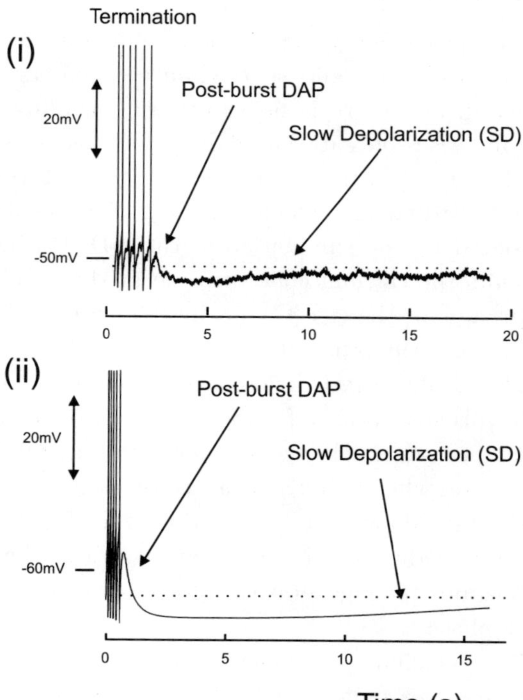

Fig. 3.8. Burst termination and the inter-burst period: (ii) whole cell electrode recording from the SON of a hypothalamic slice, and (ii) model. Note that the firing frequency remains steady until the end of the burst. The final spikes are succeeded first by a post-burst DAP, which in turn is followed by a lengthy, slow depolarization (SD). The experimental trace has been low-pass filtered to remove membrane noise and to make the general trend more evident. Spikes have been trimmed for clarity. (Reproduced from [50].

The end of the burst is characterized by a brief slowing down of the firing rate over the final few spikes, and once spiking has ceased the plateau lingers transiently as a post-burst DAP before collapsing completely. After the active phase the cell falls quiet for another 20s or so, although it can emit occasional spikes during this time. During this silent period, the membrane potential steadily depolarizes until it comes close to, or crosses, spike threshold, and the process can then repeat. Burst termination, the transient persistence of the plateau and the subsequent slow depolarization are shown in Fig. 3.8.

3.6. The Role of Calcium

AVP cells do not prominently express low-voltage gated calcium channels [26] (but see also [25]), and so calcium only enters the cell during an action potential, and there is no sub-threshold influx [51]. In consequence $[Ca^{2+}]_i$ increases only during activity and decays to its rest state ($[Ca^{2+}]_{rest} \simeq$ 113nM) when the cell is silent. Figure 3.9(i) shows simultaneous whole-cell recording and calcium imaging of two evoked bursts, each of which is initiated by the summation of three DAPs. The upper trace in each figure plots the calcium concentration at three different locations in each cell. Throughout the cell $[Ca^{2+}]_i$ initially rises as the burst develops, but long before termination it reaches an elevated steady-state that is typically >200nM above rest. The calcium concentration subsequently remains close to this steady-state for the remainder of the burst, and only decays when firing ceases. In the model, shown in Fig. 3.9(ii), the elevated calcium plateau arises when influx is balanced by clearance, and is typically >150nM supra-threshold for the full activation of the DAP. The heightened calcium concentration during the burst thus saturates the suppression of $I_{K,leak}$ and so sustains the regenerative voltage plateau for the duration of the whole active phase.

Unusually, here calcium is an agent of excitation. In other cells, *e.g.* *Aplysia* R15 bursting pacemaker cells [43], Ca^{2+} more typically mediates inhibition by activating a Ca^{2+} sensitive K^+ -current, whereas in AVP cells calcium excites by *in*activating a Ca^{2+} sensitive K^+ -current.

3.7. The Action of Dynorphin

Dynorphin and κ-opioid receptors (for which dynorphin is the endogenous ligand) are both co-localised in AVP DCGs [56]. The opioid is stored in a Zn^{2+} crystalline lattice, and whilst in the granules dynorphin is prevented from binding to its receptor by a high pH. These granules are found extra-synaptically throughout the somata and dendrites of MNCs [45], and

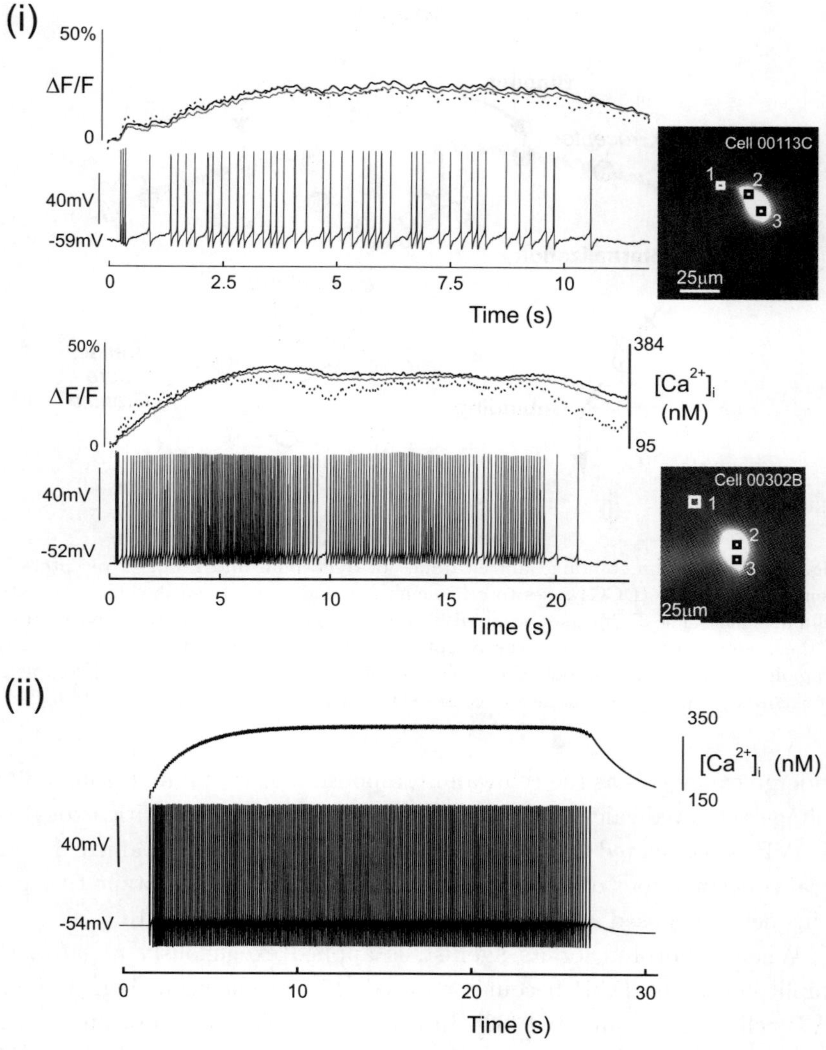

Fig. 3.9. (i) Simultaneous whole-cell recording and calcium imaging of evoked bursts *in vitro* and (ii) model of evoked burst with corresponding calcium concentration. Note that calcium initially rises rapidly until it approaches a steady state and then decays once electrical activity has ceased. The upper trace in each experimental figure plots the calcium concentration at three different locations in each cell, and these locations are shown in the photographs to the right of each figure. The trace that corresponds to each position is: (1) dashed line, (2) bold line and (3) greyscale. Reproduced from [50].

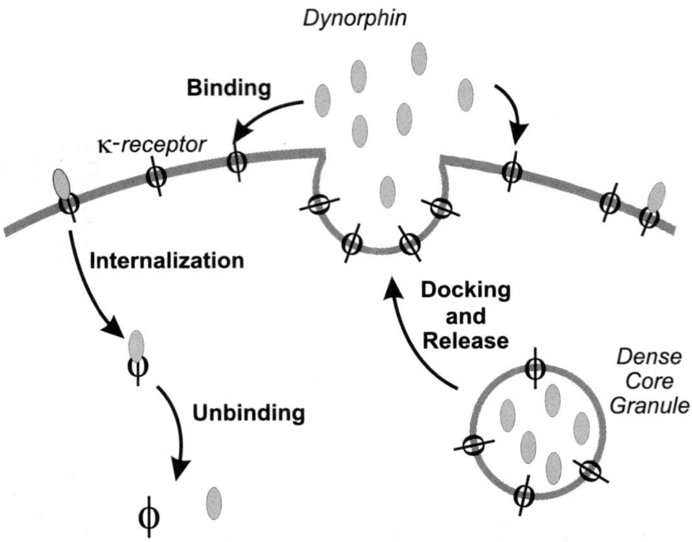

Fig. 3.10. Secretion, binding and clearance of dynorphin and κ-opioid receptors. (i) Dense-core granule (DCG) fuses to cell membrane and spills dynorphin into the extracellular space. The DCG membrane also carries κ-opioid receptors [55] and so fusion of the granule also upregulates the receptor. (ii) Extracellular dynorphin binds to the κ-opioid receptor, and the bound complex begins to signal. (iii) The bound complex is internalized, dephosphorylated, and ceases signalling (reproduced from [50]).

undergo exocytosis at the cell wall in response to Ca^{2+} influx through high-voltage-activated calcium channels [59]. Thus, somato-dendritic exocytosis of AVP is associated with electrical activity and is accompanied by high local concentrations of dynorphin over a region of cell membrane that contains newly exposed κ-opioid receptors, as shown in Fig. 3.10.

When dynorphin, or its agonist, is applied exogenously *in vitro*, the amplitude of the DAP becomes reduced [15], as shown in Fig. 3.11 and AVP cell firing is inhibited [32]. In contrast κ-opioid receptor antagonists increase DAP amplitude and prolong spontaneous and evoked bursts [15], while oxytocin and vasopressin antagonists have no significant effect. Furthermore, since dynorphin may also activate μ-opioid receptors, as well as κ-opioid receptors, we tested a μ-opioid receptor antagonist and found no significant effect. Thus activation of κ-receptors by endogenous dynorphin must both restrain burst duration, and also cause the activity dependent reduction in DAP amplitude. Furthermore, the releasable store of DCGs can be depleted with α-latrotoxin, and this also causes an increase in the DAP amplitude and a lengthening of burst duration. Prior application of a

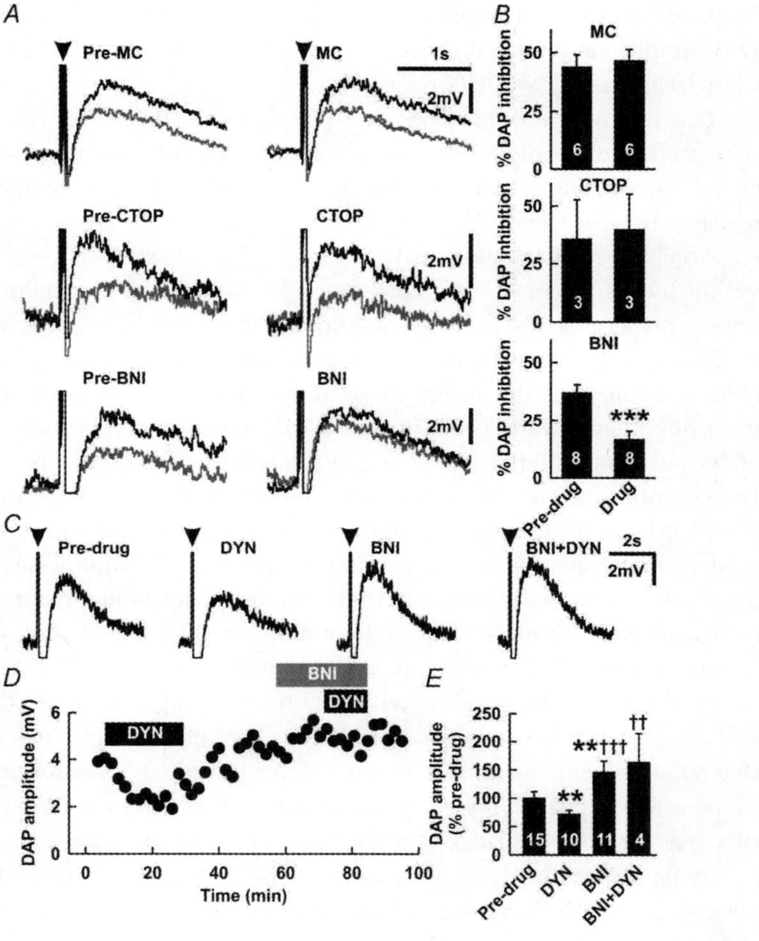

Fig. 3.11. Endogenous κ-opioids inhibit DAPs: A, paired DAPs evoked 4 seconds before (black) and 4 seconds after (grey) a 25-spike train in the presence and absence of receptor antagonists. B, mean DAP inhibition by a 25-spike train before (Pre-drug) and during superfusion (Drug) of the AVP/oxytocin antagonist, Manning Compound (MC; 10μM), the μ-opioid receptor antagonist, D-Phe-Cys-Tyr-D-Trp-Orn-Thr-Pen-Thr amide (CTOP; 1μM), or the κ-opioid receptor antagonist, *nor*-binaltorphimine (BNI; 1μM). $***P < 0.001$ versus pre-drug, paired t test. C, DAPs that each follow an 8-spike train evoked in a 12.25s cycle before and during dynorphin (1μM) and BNI (1μM) superfusion. D, time course of the opioid effects in C. E, mean DAP amplitude. $**\ P < 0.01$ versus pre-drug and $\dagger\dagger\ P < 0.01$ and $\dagger\dagger\dagger P < 0.001$ *versus* DYN, Student-Neuman-Keuls tests (see [15] for details of our statistical analysis). Reproduced from [15].

κ-opioid receptor antagonist prevents the inhibitory effect of α-latrotoxin on DAP amplitude [15], and hence endogenous dynorphin inhibition of DAPs must be mediated by DCG release.

This role of dynorphin appears to be maintained *in vivo*, and the most potent effect of κ-opioid receptor antagonists on AVP cells in anaesthetized rats is also a lengthening of burst duration [17], which is similar to that which occurs *in vitro*.

κ-opioid receptor antagonists also slightly increase AVP cell firing rate within bursts by $\sim$1 Hz [17]. However, this increase is not uniform across bursts; rather it is absent at the onset of the burst and emerges as each burst progresses [19]. Thus the inhibitory influence of endogenous dynorphin increases throughout the active phase in an activity dependent manner, and must be removed during the silent phase of the burst and prior to the onset of the subsequent burst. Resetting of the effect of dynorphin probably has two components: the first is that each bound dynorphin–κ-opioid receptor complex becomes internalized and dephosphorylated, and then ceases signalling; and secondly free extracellular dynorphin is rapidly degraded by peptidases in the brain. In fact protection of endogenous dynorphin from peptidase degradation enhances the inhibition of the DAP, and so the autocrine actions of dynorphin are limited by these enzymes [15].

Furthermore, since the activity of adjacent AVP cells is asynchronous and dynorphin inhibition is absent at the onset of bursts, we can also infer that somato-dendritic release of dynorphin acts only in an autocrine, rather than paracrine fashion under basal conditions. It would therefore seem likely that extracellular peptidases might also act as an effective barrier to the paracrine actions of dynorphin and so inhibit synchronization of activity between AVP MNCs, and maintain a smooth secretion of the peptide, from the whole population, into the blood.

3.8. The Bursting Mechanism

Although dynorphin clearly plays a role in ending a burst, the actual mechanism of termination has not yet been established. It does appear that the plateau potential progressively inactivates, and that this occurs in such a way that it eventually becomes unable to sustain firing and consequently collapses [3, 14]. In addition, the successive generation of DAPs on a timescale of several seconds significantly reduces their amplitude [12], as shown in Fig. 3.13, and their subsequent recovery is slow (τ = 4.7s) [15]. It is known that such activity-dependent inhibition can be caused by the au-

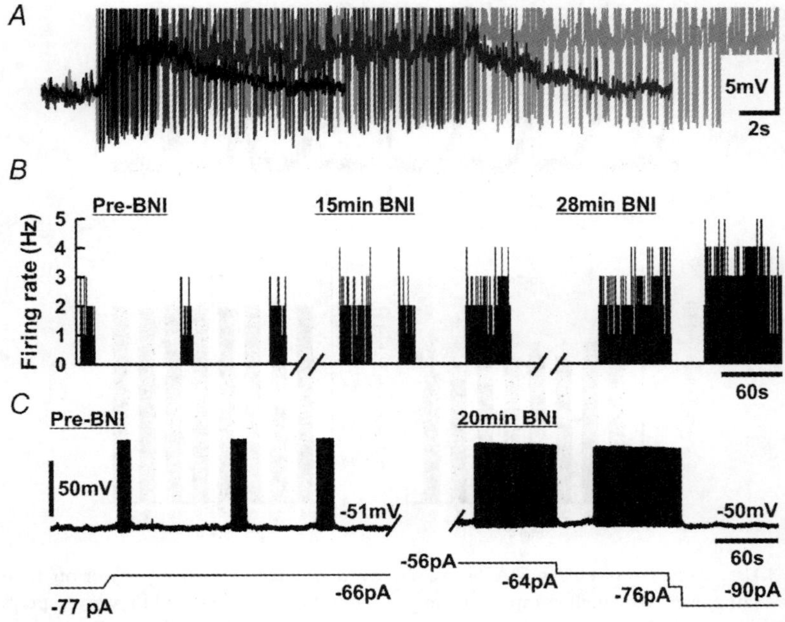

Fig. 3.12. Inhibition of autocrine κ-opioid actions prolongs spontaneous phasic bursts: A, spontaneous bursts of activity (spikes truncated) before (black) and during 1μM BNI superfusion, aligned at onset. BNI delayed plateau potential inhibition after 5 min (dark grey) and induced continuous activity after 20 min (pale grey). B, MNC spontaneous firing rate before and during BNI superfusion. BNI progressively increased the active period duration, eventually leading to continuous activity. The final period of activity shown was terminated by hyperpolarizing current injection (see C). C, membrane potential of a spontaneously phasic MNC (top trace) before (left) and during (right) superfusion of 1μM BNI. Before application of BNI, phasic activity was initiated by reducing the hyperpolarizing current injection to -66pA (bottom trace). All three Pre-BNI bursts terminated spontaneously without further manipulation of the hyperpolarizing current injection. In the presence of BNI, activity started spontaneously when the hyperpolarizing current injection was at -56pA. By contrast to activity before BNI application, in the presence of BNI activity did not spontaneously terminate; the first period of activity was terminated by increasing the hyperpolarizing current injection to -64pA. The MNC subsequently re-started firing without further adjustment of the hyperpolarizing current injection but again did not spontaneously terminate firing. Increasing the hyperpolarizing current injection to -76pA failed to terminate the second period of firing but a further increase to -90pA successfully terminated firing. Thus, during blockade of κ-opioid receptors, the MNC could spontaneously initiate activity but could not spontaneously terminate firing (as seen in 2 of 6 MNCs tested). Reproduced from [15].

tocrine action of dynorphin [16], and is prevented when dynorphin antagonists are applied (see Fig. 3.13), however it is still not clear how dynorphin exerts its effects on the membrane potential.

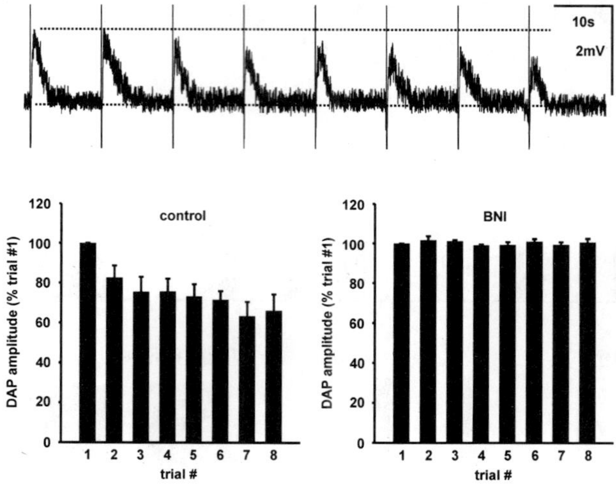

Fig. 3.13. Top: Consecutive DAPs evoked by depolarizing current injection to elicit spike trains, each of which comprised the same number of spikes. DAPs were repeatedly evoked every 12.25 seconds and show a progressive decrease in amplitude. Bottom: Mean DAP amplitude over the course of 8 consecutive trials where DAPs were evoked 12.25s apart before (left) and during (right) BNI superfusion, showing that the progressive reduction of the DAP amplitude is caused by the endogenous activation of κ-opioid receptors.

In order to keep the DAP plateau active and the cell in a repetitive firing regime, $[Ca^{2+}]_i$ needs must be maintained above the threshold for inhibiting $I_{K,leak}$. Therefore either $[Ca^{2+}]_i$ must be brought sub-threshold or the threshold must be raised for the burst to terminate. Since the calcium concentration varies little during the latter stages of the burst, see Fig. 3.9, we previously inferred [50] that termination is caused by an elevation of the threshold for triggering a calcium-dependent, self-sustaining plateau. We call this threshold, or separatrix, the DAP threshold and we model its desensitization by progressively decreasing the sensitivity of the DAP to calcium. We therefore propose that dynorphin acts to desensitize $I_{K,leak}$ by shifting the half-activation of R to higher calcium concentrations (see Fig. 3.15). Thus Equation (11) becomes

$$a_\infty(C_i) = \tanh\left(\frac{C_i - C_r - \phi D}{k_p}\right) \tag{12}$$

where $\phi = 20$nM is a scaling factor chosen to fit to data. D is a dimensionless

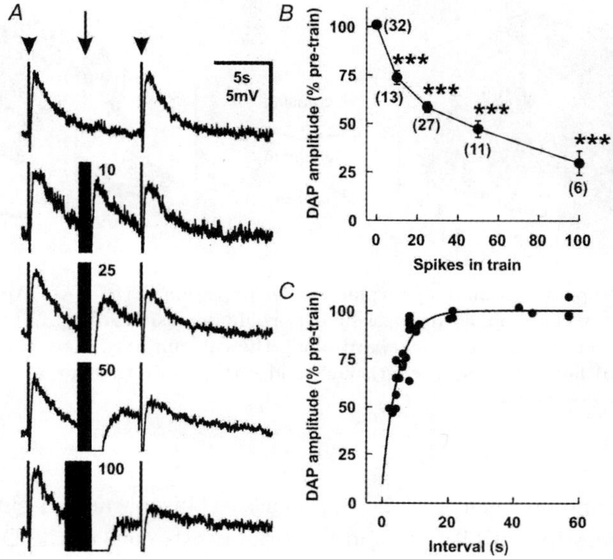

Fig. 3.14. Activity-dependent inhibition of DAPs. A, DAPs (averages of 5) that each follow a 5-spike train (arrowheads) evoked 9s apart by a 80ms depolarizing pulse (+150pA). A conditioning train (arrow) of 0 – 50 spikes over 1 s each, or 100 spikes over 2s, was evoked by a corresponding number of 5ms, +500pA DC pulses. B, DAP amplitude 4s after conditioning trains containing 0 – 100 spikes. $***P < 0.001$ *versus* pre-train, Student-Newman-Keuls tests. The number of MNCs in each group is shown in parentheses. C, DAP amplitude at various times after a 25-spike conditioning train. A single exponential function with a time constant of 4.7s was fitted to the data ($r^2 = 0.84$, data from 9 cells). Reproduced from [15].

variable that represents the indirect effect of dynorphin on the K^+-leak current, and hence on the activation of the DAP, and as such quantifies the transduction of the bound dynorphin/κ-opioid receptor complex. Therefore, although D is related to the extra-cellular concentration of dynorphin, the two are distinct.

We assume that D increases in some manner when the cell is active, and decreases when the cell is silent. If the half-activation shifts slowly as D increases, then $I_{K,leak}$ remains saturated and the firing rate remains steady until the DAP threshold approaches the calcium plateau. As this happens, $I_{K,leak}$ begins to reactivate, and this in turn reduces the plateau, which causes the firing rate to slow as the set of spiking currents (I_{spike}) approaches its saddle-node. Once the DAP threshold is brought above the calcium plateau, the de-sensitized DAP becomes unable to support repet-

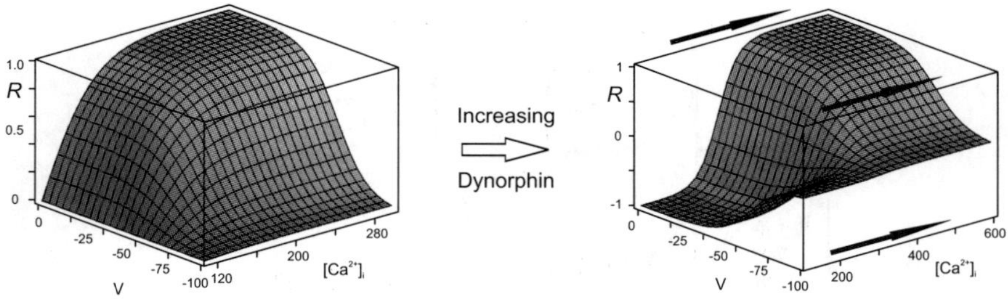

Fig. 3.15. Proposed action of dynorphin on the activation of the DAP. We suggest that the activation of the κ-opioid receptor by dynorphin desensitizes $I_{K,leak}$ to calcium and so shifts the activation curve rightward along the calcium axis. Note that the axis in the right-hand figure has been lengthened, and furthermore that for $D > 0$, R can go negative for some values of $C_i > C_r$.

itive firing and so decays and firing ceases. This paradigm closely corresponds to *in vitro* activity [2], and the brief persistence of the DAP is clear in the recording plotted in Fig. 3.8. Although the intra-cellular calcium is still elevated during this time, it is now sub-threshold for DAP re-activation and, since there is no activity, there is no further influx and it decays to rest, recall Fig. 3.9. D also decays, but if it does so more slowly than does $[Ca^{2+}]_i$, then R will remain shifted such that the cell stays sub-threshold and will not fire. While we do not know the true trajectory of D, recovery of the DAP from activity-dependent inhibition can be fit to a single exponential with time constant $\tau = 4.7$s [15] (see Fig. 3.14).

The model thus explains the temporal profile of the firing frequency throughout the burst. The initial rise and subsequent adaptation are caused first by the inaugural bootstrapping of the DAP summation and then by the ensuing activation of I_{AHP}. Since R subsequently remains saturated ($R \simeq 1$) until the end of the burst, the amplitude of the plateau, and hence the firing frequency, remains constant despite the increase in D and its attendant desensitization of $I_{K,leak}$. As the end of the burst is finally approached, R, and hence the plateau, starts to decrease until the saddle-node of I_{spike} is approached. At this time, the firing frequency starts to decrease until the saddle-node is crossed and firing ceases. Furthermore, the foreshortening of the burst by apamin [35] results from an increase in the activity-dependent secretion of dynorphin, and hence a more rapid increase of D due to the elevated firing rate within the burst.

A prolonged slow depolarization during the silent phase, shown in Fig. 3.8(i) also arises in the model and is a consequence of $[Ca^{2+}]_i$ decaying faster than does D. Recall that our hypothesis is that dynorphin desensitizes the DAP (and thus the plateau) to calcium, thus allowing $I_{K,leak}$ to re-activate even though calcium remains elevated. The burst then terminates and both $[Ca^{2+}]_i$ and D begin to decay. However if $[Ca^{2+}]_i$ decays faster than D, it approaches its rest while D is still elevated and the calcium-dependence of the DAP is still shifted. Therefore the calcium concentration temporarily lies much lower on the $I_{K,leak}$ modulation curve than it does when the cell is at rest (recall from Equation (11) that a_∞ can go negative in low $[Ca^{2+}]_i$). This therefore makes R negative, and so from Equation 9 this in turn increases the amplitude of $I_{K,leak}$ and hyperpolarizes the cell. The hyperpolarization slowly fades as dynorphin decays and $I_{K,leak}$ eventually returns to its rest state ($R = 0$). This overshoot and slow reset is manifest as a slow depolarization of the membrane potential, and is clear in Fig. 3.8(ii). The sequence of events is shown schematically in Fig. 3.16.

3.9. The Dynamics of Dynorphin

Neuromodulation by dynorphin depends not only on its extracellular concentration, but also on the interaction between dynorphin and the κ-opioid receptor, and thus also on the κ-opioid receptor density. We assume that dynorphin is secreted from the cell's dendrites when an action potential is fired, and that it also has some clearance mechanism. To model the effects of dynorphin on the membrane potential, we represent the transduction of κ-opioid receptor activation by the dimensionless variable D which increases in some manner when the cell is active, and decreases when it is silent.

The simplest model is to assume that D is zero when the cell is at rest, is augmented by an amount Δ every time the cell spikes (or the membrane potential crosses some threshold V_{thresh}), and decreases exponentially when the cell is quiet, so that

$$\frac{\mathrm{d}}{\mathrm{d}t}D = -\frac{1}{\tau_D}D \qquad \text{and} \qquad D = D + \Delta \quad \text{when} \quad V = V_{thresh}^{+} \tag{13}$$

where we set τ_D to be equal to the time constant for recovery from activity dependent inhibition of the DAP (*i.e.* $\tau_D = 4.7$s, see Fig. 3.14), and for concreteness we set the voltage threshold $V_{thresh} = 0$mV. Whilst it appears that a single spike is able to trigger somato-dendritic secretion in oxytocin cells [22], functional feedback effects of peptides thus released are only evident after clusters of spikes [19] and so Δ should be thought of as the average secretion per spike.

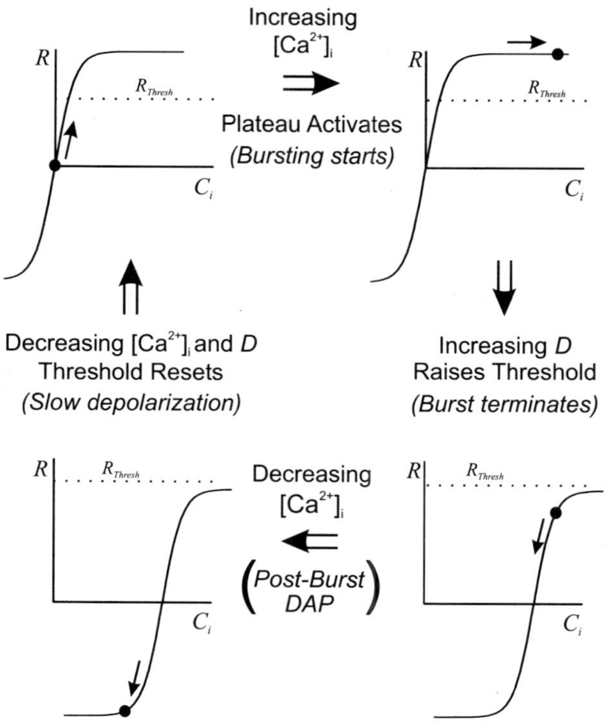

Fig. 3.16. The evolution of $[Ca^{2+}]_i$ and D throughout and between bursts, and the corresponding up- and down-modulation of $I_{K,leak}$ (shown schematically). The cycle starts from top-left and moves clockwise, and the activation of the DAP/plateau at any time is denoted by the filled circle. 'Threshold' denotes calcium threshold for triggering the plateau potential (not spike-threshold) and depends on spike-frequency. Note that the function R denotes the modulation (not activation) of $I_{K,leak}$ and so starts at zero, but can go negative if $[Ca^{2+}]_i$ decays while R is still right-shifted. This negative modulation corresponds to an upregulation of $I_{K,leak}$ and leads to a hyperpolarization of the membrane potential. The sequence of events is: (i) spike-driven Ca^{2+} influx depolarizes the cell by depressing $I_{K,leak}$. The depolarization triggers more spikes, further increasing $[Ca^{2+}]_i$ and so sustaining a plateau and initiating a burst; (ii) subsequent spikes cause further influx and so saturate the inhibition of $I_{K,leak}$; (iii) D starts to increase, desensitizing $I_{K,leak}$ to Ca^{2+} and raising the plateau threshold until it is no longer self-sustaining. Plateau then collapses and the burst terminates; (iv) D decays more slowly than Ca^{2+} and so remains elevated while Ca^{2+} decays. Thus $I_{K,leak}$ remains transiently desensitized, causing R to go negative and temporarily hyperpolarizing the membrane. Hyperpolarization decays as D is cleared, and becomes manifest as a slow-depolarization. As both $[Ca^{2+}]_i$ and D decay, the cell returns to its initial state. Reproduced from [50].

To include the effect of receptor insertion into the membrane, in [50] we assumed that Δ depends directly on D, so that

$$\Delta(D) = \xi + \gamma D \tag{14}$$

where ξ is a small constant bias term that breaks the symmetry of the $D = 0$ state.

3.10. Analysis of Bursting

A burst is driven by two slow variables: C_i, which is excitatory, and D, which is inhibitory and must have a slower time-course than C_i. This model differs significantly from that of [48] since here the slow system does not oscillate autonomously. Instead the slow variables are driven by the spiking activity since both C_i and D only increase when the cell fires an action potential.

The standard methodology for analyzing bursting models such as this one is to adiabatically decouple the full model into two disconnected subsystems [48], *FAST* and *SLOW*, such that:

- *FAST* includes all currents that have a time-course of milli-seconds, *i.e.* those that contribute to single spikes (I_{spike})
- *SLOW* comprises all processes with a time-course of seconds, such as the calcium–dynorphin oscillation and its effect on the plateau

The AHP provides a third, distinct, time-scale ($\tau_{AHP} \simeq 500$ms). However since phasic activity still occurs during pharmacological block of I_{AHP}, and further since its major role appears to be to set the steady-state firing frequency during the burst [35], here we consider this current as part of the *FAST* subsystem.

3.10.1. *FAST*

The bifurcation diagram of *FAST* is shown in Fig. 3.17, using the amplitude of the plateau, R as a bifurcation parameter. For $R < R_{thresh}$ *FAST* has a stable steady-state and the cell remains at rest. When R is increased above R_{thresh}, the system passes through a saddle node (SN) bifurcation to a stable limit cycle that underlies repetitive firing. The system is not bistable in the region of the SN, and so again reverts to the steady-state when R is brought back below R_{thresh}.

3.10.2. *SLOW*

The dissociation of *SLOW* from *FAST* is complicated by the fact that the two subsystems are not autonomous, and since *SLOW* is strongly coupled

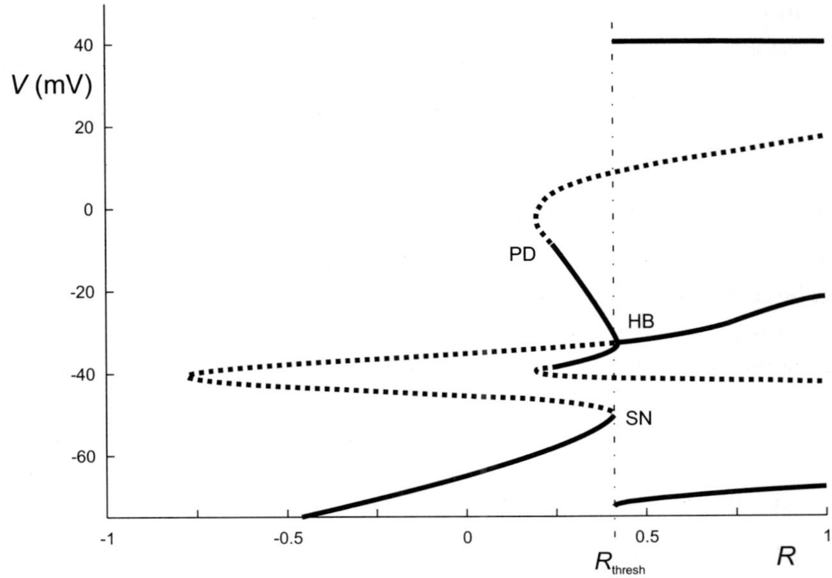

Fig. 3.17. The bifurcation diagram of FAST, for $I_{app} = 0$, using R, the relative amplitude of the plateau potential as a parameter. For $R < R_{thresh}$ $FAST$ has a stable steady-state and the cell remains at rest. The rest state loses stability *via* a saddle-node bifurcation (SN) if R is raised about R_{thresh}, and $FAST$ moves to a stable limit cycle. For larger values of R, $FAST$ does in fact exhibit a second fixed point which bifurcates to another stable limit cycle *via* a Hopf bifurcation (HB), and this branch of limit cycles in turn lose stability through a period doubling (PD) bifurcation, but for $R \in [-1, 1]$ this latter manifold is not simply connected to the former by any stable trajectory. Thus it is inaccessible within the physiological range of behaviour and so does not correspond to any observed state.

to $FAST$ their decomposition is non-trivial. A further difficulty is that the plateau activation, R, depends not only on C_i, but also on V, which introduces a second direct coupling between $SLOW$ and $FAST$. However R is saturated during most of the burst and so its voltage dependence is only effectual during the initial rise and the final fall of the plateau. Thus we may further simplify by considering only the calcium dependence.

The slow $C_i - D$ subsystem may be dissected out of the full model by using the technique of average nullclines [7, 20, 58], which necessitates a numerical integration of the spiking currents over the whole cycle of one action potential. However a simpler reduction can be obtained for this model by instead rewriting Equations (5) and (13) as a firing rate model and using this *ansatz* to decouple the subsystem (see also [49]):

$$\frac{d}{dt}C_i = \nu(R)\Delta_{Ca} - \frac{1}{\tau_{Ca}}(C_i - C_r) \tag{15}$$

$$\frac{d}{dt}D = \nu(R)\Delta_D - \frac{D}{\tau_D} \tag{16}$$

where ν is the cell's firing frequency; Δ_{Ca}, Δ_D are the incremental increases of C_i and D per spike respectively; and $\tau_{Ca} = 2.33$s and $\tau_D = 4.9$s are the decay constants of calcium and D. ν is measured as the reciprocal of the time between two consecutive spikes, and is a function of the plateau activation, *viz.* $\nu \equiv \nu(R)$. In [49] the incremental increase of the slow variable was obtained by integrating the calcium current over a single action potential cycle, however Δ_{Ca} has been measured experimentally [51], and Δ_D is not a constant, but is given by Equation (14).

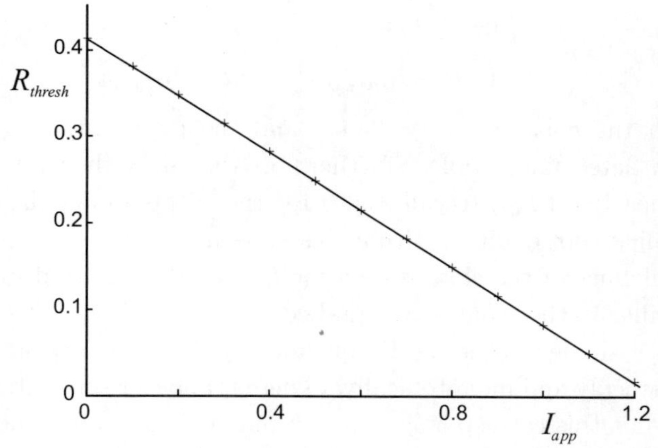

Fig. 3.18. The threshold for the activation of a regenerative plateau, R_{thresh}, depends linearly on I_{app}. Points are numerically computed values of threshold, bold line shows linear fit. Note that R_{thresh} falls below zero for $I_{app} \gtrsim 1.21$, and furthermore that since $R \equiv 0 \; \forall V$ when at rest (*i.e.* $[\mathrm{Ca}^{2+}]_i \equiv [\mathrm{Ca}^{2+}]_{rest}$, $D \equiv 0$), then this is the threshold for the onset of phasic activity.

We wish to examine how the dynamics of *SLOW* vary under depolarization, however the reduction given by Equations (15) and (16) does not explicitly include the effects of the applied current I_{app}. Nevertheless I_{app} does appear implicitly since its effect when increased is to raise the rest potential, and this in turn lowers the threshold for activation of the regenerative plateau, R_{thresh}. Numerically we find that R_{thresh} can be fit to a linear function of I_{app}, as shown in Fig. 3.18, and so increasing I_{app} simply shifts the *FAST* bifurcation diagram (recall Fig. 3.17) leftward. For large I_{app}, R_{thresh} falls below zero ($R = 0$), so that the "rest" state lies above the saddle node of the spiking currents and the cell fires continuously. However R is oscillatory during phasic activity, and so causes *SLOW* to propel *FAST* back and forth through the bifurcation. In common with the Plant model [49], each oscillation corresponds to a single burst/silent period. Since *FAST* is not bistable, there is no possibility for hysteresis and so *SLOW* here must comprise (at least) two slow variables, C_i and D. Furthermore the excitatory variable (C_i) must be significantly faster ($\tau_{Ca} = 2.33$s) than the inhibitory influence (D; $\tau_D = 4.9$s) [46].

The firing rate, ν, can be numerically determined for any given R, by evaluating Equation (2) until spike frequency adaptation is complete and then taking the reciprocal of the interspike interval. Empirically we find that ν can be fit to the function (see Fig. 3.19)

$$\nu = \begin{cases} 0 & R \leq R_{thresh} \\ \Gamma \left(R - R_{thresh}\right)^{\gamma} & R > R_{thresh} \end{cases} \tag{17}$$

where both the constant, $\Gamma = 24.63$, and the exponent, $\gamma = 0.62$, are numerically determined, and we further note that since the value of R_{thresh} depends linearly on I_{app} (recall Fig. 3.18) the effects of depolarization are indeed implicit, not explicit, within this system.

The nullclines of the slow system for $I_{app} = 0$ are plotted in Fig. 3.20, and are similar to those of the Morris-Lecar model (see *e.g.* [42, 47]): the C_i nullcline is N-shaped, while the D nullcline initially runs horizontally before increasing steeply and monotonically. (There is another symmetric nullcline for $D < 0$, but this corresponds to a non-physical solution.) The nullclines intersect at 3 fixed points, the lowest of which, $[C_i \equiv C_r,\ D \equiv 0]$, is stable; and small, transient, perturbations relax back to this point. However, as with the Morris-Lecar model, the system is excitable and a large excursion of *SLOW* – corresponding to an evoked burst in the full model – can be triggered if C_i is elevated by $\gtrsim$ 30nM. Such Ca^{2+}-transients typically arise *in vitro* after 2-3 concurrent spikes [51], and this accords with the triggering of single bursts in a non-phasic cell with a few evoked, proximal spikes (see above).

A small increase of I_{app} causes the D nullcline to shift leftward, although its shape is maintained and the fixed point remains stable. The corresponding effect on $\dot{C}_i = 0$ is twofold: the nullcline not only translates vertically, but its right-hand 'knee' moves further to the right. The

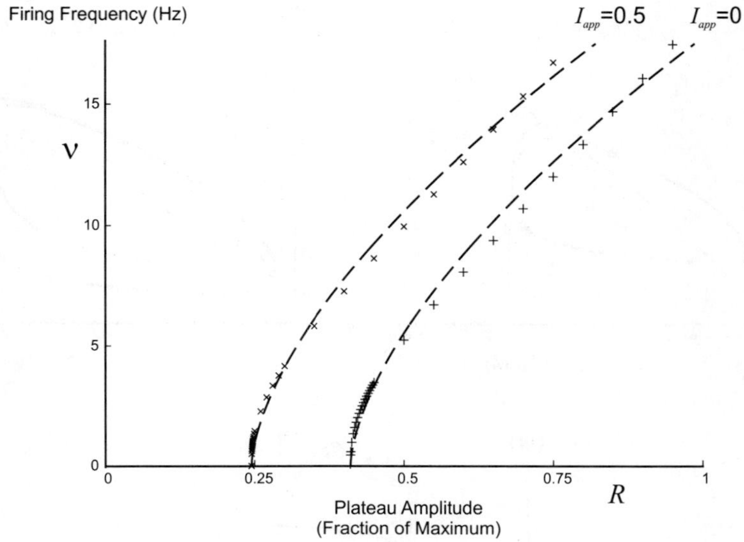

Fig. 3.19. The steady-state, intra-burst firing rate, ν, plotted as a function of R, the activation of the plateau potential, for various values of I_{app}. The intersection of $\nu(R)$ with the abscissa defines R_{thresh} for a given I_{app}, see Fig. 3.18. Symbols correspond to numerically determined values of ν for different values of I_{app}: + denotes $I_{app} = 0$, while × denotes $I_{app} = 0.5$. For any given R, $\nu(R)$ is computed by numerically evaluating Equations (2) and (9) until spike-frequency adaptation has ended and then taking the reciprocal of the interspike interval. Dashed lines show the fit to Equation (17). The non-linearity of $\nu(R)$ stems from the fact that R is not the amplitude of a constant depolarization, but is the modulation of a potassium current with a reversal potential.

sum of these effects that the system remains excitable but with a depressed threshold and an increased oscillation amplitude. (The increased amplitude translates to higher values of both C_i and D during the burst.) However, if I_{app} becomes large enough then the left knee of $\dot{C}_i = 0$ rises above the D nullcline, causing the two lower fixed points to coalesce and disappear in a saddle-node bifurcation. This loss of stability is the nascence of phasic activity, and examples of repetitive phasic bursting in both the model and *in vitro* are shown in Fig. 3.22. Thus $SLOW$ also exhibits Class I excitability: emergent, fixed-amplitude, arbitrarily low-frequency oscillations, as with the Morris-Lecar model (but *cf.* [37]). Note that, in contrast to the $FAST$ subsystem, each oscillation of $SLOW$ represents a full burst of spikes and a subsequent silent phase, rather than a single action potential.

As I_{app} increases still further, the C_i nullcline continues to rise and the right knee moves further to the right, and so $SLOW$ oscillates with

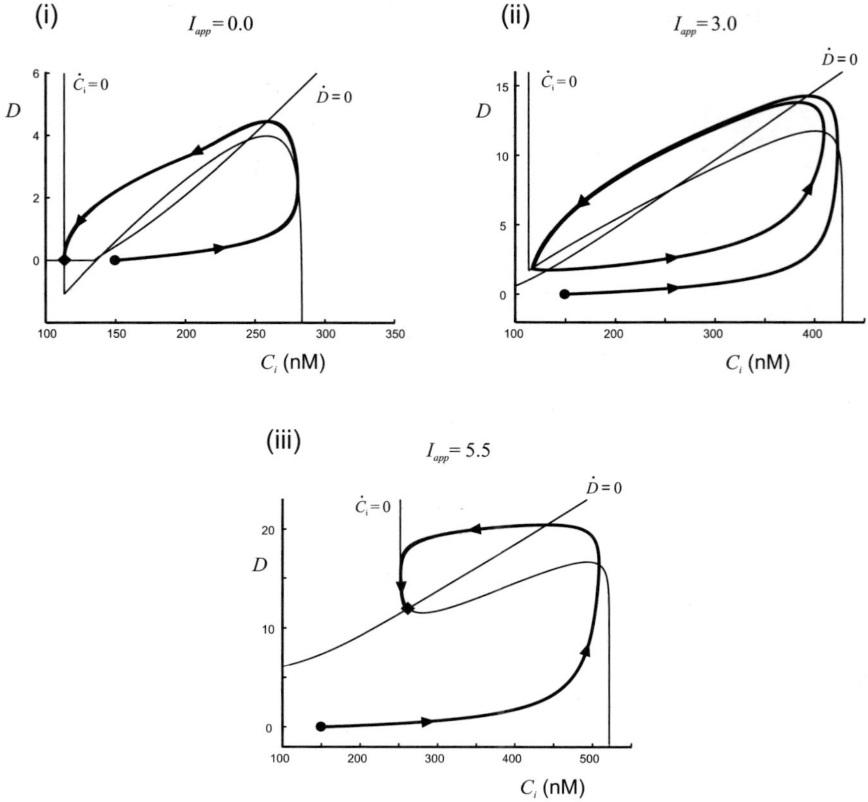

Fig. 3.20. The *SLOW* phase plane for increasing I_{app}. Bold lines show the trajectory of *SLOW* when started from an initial condition of $[C_i = 150\text{nM}, D = 0]$ (shown as a filled circle). This is equivalent to the calcium transient occurring after three concurrent evoked spikes. (i) $[I_{app} = 0]$ The C_i and D nullclines intersect thrice: a single, stable fixed-point $[C_i \equiv C_r, D \equiv 0]$ and two unstable fixed points. *SLOW* has an unstable limit cycle and is excitable for large, transient perturbations. An excitable burst is clear in the trajectory which terminates at the fixed point (filled diamond). (ii) $[I_{app} = 3.0]$ The nullclines now have only a single point of intersection. *SLOW* has a stable limit cycle and is therefore oscillatory, as shown in the trajectory. (iii) $[I_{app} = 5.5]$ The intersection of the C_i and D nullclines moves from the middle branch to the left branch, and *SLOW* stabilizes to a fixed point *via* a Hopf bifurcation. *SLOW* is still excitable when started from the initial condition $[C_i = 150\text{nM}, D = 0]$ but since C_r now lies above this point, the burst does not repeat.

a further increasing burst amplitude. Eventually the intersection of the nullclines moves from the middle branch to the left branch and so stabilizes the fixed point *via* a Hopf bifurcation. Thus *SLOW* eventually 'locks up' and ceases to oscillate, while *FAST* is supra-threshold, and this is the final transition from phasic to a fast-continuous pattern. Note that when the oscillation ceases, the plateau activation, R, tends to a constant, non-zero value. This is also seen *in vitro*, since a persistent plateau remains evident when fast-continuous cells are briefly hyperpolarized below spike threshold [2].

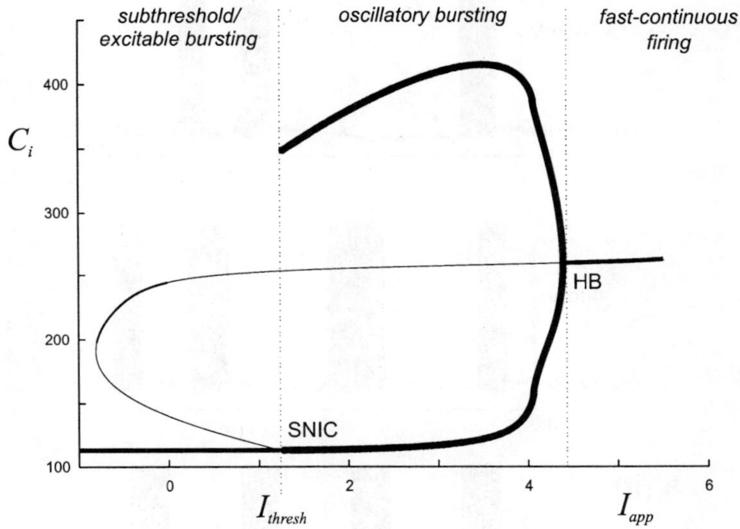

Fig. 3.21. The bifurcation diagram of the $SLOW$ subsystem. The diagram can be subdivided into three regions, and these may be related to the three modes of behaviour observed both *in vitro* and *in vivo*. The left-hand section of the diagram has a only a single stable fixed point, which is below spike-threshold and corresponds to the resting state. In this region $SLOW$ is excitable and a single burst can be evoked when C_i is transiently elevated. When I_{app} is raised above I_{thresh}, the stable fixed point collides with an unstable fixed point and they coalesce in a saddle-node bifurcation (SNIC). Thus the center of the diagram contains a stable limit cycle, which corresponds to repetitive, phasic bursting. As I_{app} increases yet further, the limit cycle disappears in a Hopf bifurcation (HB) so that the right-hand side of the diagram again has only a single, stable fixed-point. However, this fixed point is now supra-threshold for spiking, and so this mode may correspond to the fast continuous spiking seen during sustained dehydration *in vivo*.

$SLOW$ therefore has three distinct modes: a subthreshold/excitable mode, an oscillatory mode, and a steady-state that lies above spike threshold. These three modes are also enunciated on the $SLOW$ subsystem bifurcation diagram plotted in Fig. 3.21. The phasic behaviour seen both *in vitro* and *in vivo* may correspond not only to the oscillatory mode, but might also be engendered during the subthreshold/excitable mode if single bursts are repeatedly evoked, *e.g.* by strong synaptic input. Finally, the supra spike-threshold steady state may correspond to the fast-continuous discharge mode seen during prolonged dehydration *in vivo* [44].

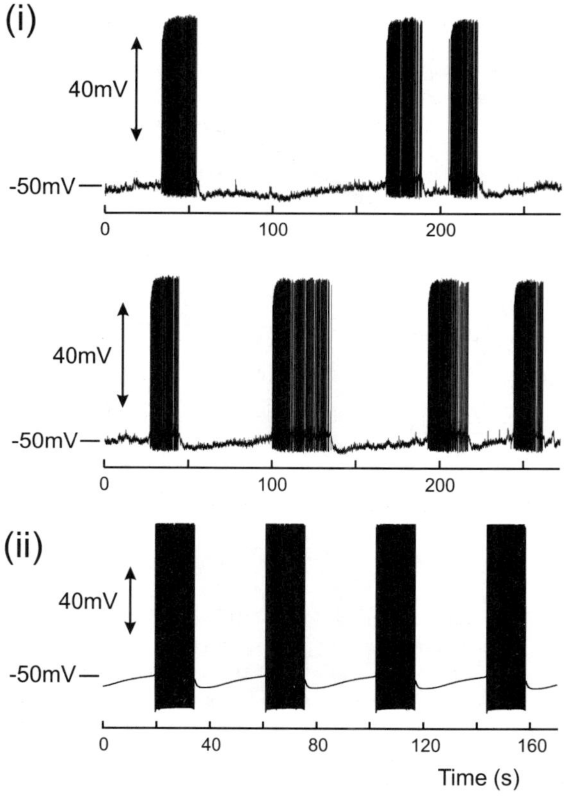

Fig. 3.22. Phasic activity occuring in MNC's during sustained depolarization: (i) experimental recordings and (ii) model. Note silent phase characterized first by post-burst DAP, and then by slow depolarization. Both active and silent phases of the burst have mean length ~20s (see text), but display a wide variability both *in vitro* and *in vivo*. Model parameters are $I_{app} = 1.28$, $\lambda = 0.6$ and $\Gamma = 0.4$. Phasic activity only occurs when the model is depolarized above spike-threshold, and the oscillation is driven by an upregulation of $I_{K,leak}$ which transiently depresses V below threshold and interrupts firing. Reproduced from [50].

When subthreshold, *SLOW* exhibits Class I excitability [31, 47] and so is directly analogous to the Morris-Lecar model for barnacle muscle fibres [42]. Excitable bursting of this sort was discussed briefly by [33] (but see also [20, 57]), and was analyzed extensively, within the context of the ghost-burster model [23] for the pyramidal cells of weakly electric fish, by [37]. However the reduction presented here is closer in spirit to the Morris-Lecar model than is the ghost-burster, since the latter is only excitable when the corresponding $FAST$ subsystem is oscillating periodically. The ghost-burster's excitability therefore depends on the phase of $FAST$ at the time of stimulation, while our AVP model shows no phase dependence, and so here the analogy with type I excitability is exact.

3.11. Discussion

3.11.1. *A dual role for calcium*

By activating the AHP, calcium is usually perceived as a messenger of electrical inhibition rather than excitation (see *e.g.* [62]). However in AVP cells it plays two opposing roles: not only does it mediate both short- and long-term inhibition *via* the activation of BK and SK channels (I_c and I_{AHP}), but it can also excite the cell by turning off the resting K^+ current, $I_{K,leak}$ [39]. Having two such antithetical functions appears at first glance to be contradictory. However there is a delicate interplay between the DAP and the AHP that is dictated by their respective time-scales, and whether the cell exhibits a depolarizing or a hyperpolarizing after-potential depends both on the stimulation frequency and also the number of spikes in the train [3]. In phasic neurones strongly expressing DAPs, prolonged low frequency stimulation (<1Hz) evokes single spikes and consequent DAPs, which then fade to the resting potential. At intermediate frequencies (>1Hz and <10Hz) the DAPs sum to form a regenerative depolarized plateau potential which can then support endogenous firing *via* positive feedback [1]. In contrast, at higher frequencies (>10Hz) the AHP becomes predominant and instead a net hyperpolarization occurs (see Fig. 3.4(b)). Thus calcium acts here both to amplify signals of a certain bandwidth, and to filter stimulation that is of too high or too low a frequency. Furthermore, since the DAP is also voltage-dependent, this signal processing is labile and depends on the membrane potential. Thus the depolarization occurring during osmotic stress magnifies the gain of the amplification, and contributes to phasic activity.

3.11.2. *Alternative mechanisms for the plateau potential*

Here we have adopted the paradigm, initially proposed by [39], that the DAP is a Ca^{2+}-mediated reduction in a resting K^+-current. Not only does this model show burst initiation and termination profiles that closely agree with experiment, but it also clarifies some more subtle features of the cells' electrical activity (*e.g.* the post-burst DAP and the intra-burst slow-depolarization). However, it is also possible that DAP is caused by a Ca^{2+}-activated non-specific cation (CAN) current [10, 27].

In [50] we also examined a model based on the activation and modulation of a CAN current, and showed that, to a first approximation, both models are equivalent since the former is the addition of a depolarizing current while the latter is the subtraction of a hyperpolarizing current. If we also assume that desensitization to Ca^{2+} causes burst termination in both cases, then both models support burst initiation, the plateau potential and burst termination, and so their active phases are indistinguishable. However, recall that R goes negative when $[Ca^{2+}]_i < [Ca^{2+}]_{rest}$ and that this causes the slow-depolarization between bursts. In our model this can be readily interpreted as an upregulation of the resting current $I_{K,leak}$, but if $I_{CAN} = 0$ at rest in the CAN model, then the corresponding mechanism is less fathomable since it should not reverse in low calcium.

We therefore proposed that if I_{CAN} were to be a persistent current, contributing to the resting membrane potential in a similar manner to that which we originally proposed for $I_{K,leak}$, then it is conceivable that it too could be both up- and down-regulated by $[Ca^{2+}]_i$ and dynorphin. Thus a CAN model can only fully explain phasic activity if it is driven by a non-specific cation current that is partially active at rest. Such a current has recently been observed by [30], but it has not yet been shown to be modulated by $[Ca^{2+}]_i$.

3.11.3. *Excitable bursting*

Is burst excitability physiologically useful, or is it merely an artefact of the dynamics? The answer probably lies in the ability of these nuclei to respond to and to integrate multifarious inputs. Recall that phasic firing is the discharge mode most efficient for release from AVP nerve terminals [8]. Thus, while some efferents, *e.g.* histaminergic inputs from the tuberomamillary nucleus [4, 38], cause a tonic and sustained depolarization and so might educe oscillatory, or supra-threshold bursting. Others, for example NMDA receptor activation [41], have a punctuate effect on the cells membrane potential and so can only elicit single spikes. Nevertheless, such discrete input can evince a phasic discharge if excitable bursts are repeatedly evoked, and this may in turn be achieved by triggering spikes with a mean rate of as low as 3Hz [44]. Thus for MNCs *in vivo*, excitable bursting might allow the SON swiftly to amplify intermittent synaptic input into the most efficient discharge mode for secretion.

Acknowledgements

We thank Chunyun (Lisa) Li (University of Tennessee, Memphis) and Ryoichi Teruyama (University of Tennessee, Memphis) for allowing us to reproduce their data, shown in Fig. 3.1, and Figs. 3.4, 3.6, 3.7, 3.8 and 3.22 respectively. We also thank Bard Ermentrout (University of Pittsburgh) for releasing, and supporting XPPaut[b], which was used for all of our numerical work. We also thank Arthur Sherman (NIDDK) both for support and guidance during this work, and for a careful critique of this chapter.

PR is supported by a fellowship from NIH/NIDDK; CB is supported by Wellcome Trust grant numbers 058040 and 070118; WEA is supported by NIH grant number NS23941; and CWB is supported by Operating and Senior Investigator Awards from the Canadian Institutes of Health Research, and by a James McGill Research Chair.

References

[1] R. Andrew and F. Dudek, Burst discharge in mammalian neuroendocrine cells involves an intrinsic regenerative mechanism, *Science*. **221** (4615), 1050–1052, (1983).

[2] R. Andrew and F. Dudek, Analysis of intracellularly recorded phasic bursting by mammalian neuroendocrine cells, *Journal of Neurophysiology*. **51**(3), 552–566, (1984).

[3] R. Andrew and F. Dudek, Intrinsic inhibition in magnocellular neuroendocrine cells of rat hypothalamus, *Journal of Physiology (London)*. **353**, 171–185, (1984).

[4] W. Armstrong and C. Sladek, Evidence for excitatory actions of histamine on supraoptic neurons *in vitro*: Mediation by an H_1-type receptor, *Neuroscience*. **16**, 307–322, (1985).

[5] W. Armstrong, B. Smith, and M. Tian, Electrophysiological characteristics of immunochemically identified rat oxytocin and vasopressin neurons *in vitro*, *Journal of Physiology (London)*. **475**(1), 115–128, (1994).

[b] http://www.math.pitt.edu/~bard/xpp/xpp.html

[6] W. Armstrong and J. Stern, Electrophysiological and morphological characteristics of neurons in perinuclear zone of supraoptic nucleus, *Journal of Neurophysiology.* **78**(5), 2427–2437, (1997).

[7] S. Baer, J. Rinzel, and H. Carrillo, Analysis of an autonomous phase model for neuronal parabolic bursting, *Journal of Mathematical Biology.* **33**, 309–333, (1995).

[8] R. Bicknell, Optimizing release from peptide hormone secretory nerve terminals, *Journal of Experimental Biology.* **139**, 51–65(September, 1988).

[9] C. Bondy, H. Gainer, and J. Russell, Dynorphin A inhibits and naloxone increases the electrically stimulated release of oxytocin but not vasopressin from the terminals of the neural lobe, *Endocrinology.* **122** (4), 1321–1327, (1988).

[10] C. Bourque, Calcium-dependent spike after-current induces burst firing in magnocellular neurosecretory-cells, *Neuroscience Letters.* **70**(2), 204–209, (1986).

[11] C. Bourque and D. Brown, Apamin and d-tubocurarine block the after-hyperpolarization of rat supraoptic neurosecretory neurons, *Neuroscience Letters.* **82**(2), 185–190, (1987).

[12] C. Bourque, K. Kirkpatrick, and C. Jarvis, Extrinsic modulation of spike afterpotentials in rat hypothalamoneurohypophysial neurons, *Cellular and Molecular Neurobiology.* **18**(1), 3–12, (1998).

[13] C. Bourque, J. Randle, and L. Renaud, Calcium-dependent potassium conductance in rat supraoptic nucleus neurosecretory neurons, *Journal of Neurophysiology.* **54**(6), 1375–1382, (1985).

[14] C. Bourque and L. Renaud, Membrane-properties of rat magnocellular neuroendocrine cells *in vivo*, *Brain Research.* **540**(1-2), 349–352, (1991).

[15] C. Brown and C. Bourque, Autocrine feedback inhibition of plateau potentials terminates phasic bursts in magnocellular neurosecretory cells of the rat supraoptic nucleus, *Journal of Physiology (London).* **557**(3), 949–960, (2004).

[16] C. Brown, M. Ghamari-Langroudi, G. Leng, and C. Bourque, κ-opioid receptor activation inhibits post-spike depolarizing after-potentials in rat supraoptic nucleus neurones *in vitro*, *Journal of Neuroendocrinology.* **11**(11), 825–828, (1999).

[17] C. Brown, M. Ludwig, and G. Leng, κ-opioid regulation of neuronal activity in the rat supraoptic nucleus *in vivo*, *Journal of Neuroscience.* **18**(22), 9480–9488, (1998).

[18] C. Brown, M. Ludwig, and G. Leng, Phasic bursts in rat magnocellular neurosecretory cells are not intrinsically regenerative *in vivo*, *European Journal of Neuroscience.* **19**(11), 2977–2983, (2004).

[19] C. Brown, M. Ludwig, and G. Leng, Temporal dissociation of the feedback effects of dendritically co-released peptides on rhythmogenesis in vasopressin cells, *Neuroscience.* **124**(1), 105–111, (2004).

[20] R. Butera, Jr., J. Clark, Jr., and J. Byrne, Transient responses of a modeled bursting neuron: analysis with equilibrium and averaged nullclines, *Biological Cybernetics.* **77**(5), 307–322, (1997).

[21] G. Dayanithi, N. Sabatier, and H. Widmer, Intracellular calcium signalling in magnocellular neurones of the rat supraoptic nucleus: understanding the autoregulatory mechanisms, *Experimental Physiology.* **85**(SISI), S75–S84, (2000).

[22] C. de Kock, K. Wierda, L. Bosman, R. Min, J. Koksma, H. Mansvelder, M. Verhage, and A. Brussaard, Somatodendritic secretion in oxytocin neurons is upregulated during the female reproductive cycle, *Journal of Neuroscience.* **23**(7), 2726–34(May, 2003).

[23] B. Doiron, C. Laing, A. Longtin, and L. Maler, Ghostbursting: a novel neuronal burst mechanism, *Journal of Computational Neuroscience.* **12**, 5–25, (2002).

[24] R. Dyball. The importance of bursting in determining secretory responses: How does a phasic firing pattern influence peptide release from neurohypophyseal vasopressin terminals. In ed. G. Leng, *Pulsatility in Neuroendocrine Systems*, chapter 10, pp. 181–196. CRC Press, Inc, Boca Raton, Florida, (1988).

[25] T. Fisher and C. Bourque, Voltage-gated calcium currents in the magnocellular neurosecretory cells of the rat supraoptic nucleus, *Journal of Physiology (London).* **486**(3), 571–580, (1995).

[26] R. Foehring and W. Armstrong, Pharmacological dissection of high-voltage-activated Ca^{2+} current types in acutely dissociated rat supraoptic magnocellular neurons, *Journal of Neurophysiology.* **76**(2), 977–983, (1996).

[27] M. Ghamari-Langroudi and C. Bourque, Flufenamic acid blocks depolarizing afterpotentials and phasic firing in rat supraoptic neurones, *Journal of Physiology (London).* **545**(2), 537–542, (2002).

[28] M. Ghamari-Langroudi and C. W. Bourque, Muscarinic receptor modulation of slow afterhyperpolarization and phasic firing in rat supraoptic nucleus neurons., *Journal of Neuroscience.* **24**(35), 7718–7726(September, 2004).

[29] W. Greffrath, E. Martin, S. Reuss, and G. Boehmer, Components of after-hyperpolarization in magnocellular neurons of the rat supraoptic nucleus *in vitro*, *Journal of Physiology (London).* **513**(2), 493–506, (1998).

[30] J. Han, C. Gnatenco, C. Sladek, and D. Kim, Background and tandem-pore potassium channels in magnocellular neurosecretory cells of the rat supraoptic nucleus, *Journal of Physiology.* **546**, 625–639, (2003).

[31] A. Hodgkin, The local electric changes associated with repetitive action in a non-medullated axon, *Journal of Physiology (London).* **107**, 165–181, (1948).

[32] K. Inenaga, H. Imura, N. Yanaihara, and H. Yamashita, κ-selective opioid receptor agonists leumorphin and dynorphin inhibit supraoptic neurons in rat hypothalamic slice preparations, *Journal of Neuroendocrinology.* **2**, 389–396, (1990).

[33] E. Izhikevich, Neural excitability, spiking, and bursting, *International Journal of Bifurcation and Chaos.* **10**(6), 1171–1266, (2000).

[34] K. Kirkpatrick. *Functional role and modulation of a calcium-activated potassium current in rat supraoptic neurons in vitro.* PhD thesis, Department of Neurology and Neurosurgery, McGill University, Montreal, (1997).

[35] K. Kirkpatrick and C. Bourque, Activity dependence and functional role of the apamin-sensitive K^+ current in rat supraoptic neurones *in vitro*, *Journal of Physiology (London).* **494**(2), 389–398, (1996).

[36] S. Kombian, D. Mouginot, M. Hirasawa, and Q. Pittman, Vasopressin preferentially depresses excitatory over inhibitory synaptic transmission in the rat supraoptic nucleus *in vitro*, *Journal of Neuroendocrinology.* **12**(4), 361–367, (2000).

[37] C. Laing, B. Doiron, and A. Longtin, Type I burst excitability, *Journal of Computational Neuroscience.* **14**(3), 329–342, (2003).

[38] Z. Li and G. Hatton, Histamine-induced prolonged depolarization in rat supraoptic neurons: G-protein-mediated, Ca^{2+}-independent suppression of K^+ leakage conductance, *Neuroscience.* **70**(1), 145–158, (1996).

[39] Z. Li and G. Hatton, Reduced outward K^+ conductances generate depolarizing after-potentials in rat supraoptic nucleus neurones, *Journal of Physiology (London).* **505**(1), 95–106, (1997).

[40] W. Mason, Supraoptic neurones of rat hypothalamus are osmosensitive, *Nature.* **287**(11), 154–157(September, 1980).

[41] R. Meeker, S. McGinnis, R. Greenwood, and J. Hayward, Increased

hypothalamic glutamate receptors induced by water deprivation, *Neuroendocrinology.* **60**(5), 477–485, (1994).

[42] C. Morris and H. Lecar, Voltage oscillations in the barnacle giant muscle fiber., *Biophysical Journal.* **35**(1), 193–213(July, 1981).

[43] R. Plant and M. Kim, On the mechanism underlying bursting in the Aplysia abdominal ganglion R15 cell, *Mathematical Biosciences.* **26**, 357–375, (1975).

[44] D. Poulain, D. Brown, and J. Wakerley. Statistical analysis of patterns of electrical activity in vasopressin- and oxytocin-secreting neurones. In ed. G. Leng, *Pulsatility in Neuroendocrine Systems*, chapter 8, pp. 119–154. CRC Press, Inc, Boca Raton, Florida, (1988).

[45] D. Pow and J. Morris, Dendrites of hypothalamic magnocellular neurons release neurohypophyseal peptides by exocytosis, *Neuroscience.* **32**(2), 435–439, (1989).

[46] J. Rinzel. A formal classification of bursting mechanisms in excitable systems. In eds. E. Teramoto and M. Yamaguti, *Mathematical Topics in Population Biology, Morphogenesis and Neurosciences*, number 71 in Lecture Notes in Biomathematics, pp. 267–281. Springer-Verlag, (1987).

[47] J. Rinzel and B. Ermentrout. Analysis of neural excitability and oscillations. In eds. C. Koch and I. Segev, *Methods in Neuronal Modeling: From Ions to Networks*, chapter 7, pp. 251–291. MIT Press, Inc, Cambridge, Massachusetts, 2nd edition, (1998).

[48] J. Rinzel and Y. Lee, Dissection of a model for neuronal parabolic bursting, *Journal of Mathematical Biology.* **25**, 653–675, (1987).

[49] J. Rinzel and Y. S. Lee. On different mechanisms for membrane potential bursting. In ed. H. Othmer, *Nonlinear Oscillations in Biology and Chemistry*, number 66 in Lecture Notes in Biomathematics, pp. 19–33. Springer-Verlag, (1986).

[50] P. Roper, J. Callaway, and W. Armstrong, Burst initiation and termination in phasic vasopressin cells of the rat SON, *Journal of Neuroscience.* **24**(20), 4818–4831, (2004).

[51] P. Roper, J. Callaway, T. Shevchenko, R. Teruyama, and W. Armstrong, AHP's, HAP's and DAP's: How potassium currents regulate the excitability of rat supraoptic neurones, *Journal of Computational Neuroscience.* **15**(3), 367–389, (2003).

[52] P. Roper and A. Sherman, Mathematical analysis of firing pattern transitions in rat SON magnocellular neurosecretory cells subject to osmotic stress, *Society for Neuroscience Abstracts.* **28**(273.3), (2002).

[53] K. Rusin, D. Giovannucci, E. Stenkel, and H. Moises, κ-receptor activation modulates Ca^{2+} currents and secretion in isolated neuroendocrine nerve terminals, *Journal of Neuroscience.* **17**(17), 6565–6574, (1997).

[54] N. Sabatier, C. Brown, M. Ludwig, and G. Leng, Phasic spike patterning in rat supraoptic neurones *in vivo* and *in vitro*, *Journal of Physiology (London).* **558**, 161–180, (2004).

[55] S. Shuster, M. Riedl, X. Li, L. Vulchanova, and R. Elde, Stimulus-dependent translocation of κ opioid receptors to the plasma membrane, *Journal of Neuroscience.* **19**(7), 2658–2664, (1999).

[56] S. Shuster, M. Riedl, X. Li, L. Vulchanova, and R. Elde, The κ opioid receptor and dynorphin co-localize in vasopressin magnocellular neurosecretory neurons in guinea-pig hypothalamus, *Neuroscience.* **96**(2), 373–383, (2000).

[57] E. Sivan, L. Segel, and H. Parnas, Modulated excitability: a new way to obtain bursting neurons, *Biological Cybernetics.* **72**(5), 455–461, (1995).

[58] P. Smolen, D. Terman, and J. Rinzel, Properties of a bursting model with two slow inhibitory variables, *SIAM Journal on Applied Mathematics.* **53**(3), 861–892, (1993).

[59] B. Soldo, D. Giovannucci, E. Stuenkel, and H. Moises, Ca^{2+} and frequency dependence of exocytosis in isolated somata of magnocellular supraoptic neurones of the rat hypothalamus, *Journal of Physiology (London).* **555**(Pt 3), 699–711(March, 2004).

[60] J. Summy-Long, L. Rosella-Dampman, G. McLemore, and E. Koehler, Kappa opiate receptors inhibit release of oxytocin from the magnocellular system during dehydration, *Neuroendocrinology.* **51**(4), 376–84(April, 1990).

[61] R. Teruyama and W. Armstrong, Changes in the active membrane properties of rat supraoptic neurons during pregnancy and lactation, *Journal of Neuroendocrinology.* **14**, 1–17, (2002).

[62] C. Vergara, R. Latorre, N. Marrion, and J. Adelman, Calcium-activated potassium channels, *Current Opinion in Neurobiology.* **8**(3), 321–329, (1998).

[63] J. Wakerley, D. Poulain, and D. Brown, Comparison of firing patterns in oxytocin- and vasopressin-releasing neurones during progressive dehydration, *Brain Research.* **148**, 425–440, (1978).

CHAPTER 4

BIFURCATIONS IN THE FAST DYNAMICS OF NEURONS: IMPLICATIONS FOR BURSTING

John Guckenheimer
Joseph H. Tien
Mathematics Department, Cornell University
Ithaca, NY 14853, USA
e-mail: gucken@cam.cornell.edu

Allan R. Willms
Department of Mathematics and Statistics, University of Guelph
Guelph, ON, Canada, N1G 2W1
e-mail: awillms@uoguelph.ca

Singular perturbation analysis of models for bursting neural rhythms relies upon decomposition of models into slow and fast time scales. Transitions between spiking and quiescent dynamics correspond to bifurcations of the fast subsystems. We observe that the fast subsystems of bursting models also have two time scales. Consequently, the bifurcation analysis of the fast subsystems is surprisingly complex. This is illustrated by a complete two parameter bifurcation analysis of a model that combines just sodium and leak currents. The very fast time scale in bursting models is frequently dominated by a sodium current, suggesting that the bifurcation diagram presented here is representative of that found for large classes of systems. The second part of this chapter explores further the relationship between transitions in several bursting models with bifurcations of reduced subsystems. Slow currents are combined into a pair of parameters for an "effective" leak conductance, and the bifurcations of these reduced models are compared with the transitions in the bursting rhythms.

4.1. Introduction

Models of neuronal bursting have been studied extensively as illustrated throughout this volume. Different types of periodic bursting have been observed and classified according to criteria related to bifurcation theory [3, 19, 25]. From the perspective of (geometric) singular perturbation theory [20], bursting is viewed within the context of systems with multiple time scales – normally a slow time scale and a fast time scale. Most work has focused upon the "slow motion" of the system during quiescent and active portions of a bursting cycle. During these epochs, the system state is described by attractors that evolve on the slow time scale. The transitions between quiescent and active states are marked by bifurcations of the "fast subsystem." In the singular limit of an infinite separation of time scales, the slow variables of a system remain fixed on the fast time scale and become parameters in the fast subsystem. Singular perturbation theory describes how this picture applies to situations in which the time scales are well, but not infinitely, separated. The separation of time scales is not always apparent in the equations themselves, so we seek computational methods that perform slow-fast decompositions of the dynamics.

The focus of this chapter is upon the bifurcation analysis of the fast subsystems of neuronal models of bursting. Because these bifurcations mark the transitions between active and quiescent states in bursting rhythms of model neurons, they play a key role in determining which types of bursting can occur in the model. The hypothesis we explore in this chapter is that there are widespread similarities among the fast subsystems of many models. The basis for this hypothesis is that spike generating sodium currents are often the largest and fastest currents in neurons, consequently representing a central part of the fast subsystem. Moreover, less variability has been found in fast sodium channels than in other common types of channels [17]. This prompts us to study a model with only a fast sodium current and a passive leak conductance. Using the Hodgkin-Huxley representation of the sodium conductance and making the familiar assumption that the activation of this current is "instantaneous" yields a two dimensional vector field. The bifurcations of this model can be studied thoroughly, although the numerical analysis must confront issues arising from multiple time scales. These issues were already apparent in early work of FitzHugh [11] . His work depicts a "no man's land" in the phase space of a reduced Hodgkin-Huxley model that foreshadows numerical issues in determining the bifurcation diagrams of these systems. The "cusp and loop" structure for bifurcations of equilibrium points in this model form a paradigm for the bifurcations of many neural models.

Classifications of bursting oscillations have not yet produced a good understanding of how to "tune" models to produce different types of oscillations. Parameter space maps [13] obtained from bifurcation analysis and/or systematic variation of parameters in neural models display how parameters such as maximal conductances of different channels interact to produce different oscillatory rhythms. Numerical computations answer questions about the types of bursting for any chosen set of parameter values without yielding a clear intuition of what will happen in a new model or in different parameter ranges. By investigating how our analysis applies to several bursting models, we take a step here towards the development of predictive guidelines describing which characteristics of a model lead to different kinds of bursting.

4.2. A Two Dimensional Model of Spiking Sodium Currents

In this section, we study the following two dimensional vector field:

$$
\begin{aligned}
\dot{v} &= -(g_{Na} m^3 h(v - v_{Na}) + g_l(v - v_l)) \\
\dot{h} &= \alpha_h(v)(1-h) - \beta_h(v)h \\
\alpha_h(v) &= 0.07\exp\left(\frac{-60-v}{20}\right) \\
\beta_h(v) &= \frac{1}{1+\exp(\frac{-30-v}{10})} \\
m &= \frac{1}{1+\exp(\frac{-(v+35)}{9})}
\end{aligned}
\tag{1}
$$

This vector field is derived from the Hodgkin-Huxley model for squid giant axon [18] by

- assuming that the gating variable m is at its steady state,
- eliminating the potassium current,
- replacing the steady state curve of m by a sigmoidal "Boltzmann" that is a good approximation to the Hodgkin-Huxley representation but analytically simpler, and
- assuming that the capacitance and temperature dependent parameters in the model are both 1

We shall set $g_{Na} = 120$, the value used by Hodgkin-Huxley, in these equations.

We regard this as a minimal model for action potentials, representative of the fast dynamics of more complex model neurons containing additional conductances. In such models, if the gating of other conductances is sufficiently slow, then we examine the singular limit in which they are constant. The sum of these currents then has the form of a "leak" conductance, the term $g_l(v - v_l)$ in equation (1) for $\dot{v}$. Modulation of the slow currents or changes in their values on slow time scales can be represented as variations of these parameters. Thus, crossing bifurcation boundaries in the model is correlated with changes in the firing properties of the neuron. This is the conceptual basis for the multiple time scale analysis of neuronal bursting. Our primary interest in this section is to investigate how the dynamics of system (1) depend on the parameters g_l and v_l. The two parameter bifurcation diagram of system (1) yields predictions about the types of transitions that could occur at the initiation or termination of a burst of action potentials in neurons for which the sodium current is the dominant fast current. We analyze several bursting model neurons in section 4.3 from this perspective.

The bifurcation theory of two parameter families of two dimensional vector fields has been thoroughly studied [28]. We employ the classification of codimension one and two bifurcations in generic families of planar vector fields to describe the bifurcation diagram of Eq. (1). This turns out to be a more difficult enterprise than initially might be expected, due to the fact that system (1) itself has two time scales. The insights of geometric singular perturbation theory point to phenomena that occur on tiny length scales in parameter space, making it difficult to numerically resolve some aspects of the bifurcation diagram. In particular, we find thin parameter regions in which periodic orbits contain "canards," segments that track unstable slow manifolds of the system in FitzHugh's no man's land. Some bifurcation curves lie very close together in these regions.

There are four types of codimension one bifurcations in planar vector fields with at most one saddle point:

(1) Hopf bifurcation - an equilibrium has Jacobian with trace 0 and positive determinant.
(2) Saddle-node bifurcation - an equilibrium has Jacobian with 0 determinant.
(3) Homoclinic bifurcation - a stable and unstable separatrix of a saddle point coincide.
(4) Saddle-node bifurcation of a periodic orbit - the return map of the

periodic orbit has derivative 1 at its fixed point.

Normal forms and unfoldings of these bifurcations characterize the types of qualitative changes occurring in the phase portraits near the bifurcations [14]. There are several different types of codimension two bifurcations that occur in this system. We introduce them as they are encountered in our description of the bifurcation diagram.

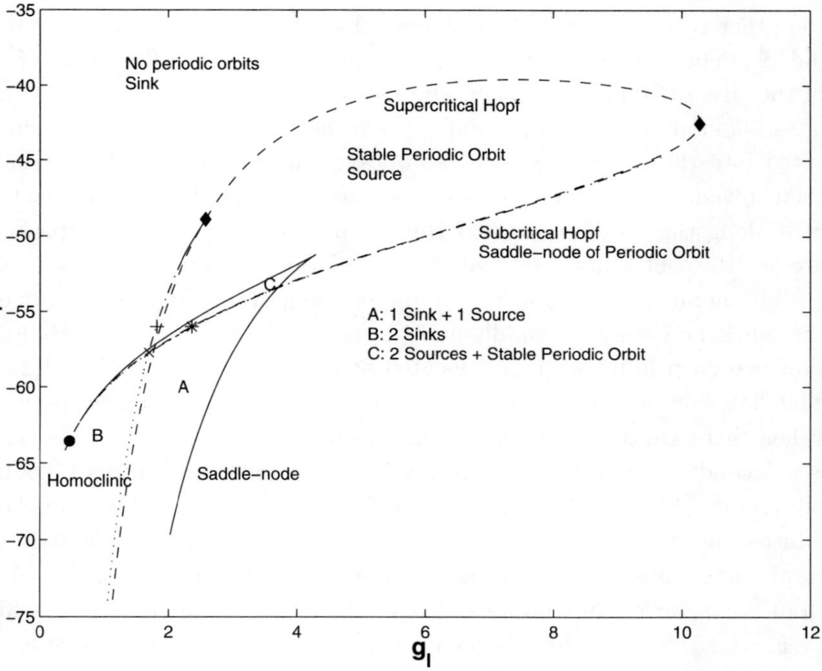

Fig. 4.1. Bifurcation diagram of the system (1) in the (g_l, v_l) plane of parameters. Saddle-node bifurcations are shown as a solid curve, Hopf bifurcations as a dashed curve, saddle-node of periodic orbit bifurcations as dash-dotted curves and homoclinic bifurcations as dotted curves. The two degenerate Hopf bifurcations are marked with diamonds and the Takens-Bogdanov point with a filled circle. The plus, cross and asterisk mark parameter values for which the phase portraits are displayed below.

Figure 4.1 shows a numerically computed bifurcation diagram in the (g_l, v_l) parameter plane. The curves of saddle-node bifurcations drawn as solid curves and Hopf bifurcations drawn as dashed curves were computed explicitly with the symbolic computer package Maple. Writing $J(v, h, g_l, v_l)$ for the Jacobian of the vector field, the defining equations for Hopf bifurcation are $\dot{v} = \dot{h} = tr(J) = 0$ and the defining equations for saddle-node bifurcations are $\dot{v} = \dot{h} = \det(J) = 0$. These equations depend upon v in a complicated manner, but their dependence upon h and the parameters is simpler. Therefore, we make v the continuation parameter in our calculations. This means that we obtain h, g_l, v_l as functions of v along each bifurcation curve. This is done as follows. The equation $\dot{h} = 0$ is independent of the parameters and linear in h, so we solve $\dot{h} = 0$ first to obtain h as a function of v at equilibrium points. This value of h is substituted into the other equations. Next, we observe that $tr(J) = 0$ and $\det(J) = 0$ are independent of v_l and depend linearly on g_l, so $tr(J) = 0$ is solved for g_l in the case of Hopf bifurcation, and $\det(J) = 0$ is solved for g_l in the case of saddle-node bifurcation. Finally, when the values of g_l and h are substituted into the equation $\dot{v} = 0$, we obtain a linear equation for v_l that is then solved. Solving these successive equations gives (h, g_l, v_l) as functions of v along the saddle-node and Hopf bifurcation curves. The expressions are lengthy, but Maple performs the calculation readily.

The number of equilibrium points of the system changes from one to three upon crossing the saddle-node curve [14]. This curve has a codimension two cusp bifurcation [14] located near $(g_l, v_l) = (4.29367, -51.2428)$. The "interior" of the cusp is the region in which there are three equilibria. When there are three equilibria, exactly one of the three is a saddle. There is a second codimension two bifurcation point, called a Takens-Bogadnov bifurcation [14], near $(g_l, v_l) = (0.46387, -63.5318)$. The Takens-Bogdanov bifurcation is located by a filled circle in Fig. 4.1. The saddle-node and Hopf curves intersect tangentially at the Takens-Bogdanov point, and the Hopf curve terminates because $\det(J)$ changes sign on the curve defined by $\dot{v} = \dot{h} = tr(J) = 0$ at this point. Theoretical analysis [14] demonstrates that there is also a curve of homoclinic bifurcations that terminates at the Takens-Bogdanov point.

Periodic orbits emerge from equilibrium points undergoing Hopf bifurcation [14]. There is a "Lyapunov" quantity determined by the third degree Taylor expansion of the vector field at each Hopf bifurcation point which determines the stability of the orbits. The Lyapunov quantity of supercritical Hopf bifurcations is negative and the periodic orbits are stable. At subcritical Hopf bifurcations the Lyapunov quantity is positive and the periodic orbits are unstable. In the system (1), there are a pair of codimension two bifurcation points called degenerate Hopf bifurcations, where the Lyapunov quantity is zero. These two points, shown with filled diamonds in Fig. 4.1, bound a segment of supercritical Hopf bifurcations, with the remainder of the Hopf bifurcation curve consisting of subcritical bifurcations. The Hopf curve also has a point of self-intersection where the two equilibrium points that are not saddles simultaneously undergo subcritical Hopf bifurcation.

The properties of a structurally stable planar vector field are characterized by its equilibrium points and their stability, its periodic orbits and their stability, and by the limit sets of saddle separatrices. Thus we want to locate periodic orbits and saddle separatrices and see how they change as the parameters (g_l, v_l) vary. We have pointed out that periodic orbits emerge at Hopf bifurcations. Families of periodic orbits in planar vector fields can also terminate in three other ways.

(1) At saddle-nodes (also called folds) of periodic orbits, a stable periodic orbit and an unstable periodic orbit coalesce into a single orbit that is stable from one side and unstable from another.
(2) At homoclinic bifurcations a family of periodic orbits terminates as it approaches a saddle point and its period grows without bound.
(3) A periodic orbit may approach a saddle-node equilibrium point at a saddle-node bifurcation of a parameter. The equilibrium emerges "astride" the periodic orbit, and once again the period of the periodic orbit grows unbounded as the bifurcation is approached. Rinzel and Ermentrout [26] call these bifurcations saddle-nodes in cycles (SNIC).

We seek to compute the bifurcation curves for saddle-nodes of periodic orbits and homoclinic bifurcations. Homoclinic orbits can only exist when there is a saddle equilibrium; i.e., inside the cusp. We used a "shooting" strategy to compute parameter values for homoclinic bifurcations. The defining equation for homoclinic bifurcation can be expressed in terms of a cross-section Γ to the homoclinic orbit. As a parameter is varied, the intersections of the stable and unstable manifolds of the saddle with Γ smoothly switch sides, coinciding at the bifurcation value of the parameter. In terms of a coordinate along Γ, the difference between the intersection of the stable and unstable manifolds of the saddle with Γ is a defining function for the homoclinic bifurcation. We begin with parameter values that straddle the bifurcation and employ a secant method to converge to a bifurcation value. A bisection algorithm could also be used. Beginning with two nearby points on a curve of homoclinic bifurcations, a simple extrapolation procedure is used to search for new starting parameter values that straddle the bifurcation curve. This procedure readily detects two intersecting curves of homoclinic bifurcations in which the interior of the homoclinic orbit makes a convex angle at the saddle point. In addition to these "small" homoclinic orbits, there are two families of "large" homoclinic orbits in which the angle made by the interior of the homoclinic orbits is larger than π. In generic families, the two bifurcation curves of large homoclinic orbits terminate at the intersection of the bifurcation curves of small homoclinic orbits. This intersection is a codimension two "gluing bifurcation" where the stable and unstable manifolds of the saddle form a figure eight [12]. The large homoclinic orbits closely follow branches of small homoclinic bifurcation[a]. If one varies parameters and solves the initial value problem, it can be difficult or impossible to locate parameter values in the very narrow strip between the large and small bifurcation curves.

Figure 4.2 is a qualitative depiction of the region around the gluing bifurcation in Fig. 4.1. This is one region in which we need to rely upon theoretical insight to develop a consistent bifurcation diagram. The figure shows the relative position of the large and small homoclinic bifurcation curves as well as the location of the curve of saddle-node of periodic orbit bifurcations discussed below. At each homoclinic bifurcation curve, there is one family of periodic orbits that terminates. Periodic orbits that surround the right hand equilibrium point (i.e. the equilibrium with larger h) exist in the strip between the Hopf bifurcation of the right-hand equilibrium and the curve of small homoclinic bifurcations for loops that surround this equilibrium. Similarly, periodic orbits surrounding the left-hand equilibrium occur in a strip between the Hopf bifurcations of this equilibrium and a small homoclinic curve. Unstable periodic orbits appear to the left and below the two curves of large homoclinic bifurcations. Figures 4.4, 4.5 and 4.6 lie in the region to the right of the left Hopf curve. Figure 4.4 lies in the region labelled with *1 between the right Hopf and the right homoclinic curve, Fig. 4.5 lies in the region labelled with *2 between the right homoclinic curve and the large homoclinic curve, and Fig. 4.6 lies in the region labelled with *3 below the curve of saddle-nodes of periodic orbits. The strip between the large homoclinic curve and the saddle-node of periodic orbits curve is so thin that we were unable to locate parameter values inside it.

Computation of approximate parameter values for saddle-node (or fold) bifurcations of periodic orbits in the system (1) is easier than locating the orbits themselves. At these bifurcations, there is a periodic orbit that is

[a]To reliably compute the large homoclinic bifurcations with a shooting algorithm, it is important to choose a cross-section for which the intersections with the appropriate branches of the stable and unstable manifolds of the saddle vary smoothly in a substantial neighborhood of the bifurcation.

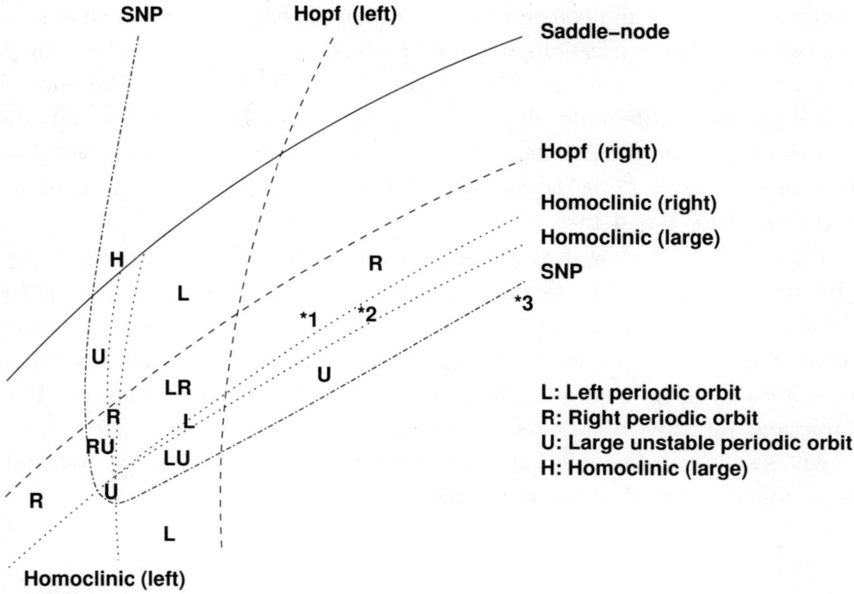

Fig. 4.2. Qualitative depiction of the bifurcation diagram of the system (1) near the codimension two gluing bifurcation where homoclinic curves cross. Regions are labelled with the type(s) of periodic orbits found at parameter values in the region. R and L indicate periodic orbits surrounding a single equilibrium point on the right or left in Figs. 4.4, 4.5 and 4.6; U indicates that there is an unstable periodic orbit surrounding all three equilibria. Above and to the right of the saddle-node of periodic orbits bifurcation curve (labelled SNP), there is also a stable periodic orbit surrounding all of the equilibrium points. The labels *1, *2 and *3 show the regions to which Figs. 4.4, 4.5 and 4.6 belong, respectively.

(weakly) stable from one side and (weakly) unstable from the other. Expressed in terms of a return map θ, the defining equations are $\theta(x) = x$ and $\theta'(x) = 1$ where x is constrained to the cross-section. However, it is difficult to compute the return map close to the bifurcating periodic orbit because one segment of the periodic orbit is highly stable and another segment is highly unstable. We discuss this behavior below in relation to the phase portrait shown in Fig. 4.5. Therefore, we use indirect methods to locate the saddle-node of periodic orbit bifurcations. To one side of the bifurcation in the parameter space, there is a pair of nearby periodic orbits, one stable and one unstable. To the other side of the bifurcation, there are no nearby periodic orbits. Outside the cusp of saddle-nodes of equilibria, we followed the curves of saddle-nodes of periodic orbits by searching for the boundary between parameter regions with and without periodic orbits.

This procedure is time consuming, but accomplishes the desired task reasonably well. The curves extend into the interior of the cusp where they lie very close to the curves of large homoclinic bifurcations. The end of each curve of saddle-node bifurcation of periodic orbits that lies outside the cusp region terminates at a degenerate Hopf bifurcation, near parameter values $(g_l, v_l) = (2.5851, -48.870), (10.277, -42.513)$. These are marked by diamonds in Fig. 4.1.

Figures 4.3–4.7 show five phase portraits from different regions in the bifurcation diagram, illustrating varied aspects of this system. Referring to Fig. 4.1, the locations of these parameter values are marked on this bifurcation diagram. We use the following conventions in these phase portraits: sinks are drawn as triangles, saddles as +'s and sources as squares. The stable and unstable manifolds of the saddles and the periodic curves are drawn as solid curves, while the h nullclines are drawn as dotted curves and the v nullclines are dash-dotted curves.

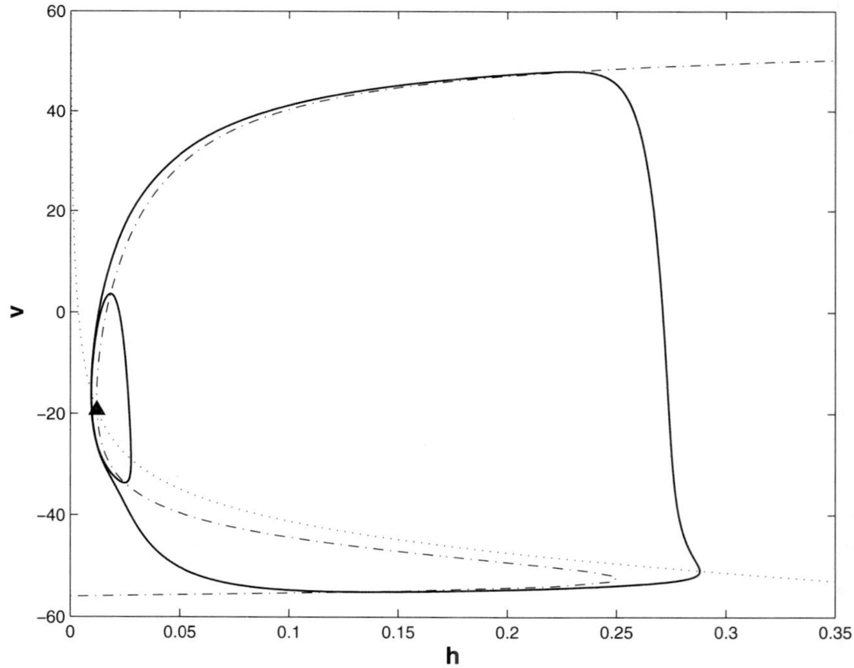

Fig. 4.3. Phase portrait of the system (1) for $(g_l, v_l) = (1.82, -56)$. There is a sink, unstable periodic orbit (small) and stable periodic orbit (large). Nullclines are plotted as dotted and dash-dotted curves.

Figure 4.3 shows a phase portrait for parameters $(g_l, v_l) = (1.82, -56)$, depicted by the + on the bifurcation diagram in Fig. 4.1. These parameter values lie outside the cusped region bounded by the saddle-node bifurcation curve, and it lies between the Hopf curve and the curve of saddle-nodes of periodic orbits. As shown in the phase portrait, there is a stable equilibrium, a small unstable periodic orbit and a large stable periodic orbit. The unstable periodic orbit divides the basin of attractions of the equilibrium and the stable periodic orbit.

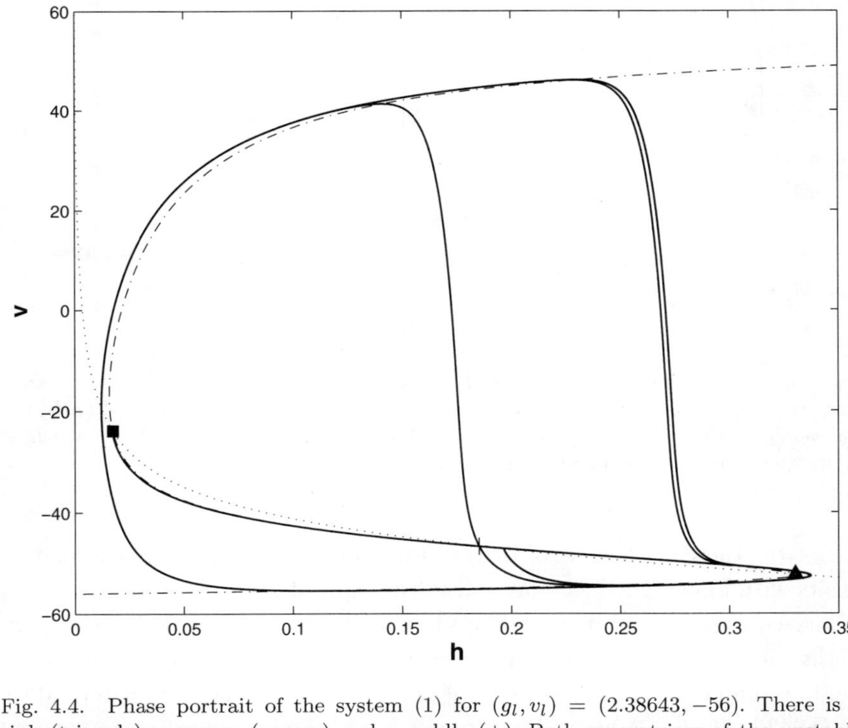

Fig. 4.4. Phase portrait of the system (1) for $(g_l, v_l) = (2.38643, -56)$. There is a sink (triangle), a source (square) and a saddle (+). Both separatrices of the unstable manifold of the saddle tend to a stable periodic orbit and the right separatrix of the stable manifold limits on an unstable periodic orbit. In this and the subsequent figures, the unstable manifold leaves the saddle more vertically than the stable manifold.

The three phase portraits in Figs. 4.4, 4.5 and 4.6 correspond to parameter values $(2.38643, -56)$, $(2.3864443369, -56)$, and $(2.386444337, -56)$. These nearby parameter values are located at the asterisk in Fig. 4.1. There are four bifurcation curves that pass through this region of Fig. 4.1: from top

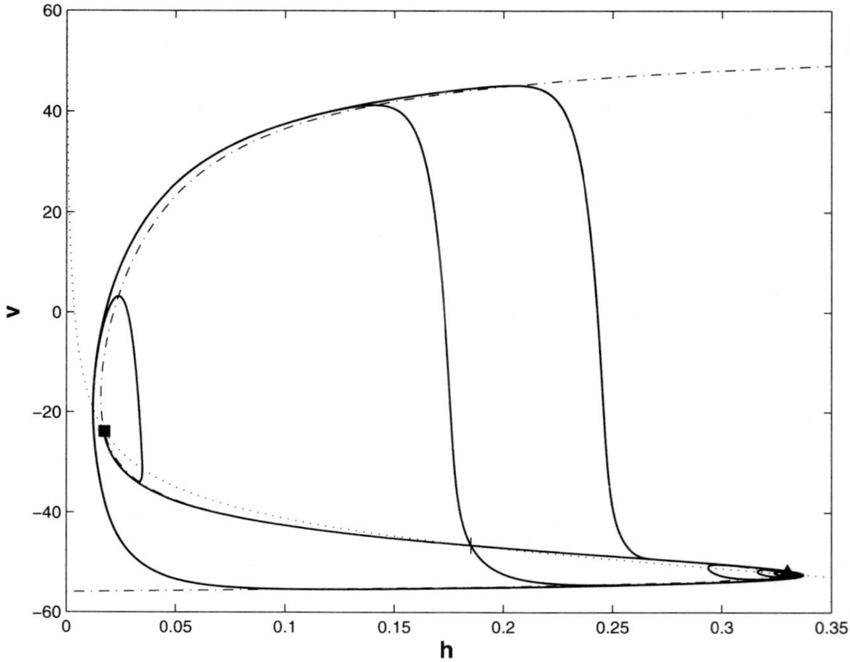

Fig. 4.5. Phase portrait of the system (1) for $(g_l, v_l) = (2.3864443369, -56)$. The change that has occurred from Fig. 4.4 is that the lower separatrix of the unstable manifold of the saddle and the right separatrix of the stable manifold have crossed in a homoclinic bifurcation, annihilating the unstable periodic orbit in the process.

to bottom these are a curve of Hopf bifurcations, a curve of small homoclinic orbits with loops that lie below and to the right of the saddle point, a curve of large homoclinic orbits with loops in which the upper unstable separatrix of the saddle returns to the saddle along the right branch of the stable manifold, and a curve of saddle-nodes of periodic orbits. The parameter values $(2.38643, -56)$ lie between the Hopf curve and the first curve of homoclinic bifurcations; the parameter values $(2.3864443369, -56)$ lie between the two homoclinic curves, and the parameter values $(2.386444337, -56)$ lie below the curve of saddle-nodes of periodic orbits. Phase portraits above the Hopf curve lie in region C of the bifurcation diagram and have two sources and a stable periodic orbit. In region C, each branch of the stable manifold of the saddle comes from a source. Fig. 4.4 depicts a phase portrait below the Hopf curve: there is a sink, a saddle and a source. The stable manifold of the saddle has one separatrix that comes from the source, while the other

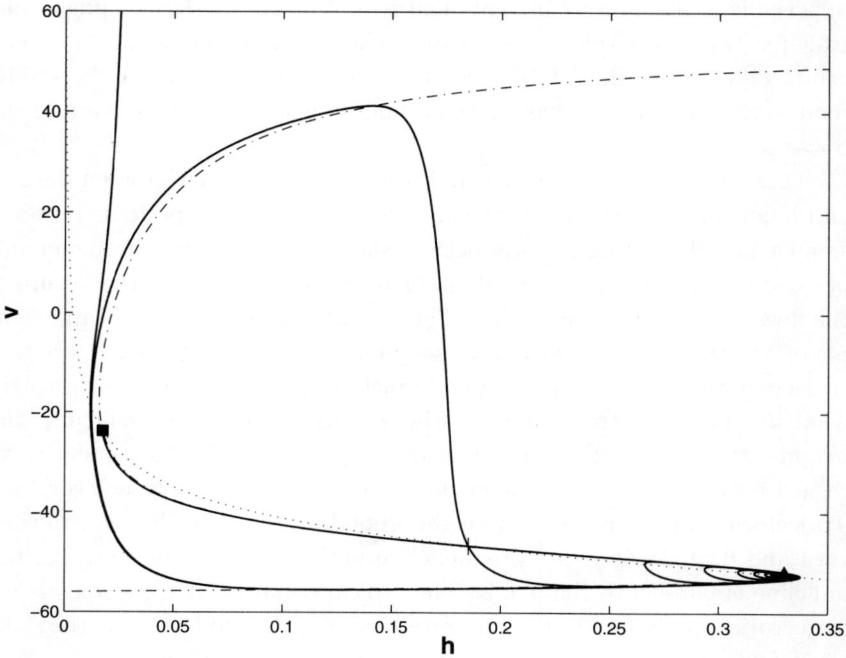

Fig. 4.6. Phase portrait of the system (1) for $(g_l, v_l) = (2.386444337, -56)$. The changes that have occurred from Fig. 4.5 are that the upper separatrix of the unstable manifold of the saddle and the right separatrix of the stable manifold have crossed in a homoclinic bifurcation, recreating an unstable periodic orbit that then coalesced with the stable periodic orbit in a saddle-node of periodic orbits.

comes from an unstable periodic orbit that bifurcated from the right-hand equilibrium point at its (subcritical) Hopf bifurcation. For the parameter values shown, this periodic orbit is close to forming a homoclinic orbit with the saddle. Both branches of the unstable manifold tend to the stable periodic orbit surrounding all three equilibrium points. As one passes the first homoclinic curve between the phase portraits of Fig. 4.4 and Fig. 4.5, the unstable periodic orbit disappears, the lower branch of the unstable manifold of the saddle tends to the sink and the right branch of the stable manifold comes from the source. As g_l increases slightly from 2.3864443369, the right branch of the stable manifold of the saddle and the upper branch of its unstable manifold coalesce into a homoclinic orbit. Crossing this homoclinic orbit generates a new unstable periodic orbit surrounding all three equilibrium points because the trace at the saddle is positive. This unstable periodic orbit quickly collides with the stable periodic orbit in a saddle-node of periodic orbits bifurcation, annihilating both. Fig. 4.6 shows a phase portrait for parameter values just to the right of the saddle-node of periodic orbits bifurcation. Both branches of the unstable manifold of the saddle tend to the sink in this phase portrait and no periodic orbits remain in the phase portrait.

These numerical calculations indicate that the distance between the second homoclinic bifurcation curve and the saddle-node of periodic orbits is smaller than 10^{-9}, and we have been unsuccessful in finding parameter values between these two curves. This is hardly surprising given the nature of the flow in this parameter region. The second homoclinic orbit is an example of a "canard". This term from singular perturbation theory refers to a trajectory that follows an unstable branch of a slow manifold. We explain what this means in the context of Fig. 4.5. Away from the v nullcline, the magnitude of $\dot{v}$ is much larger than the magnitude of $\dot{h}$. Consequently, we regard v as the "fast" variable of the system and h as the "slow" variable. Trajectories are attracted to a neighborhood of the v nullcline where they turn and flow slowly along this nullcline until reaching a place where the nullcline is parallel to the v axis. The typical behavior at these folds is for trajectories to "jump" to the opposite branch of the nullcline. At the right hand fold, this does not happen for the unstable manifold of the saddle in the small parameter range we are investigating. Instead, the unstable manifold tends back along the middle, unstable branch of the v nullcline. Only later does it jump. This branch of the nullcline closely approximates the stable manifold of the saddle. The eigenvalues at the saddle are approximately -0.05 and 3, so the exponential rate of divergence away from the stable manifold is 60 times faster than the exponential rate of attraction to the saddle along the manifold. In order to approach the saddle along the stable manifold, a trajectory must be extremely close to the stable manifold. Using estimates from the linear approximation at the saddle, the distance from the stable manifold grows by a factor $2^{60} \approx 10^{18}$ as the distance from the saddle decreases by a factor of only $1/2$. Consequently, even the round-off errors of floating point arithmetic preclude integration of the unstable manifold back close to the saddle. The region near the stable manifold is FitzHugh's "no man's land" – numerical integration of trajectories starting outside the region do not enter it. As the parameter g_l changes, the unstable and stable manifolds of the saddle sweep past each other. The "take off" point for where the unstable manifold diverges from the stable manifold changes so rapidly that it appears discontinuous in the numerical integrations when the manifolds cross. The second homoclinic orbit bifurcation and the saddle-node of periodic orbit bifurcation both come from trajectories containing segments inside this "no man's land," that bounds the apparent discontinuity. The bifurcations are too close together in parameter space to resolve without greatly extended precision for the calculations.

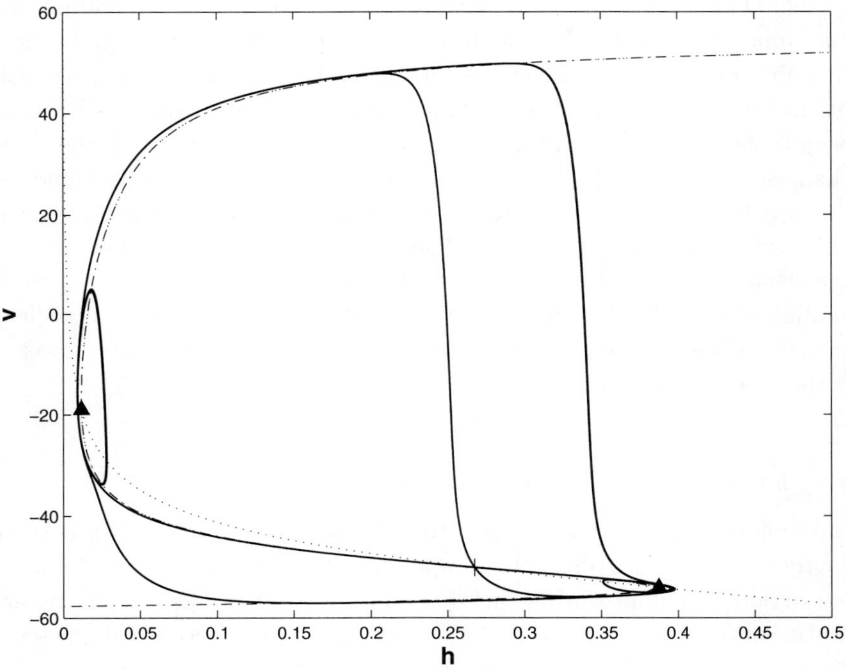

Fig. 4.7. Phase portrait of the system (1) for $(g_l, v_l) = (1.7, -57.75)$. There are two sinks (triangles), a saddle, a stable periodic orbit and two unstable periodic orbits. The system is tristable with three attractors.

Finally, Fig. 4.7 shows the phase portrait of (1) for parameter values $(g_l, v_l) = (1.7, -57.75)$, marked by the cross in Fig. 4.1 near the intersections of the homoclinic curves. This phase portrait shows *tristability*: there are two stable equilibria and a stable periodic orbit representing tonic spiking of the system. The domains of attraction of the stable equilibria are bounded by unstable periodic orbits that emerged from the equilibria at subcritical Hopf bifurcations. Note that the parameter values are also close to the self intersection of the Hopf curve in Fig. 4.1. At the codimension two gluing bifurcation, both of the unstable periodic orbits grow to homoclinic orbits. The stable and unstable manifolds of the saddle point form a figure eight at the gluing bifurcation. In the parameter space, all of the homoclinic bifurcation curves meet at this gluing bifurcation.

We note that the global homoclinic and saddle-node of periodic orbit bifurcation curves in Fig. 4.1 lie close to the steady state Hopf bifurcation curves. This property of the system can be attributed to the stiffness of system (1) in which v is a fast variable relative to h. Hopf bifurcation in a two dimensional fast-slow system occurs when equilibrium points lie close to a fold of the slow manifold. As analyzed by Dumortier and Roussarie [9] and others [1, 10], the periodic orbits growing from these bifurcation acquire canards and pass through a parameter regime in which their size changes extremely rapidly. Global bifurcations are likely to be found, as they are here, in the canard regions. In the next section, we analyze models of bursting neurons and encounter higher dimensional fast subsystems than the one described in this section. Although we do not show the global bifurcations of these models, we expect, and preliminary calculations confirm, that many will be found close to curves of equilibrium point bifurcation as is the case in this model.

4.3. Fast-Slow Analysis of Bursting

Bursting in neuronal models refers to compound oscillations which have an "active" phase consisting of action potentials and a quiescent phase without action potentials during each period of oscillation. Geometric singular perturbation theory interprets the transitions between active and quiescent phases as bifurcations in a fast subsystem of the model, occurring as the parameters of the fast subsystem change on the slow time scale. We investigate when the results of the previous section can be applied directly to models of bursting, assuming that time constants of gating variables for other currents are slower than the inactivation time scales of the sodium current. Although this requirement is seldom satisfied (even in the original Hodgkin-Huxley model), this analysis gives insight into the role that additional currents play in the initiation or termination of action potentials.

This section examines these ideas within the context of several models of neuronal bursting. We approach the separation of fast and slow components of a system in different ways. Most of the mathematical theory is formulated in terms of systems in which some phase space variables are slow and others are fast. This is made explicit by a small parameter ε that is the ratio of time scales, and ε approaching 0 gives a singular limit in which the slow variables no longer change on the fast time scale. Here we take a somewhat different approach based upon the representation of transmembrane current as a sum of currents associated with different channels. We separate currents into ones we regard as fast and ones we regard as slow because this allows us to map the slow dynamics of the system into variations of the leak parameters in the fast subsystem. However, the phase space variables are gating variables of the currents and currents with fast activation and slow inactivation are not readily assigned to the slow or fast categories.

The currents in all the models that we investigate have the Hodgkin-Huxley representation

$$I_y = g_y m_y^p h_y \left(V - V_y\right),$$

where g_y is a constant conductance, V_y is the reversal potential, p is a positive integer, and m_y and h_y are activation/inactivation variables or functions that take values in the range $[0, 1]$. Non-inactivating currents can be written in this form with h_y set to be identically equal to 1; a passive leak current has both m_y and h_y set identically to 1. The voltage equation in these models may be then written as

$$C_m \frac{dV}{dt} = -\sum_y I_y,$$

where C_m is the membrane capacitance. We do not consider directly the effects of an "injected" current in these neuronal models, but this can be investigated indirectly as a change in the reversal potential of a leak conductance. Our strategy is to map the slow currents into an "effective" leak current of the fast subsystem, regarding the reversal potential and conductance of this leak current as slowly varying variables. Specifically, we define the effective leak parameters as

$$g_{L_{\text{eff}}} = \sum_y g_y m_y^p h_y$$

$$V_{L_{\text{eff}}} = \left(\sum_y g_y m_y^p h_y V_y\right) / g_{L_{\text{eff}}}$$

the sum being taken over the slow currents. The ranges of the activation/inactivation functions yield a region in the $(g_{L_{\text{eff}}}, V_{L_{\text{eff}}})$ plane inside which the effective leak parameters are confined.

Analysis of bifurcations of the fast subsystems as the effective leak conductance and reversal potential are varied must be repeated for each model. Methods like those described in the previous section readily yield the bifurcation curves for saddle-node and Hopf bifurcations of equilibria. When the dimension of a fast subsystem is larger than two, computation of the global bifurcations are problematic for two reasons. First, the methods for computing these curves in multiple time scale systems discussed in the previous section were specific to planar vector fields, and robust algorithms that address these numerical issues in the context of higher dimensional vector fields are not as well developed. Second, more complicated limit sets can and do occur, even in the context of the original Hodgkin-Huxley model for squid axon [15]. Consequently, we show only the equilibrium point bifurcation curves in the examples discussed below.

4.3.1. *Aplysia*

The R15 neuron of *Aplysia* is a bursting neuron whose electrophysiology has been studied by many researchers [4, 21]. One of the simplest models of bursting in this neuron is given by Rinzel and Lee [27], which is based on a model by Plant. [24] Their model involves a sodium current I_{Na} with instantaneous activation; a potassium current, I_{K}; a passive leak current, I_L; a slow calcium current, I_{Ca}; and a calcium-activated potassium current, $I_{\mathrm{K-Ca}}$. Their work is a paradigm for the application of singular perturbation methods to analyze bursting. They chose fast subsystem variables to be the membrane potential, the sodium inactivation gating variable, and the potassium activation gating variable. The activation of the calcium current and the intra-cellular calcium concentration constitute the slow subsystem, giving a five dimensional phase space.

Here we regard the calcium and calcium-activated potassium currents as slow, and the sodium and potassium currents as part of the fast subsystem. We combine the calcium, calcium-activated potassium currents and leak currents of the full model to obtain the effective leak parameters of the fast subsystem. The region in the (g_L, V_L) plane in which the effective leak parameters are confined is shown in gray in Fig. 4.8(B) and (D).

Figure 4.8(A) shows a typical bursting trajectory from which we calculate the effective leak parameters for a bursting cycle. These effective leak parameters are plotted in Fig. 4.8(B) along with the bifurcation curves. Figure 4.8(C) shows a plot of v vs. $g_{L_{\mathrm{eff}}}$ and Fig. 4.8(D) is a magnified view of the region in the $(g_{L_{\mathrm{eff}}}, V_{L_{\mathrm{eff}}})$ plane where the burst cycle terminates.

Rinzel and Lee described the bursting mechanism in their model as parabolic. The bursts are apparently terminated by homoclinic bifurcations that lie close to the curve of saddle-nodes in Fig. 4.8(B). The separation between these curves is smaller than 0.1 mV in the region where the bursting

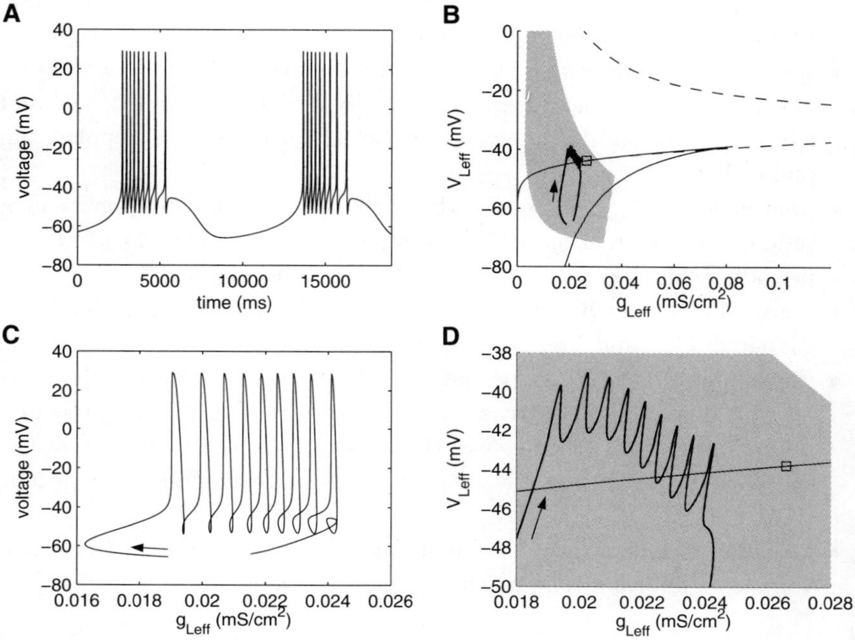

Fig. 4.8. Mapping of the Rinzel-Lee model to leak parameters of its fast subsystem. A: The full model's bursting trajectory. B: The effective leak parameters and equilibrium bifurcation curves. The envelope of possible leak parameters is shaded gray. The saddle-node curve is a solid line, and the Hopf curve is a dashed line that originates at a Takens-Bogdanov bifurcation (square) and extends to the right out of the panel and then passes through the panel once more on the upper right. The image of the bursting trajectory (thick solid line) lies to the left of the Takens-Bogdanov point and passes through the saddle-node curve. Arrows indicate the direction of traversal. C: Voltage vs. effective leak conductance for the burst cycle. D: Close up of B showing the region where bursting terminates.

stops. Note that the burst does not cease when the $(g_{L_{\text{eff}}}, V_{L_{\text{eff}}})$-trajectory first crosses the bifurcation curves, but rather the trajectory crosses and re-crosses these curves several times during the last few spikes. Although the time scales of the slow currents are more than a factor of two separated from the fast currents, this separation is insufficient to exactly obtain the behavior dictated by the singular limit of slow currents that do not vary. This phenomenon is also apparent in the figures of Rinzel and Lee's work [27]. We make the following additional observations about these bursting oscillations:

- during the quiet phase the system inhabits a region where the fast subsystem has a stable equilibrium
- slowly the effective leak reversal potential increases due to (i) reduction of Ca^{++} (which reduces I_{K-Ca} and the hyperpolarizing pull of V_K) and (ii) slow increase of I_{Ca} activation (which increases the depolarizing pull of V_{Ca})
- eventually, as $V_{L_{\text{eff}}}$ increases, the stable equilibrium disappears in a saddle-node bifurcation and the system is immediately attracted to a periodic orbit that was born in a homoclinic bifurcation
- Figure 4.8(B) and (C) show that V rapidly increases with virtually no change in $g_{L_{\text{eff}}}$ and $V_{L_{\text{eff}}}$
- the spiking eventually stops as Ca^{++} slowly increases during the spiking, yielding a slow decrease in $V_{L_{\text{eff}}}$ (due to the calcium-activated potassium current) that causes the trajectory to once again cross the saddle-node curve and the nearby curve of homoclinic bifurcations (Fig. 4.8(D))
- following termination of the burst, the trajectory jumps to the stable voltage equilibrium to start the cycle once again.

Thus the saddle-node and nearby homoclinic curves of the fast subsystem are of primary importance for the Rinzel-Lee bursting model.

4.3.2. *Thalamic relay neurons*

We next investigate a bursting model of thalamocortical relay neurons introduced by Wang [29] (and see also chapter 1, section 1.5, of this volume) This four-dimensional model includes three fast currents: a sodium current, I_{Na}, a persistent sodium current, $I_{Na(P)}$, and a potassium current, I_K. Both sodium currents are assumed to activate instantaneously. The sodium inactivation, h, and potassium activation, n, are assumed to be related by $h = (0.85 - n)$ in accord with FitzHugh's observation [11]. The model also includes a passive leak current, I_L, and two slow currents: a T-type calcium current, I_T, and a sag current, I_h, with reversal potential $V_h = -40$ mV. The calcium inactivation, h_T, and sag current activation, h_H, are the slow variables, although the sag current activation is rapid at high voltages so that it changes value substantially during an action potential. The calcium activation is assumed to be instantaneous. Thus I_T has a fast activation but slow inactivation, and I_h is rapid at high voltages but slow when the membrane is polarized; nonetheless, we classify both of these as slow currents. In addition, the model incorporates an injected current, which we have set at -0.8 μA; this is equivalent to a decrease in the leak reversal potential. The leak current (and injected current) along with I_T and I_h are combined to obtain the effective leak parameters of the fast subsystem.

Figure 4.9 shows the same information for the Wang model as Fig. 4.8 did for the Rinzel-Lee model. The gray region in Fig. 4.9(B) is a wedge

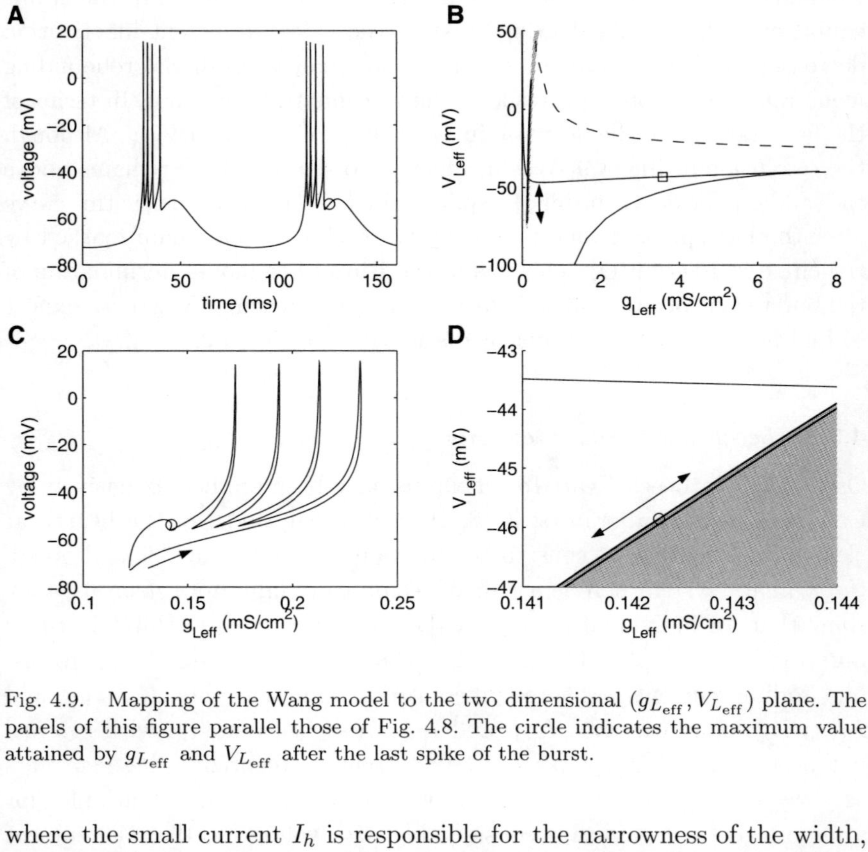

Fig. 4.9. Mapping of the Wang model to the two dimensional $(g_{L_{\text{eff}}}, V_{L_{\text{eff}}})$ plane. The panels of this figure parallel those of Fig. 4.8. The circle indicates the maximum value attained by $g_{L_{\text{eff}}}$ and $V_{L_{\text{eff}}}$ after the last spike of the burst.

where the small current I_h is responsible for the narrowness of the width, and changes in the large I_T current are responsible for movement along the length of the wedge. During the burst cycle, the effective leak parameters run along the left edge of the confining region, indicating that I_h remains very small and is not a substantial player in the bursting cycle.

Note that in comparison to the Rinzel-Lee model, where there was very little variation of $g_{L_{\text{eff}}}$ between successive spikes, Fig. 4.9(C) shows that $g_{L_{\text{eff}}}$ varies substantially for the Wang model. This is a manifestation of the fact that I_T is not a completely slow current, having an instantaneous activation with a half activation value of -65 mV and saturating at about -30 mV. For this reason, the trajectory in Fig. 4.9(C) has substantial horizontal movement during the spikes when the voltage is below -30 mV.

In the quiescent stage of the burst cycle, the system lies near the stable equilibrium of the fast subsystem. I_T (and less importantly I_h) both slowly increase pushing the voltage upward to the spiking threshold which corresponds to the saddle-node curve of the fast subsystem where the stable equilibrium disappears. During spiking, the calcium current inactivation decreases until eventually I_T becomes too small to push the rebounding membrane above spiking threshold, thus terminating the burst. In terms of the fast subsystem, the decrease in I_T causes a decrease in $V_{L_{\rm eff}}$. Although the resolution in Fig. 4.9(B) is insufficient to see this, $V_{L_{\rm eff}}$ remains above the saddle-node curve during the spike train and only drops below this curve after the last spike. It then rises slightly, reaching a maximum marked by the circle in Fig. 4.9(D). Thus, as in the Rinzel-Lee model, termination of the burst cycle occurs a little below the saddle-node curve where we expect to find homoclinic bifurcations as discussed in section 4.2.

4.3.3. *Leech heart interneurons*

Oscillations in Leech Heart Interneurons have been studied extensively by Calabrese and collaborators; [6, 8, 16] a detailed model of the heartbeat elemental oscillator was constructed by Nadim *et al.* [22] in 1995. Although the primary system here is a pair of reciprocally inhibitory neurons, they show that an individual neuron in their model can also exhibit intrinsic bursting behavior [23]. This leech heartbeat model includes $I_{\rm Na}$, a persistent sodium current, I_P, three different potassium currents, $I_{\rm K1}$, $I_{\rm K2}$, and I_A, two calcium currents, $I_{\rm CaF}$ and $I_{\rm CaS}$, a sag current, I_h, with reversal potential -21 mV, and a passive leak current. Categorizing these currents as slow or fast is not easy. The activation and inactivation variables for some of these currents vary considerably with voltage so that the current is fast in some regimes and slow in others. For example, the activation of $I_{\rm CaS}$ has a time constant of about 140 ms at voltages above -40 mV, but this reduces to a fast 5 ms at voltages below -60 mV. Also a number of the currents, particularly $I_{\rm CaF}$ and $I_{\rm K1}$, have a rapid activation but slow inactivation. In order to obtain a fast subsystem which includes all currents with fast components, we classified only I_h, $I_{\rm K2}$, and $I_{\rm CaS}$ as slow (despite the fact that the activation for $I_{\rm CaS}$ is fast at hyperpolarized voltages). It should also be noted that the fast subsystem includes some components, for example the inactivations of I_{K1} and I_{CaF}, that are slower than some of the slow current components.

Figure 4.10 shows the same information for the leech heartbeat model as Fig. 4.8 did for the Rinzel-Lee model. The number of spikes per burst

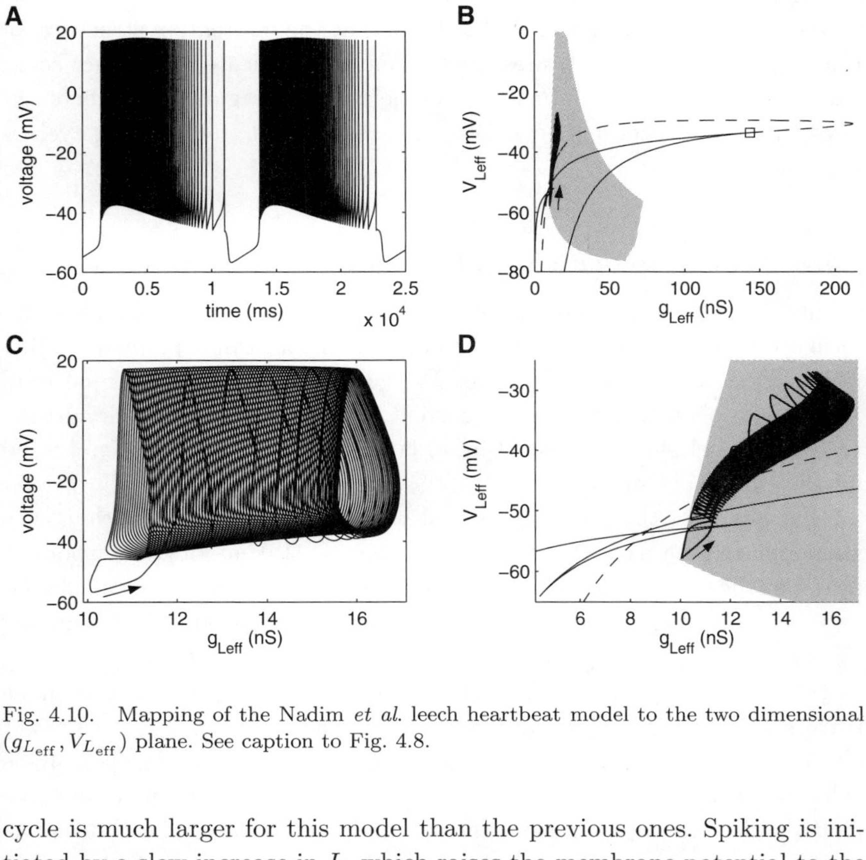

Fig. 4.10. Mapping of the Nadim *et al.* leech heartbeat model to the two dimensional $(g_{L_{\mathrm{eff}}}, V_{L_{\mathrm{eff}}})$ plane. See caption to Fig. 4.8.

cycle is much larger for this model than the previous ones. Spiking is initiated by a slow increase in I_h which raises the membrane potential to the point where I_{CaS} turns on and an action potential is generated. This can be seen in Fig. 4.10(D) where the trajectory, starting in the lower left corner of the confining region, first moves into the region, up and to the right (I_h increasing), and then abruptly turns parallel to the left boundary of the confining region and $V_{L_{\mathrm{eff}}}$ increases due to I_{CaS} turning on. After about eight spikes, $g_{L_{\mathrm{eff}}}$ and $V_{L_{\mathrm{eff}}}$ reach their maxima and then I_{CaS} slowly inactivates, reducing both effective leak parameters. The horizontal movement of the trajectory in the $(g_{L_{\mathrm{eff}}}, V_{L_{\mathrm{eff}}})$ plane is caused primarily by changes in the activation gating variable for I_{K2} which, being only moderately slow, reacts relatively quickly to changes in the membrane potential.

Termination of the burst cycle occurs shortly after I_{CaS} decreases sufficiently to cause the trajectory in the $(g_{L_{eff}}, V_{L_{eff}})$ plane to cross the saddle-node curve. Although the gross features of the saddle-node and Hopf bifurcation curves (Fig. 4.10(B)) are similar in this model to the system we studied in section 4.2, Fig. 4.10(D) shows that the bifurcation structure for this nine-dimensional fast subsystem is more complicated at a finer scale. The saddle-node curve forms a "bow-tie" shaped region near where the hopf curve intersects it, and it is in this region that the bursting cycle is terminating.

4.3.4. *Plateau oscillations in leech heart interneurons*

Cymbalyuk and Calabrese [7] present simpler models of leech heart interneurons than the model described above, which exhibit plateau oscillations. Their minimal model (model IV) consists of a fast sodium current, I_{Na}, a slow persistent potassium current, I_{K2}, and a passive leak current, I_L. Figure 4.11 shows the same information for this model as Fig. 4.8 did for the Rinzel-Lee model.

The shape of the saddle-node and hopf curves is similar to the "cusp and loop" structure of system (1) except that the Takens-Bogdanov point is nearly at the cusp of the saddle-node bifurcation curve. Since this model has only one slow current defined by a single activation variable, the confining region in the $(g_{L_{eff}}, V_{L_{eff}})$ plane is a one-dimensional curve (shown in gray in Fig. 4.11(B) and (D)). The bursting trajectory mapped to this plane traverses a portion of this curve back and forth.

During the quiescent (low voltage) phase of the burst cycle, the voltage value lies close to the low voltage fixed point in the fast subsystem, the model's effective leak parameters lie just underneath the saddle-node curve, and I_{K2} is slowly deactivating causing a decrease in $g_{L_{eff}}$ and increase in $V_{L_{eff}}$. As $V_{L_{eff}}$ continues to increase, the system crosses the saddle-node curve, where the low voltage fixed point disappears, and the system quickly approaches the high voltage fast subsystem fixed point. This corresponds to the start of the voltage plateau. The high voltage value now activates I_{K2} and the trajectory proceeds down and to the right in the $(g_{L_{eff}}, V_{L_{eff}})$ plane. At about $g_{L_{eff}} = 14$, the path crosses a supercritical Hopf curve, where the high voltage fixed point becomes unstable and an attracting periodic orbit is born. This corresponds to the small amplitude plateau oscillations in

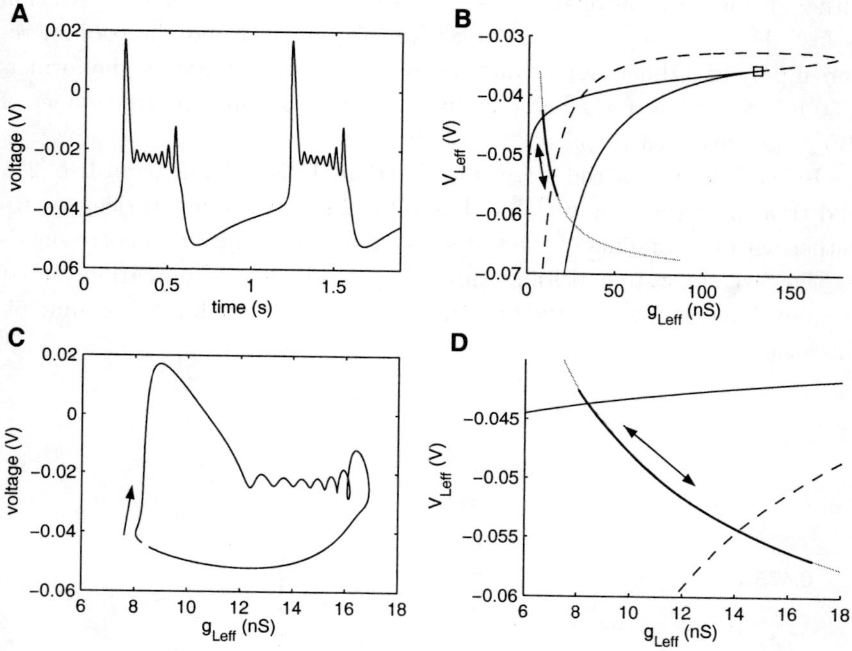

Fig. 4.11. Mapping of the Cymbalyuk-Calabrese simplified leech heart model to the two dimensional $(g_{L_{\text{eff}}}, V_{L_{\text{eff}}})$ plane. See caption to Fig. 4.8.

Fig. 4.11(A). Eventually the attracting periodic orbit is destroyed via a saddle-node of orbits, terminating the plateau, and the system collapses to the low voltage fixed point of the fast subsystem to begin the cycle anew.

4.3.5. *Neurons of the pre-Bötzinger complex*

Butera *et al.* [5] have proposed Hodgkin-Huxley type models of neurons in the pre-Bötzinger complex, a region of the brainstem essential to generating the breathing rhythm. Model I of Butera *et al.* [5] consists of fast sodium and potassium currents I_{Na} and I_{K}, a persistent sodium current $I_{\text{Na(P)}}$, and a passive leak current I_L (see also chapter 12 of this volume). Both sodium currents are assumed to activate instantaneously. Inactivation of I_{Na} is approximated by $1 - n$. The inactivation h of $I_{\text{Na(P)}}$ occurs on a much slower time scale than that of the other variables.

Despite the slow time scale of h, incorporating $I_{\text{Na(P)}}$ into an effective leak current does not work well here. This is partly due to the fact that, although inactivation of the persistent sodium current is slow, activation is fast. Furthermore, the true leak reversal potential and the sodium reversal potential differ significantly (approximately −60 mV for the former, +50 mV for the latter). These factors combine to result in large values of $dV_{L_{\text{eff}}}/dt$ during each spike.

Instead, we follow the more traditional analysis of Rinzel and Lee [27], and treat h as the slow variable. Figure 4.12 shows a burst trajectory, together with fixed points of the fast subsystem. Burst initiation corresponds to the fast subsystem passing through a saddle-node bifurcation. Burst termination occurs when the fast subsystem goes through a homoclinic bifurcation.

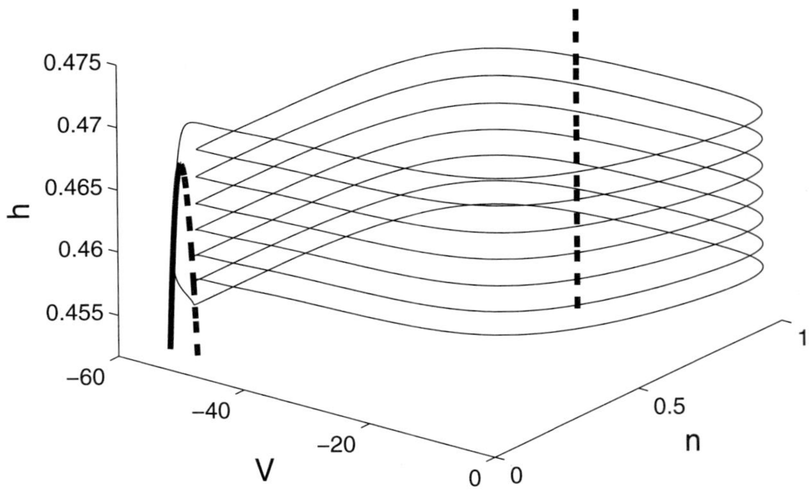

Fig. 4.12. A burst trajectory for Model I of Butera *et al.*, together with fixed points of the fast subsystem. Membrane potential V and potassium activation n are the fast variables, and inactivation of persistent sodium current h the slow variable. Equilibrium points of the fast subsystem for different values of h are plotted as bold curves. Stable equilibria are plotted as the solid curve, unstable equilibria are plotted as dashed curves.

In addition to the leak conductance and reversal potential that we have been examining throughout this chapter, we can also include the slow variable h and examine the bifurcations in the fast subsystem which result as these three parameters are varied. Note that the leak conductance and reversal potential here correspond to the true leak current in model I of Butera *et al.*, [5] not to an effective leak current. Figures 4.13(a) and (b) show the resulting hopf and saddle-node bifurcation surfaces. The shape of the hopf surface changes significantly as h is varied. On the other hand, the surface of saddle-nodes does not change much with h. Figures 4.13(c) and (d) show the $g_L - V_L$ bifurcation diagrams for $h = 0.21$ and $h = 0.95$, respectively. Note that Fig. 4.13(c) resembles the bifurcation diagrams for the Rinzel-Lee, Wang, and Cymbalyuk-Calabrese models, while Fig. 4.13(d) is similar to the bifurcation diagram of Nadim *et al.* The similarities in the shapes of the bifurcation curves for these different models suggest that a small number of qualitatively distinct bifurcation diagrams may predominate in the fast subsystems of Hodgkin-Huxley type models.

4.4. Discussion

Conductance based models for neurons with voltage gated currents based on the Hodgkin-Huxley formalism combine an equation for membrane potential with differential equations for the gating variables. Chemical concentrations of ligands or second messengers lead to a somewhat more general class of models, but the model structure is still highly constrained. We would like to determine the generality and limitations of these models in explaining observed electrical activity of neurons. Thus, we ask two complementary questions

- What types of dynamical behavior occur (generically) within this class of models?
- Are there principles that can be used to construct models and families of models that display specific types of dynamics?

The second question is often addressed in the context of fitting models to experimental data. The first question is more abstract, but even partial answers provide a framework that help us tackle the second. The questions are difficult because the dynamical behaviors we study are complex, the models have large numbers of parameters and multiple time scales bring additional challenges for the analysis. Systematically simulating models throughout biologically plausible regions of their parameter spaces is hardly feasible. Nonetheless, we speculate about generalizations in the hope that our computational and analytical studies of models will help sharpen understanding

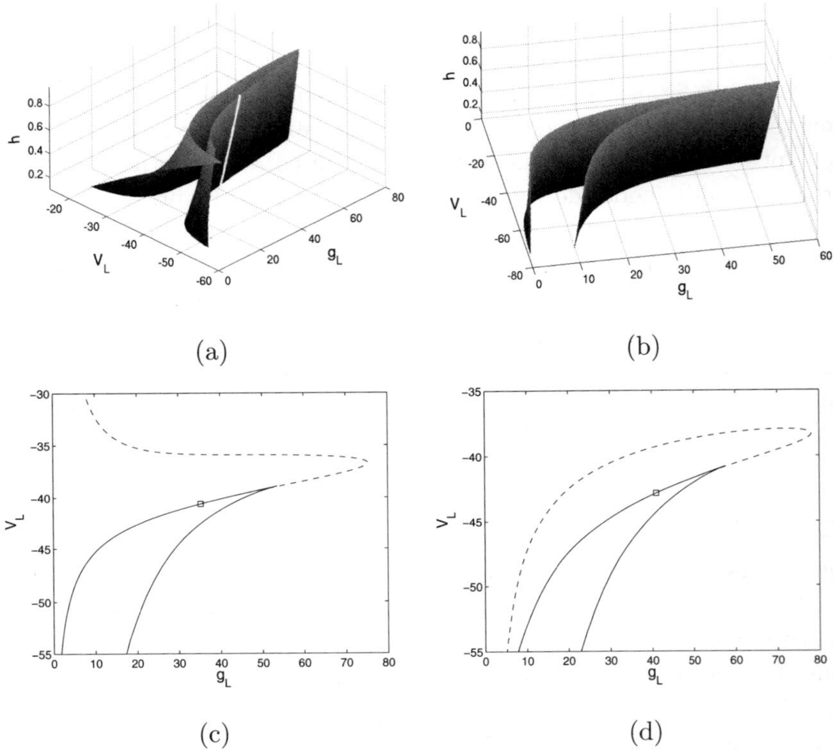

Fig. 4.13. Equilibrium point bifurcation diagrams of a three parameter fast subsystem (Model I of Butera *et al.*) with parameters (g_L, V_L, h). (a) Hopf bifurcations, Takens-Bogdanov points, and neutral saddles. The white curve separating the two dimensional surface into two components denotes Takens-Bogdanov points. The component with larger values of V_L consists of Hopf points, while the smaller V_L component consists of neutral saddles. (b) Saddle-node bifurcations. (c) Saddle-node (solid) and Hopf (dashed) bifurcation curves in the (g_L, V_L) plane with $h = 0.21$. (d) Saddle-node and Hopf bifurcation curves in the (g_L, V_L) plane with $h = 0.95$.

of how neural systems function.

Theories and models of bursting [3, 19, 25] point to multiple time scales as a key factor in the generation of neural rhythms. We present here an analysis of neuronal bursting that makes use of three time scales. We call these time scales slow, fast and very fast. Currents that change on the slow time scale bring a neuron into and out of regimes in which it fires action potentials. The thresholds and characteristics of the action potentials are determined by dynamics of the fast and very fast time scales. The bifurcations that occur in the subsystems that incorporate the fast and very fast dynamics are shaped by the separation between the fast and very fast time scales. These bifurcations are found close to parameter values at which the subsystem has degenerate slow-fast decompositions. The proximity of various bifurcation curves to one another is explained by the extreme sensitivity of limit sets containing canards to parameter variations. Consequently, information about Hopf and saddle-node bifurcations of equilibria together with a picture of the slow manifolds in these subsystems can be used to predict information about global bifurcations. As an example, inside the cusp region of the planar vector field studied in section 4.2, all the periodic orbits undergoing saddle-node bifurcations contain canards. These bifurcations lie extremely close to homoclinic bifurcations and very close to Hopf bifurcations.

We observe that the very fast subsystems of large classes of neural models are very similar to one another, describing changes in membrane potential and the rapid activation of certain currents. Typically, these activations are treated as instantaneous, removing them from the dynamical variables of the model and leaving only the membrane potential as a very fast variable. This perspective suggests that there are similarities in the bifurcation mechanisms among large classes of conductance based models for neurons. Due to their stiffness, the bifurcation diagrams of these models are difficult to determine completely, but the equilibrium point bifurcations that are easy to determine provide a backbone on which to base further study. Section 4.2 presents an analysis of one such model that contains only a fast sodium and a leak current. Reductions of the Hodgkin-Huxley model embody a frequent modification of this model by including a non-inactivating potassium current whose activation is correlated with the inactivation of the sodium current. The first equation in system (1) is replaced by

$$\dot{v} = -(g_{Na}m^3h(v - v_{Na}) + g_K n^4(v - v_K) + g_l(v - v_l))$$

with $n = h_m - h$, where h_m is often taken in the range $[0.85, 1]$. By treating g_K as a secondary parameter, we obtain a one parameter family of bifurcation diagrams. There are two notable changes in these bifurcation diagrams:

- The cusp region of saddle-nodes moves to smaller values of g_l, exiting the region where $g_l > 0$ for modest values of g_K.
- The Hopf curve undergoes a transition in which the self intersection point disappears and the curve extends upward along the positive v_l axis.

Figure 4.14 illustrates these changes, displaying the equilibrium point bifurcation diagram of this system with $g_K = 3$ and $h_m = 1$. These changes in the equilibrium point bifurcation structure are also associated with changes in the global bifurcation structure (saddle-nodes of orbits and homoclinics). In particular, there is no longer a crossing of the two small homoclinic curves and consequently no gluing bifurcation. Further, stable periodic orbits persist at high v_l values all the way to $g_l = 0$. Nonetheless, the curves of large homoclinic bifurcations and saddle-nodes of orbits still appear to be located extremely close to the equilibrium saddle-node curve, so that this curve remains a good indicator of where bursting will terminate.

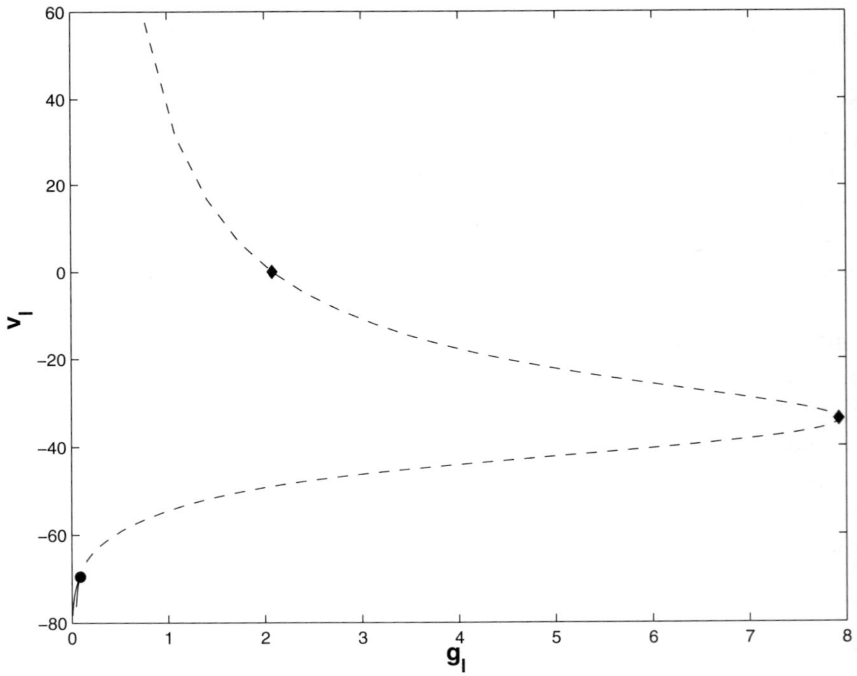

Fig. 4.14. The equilibrium point bifurcation diagram for the modified system (1). The conductance of the potassium current is $g_K = 3$ and $h_m = 1$. Degenerate Hopf bifurcations that bound a segment of supercritical Hopf bifurcation are marked by diamonds. The Takens-Bogdanov bifurcation is marked by a filled circle.

The examples described in section 4.3 illustrate two approaches to the slow-fast decomposition of neuronal models, each with advantages and disadvantages. Our results demonstrate that the equilibrium point bifurcations of a fast subsystem provide a guide to locating the transitions between spiking and quiescent dynamics in bursting rhythms. As we observe and others before us have demonstrated, some transitions between spiking and quiescent dynamics are associated with global bifurcations. However, we observe that these global bifurcations are often located close to equilibrium point bifurcations due to multiple time scales within the fast subsystems. Since the theoretical foundations for the analysis of bursting assume a large separation between slow and fast time scales, we do not expect to obtain definitive results about models in which these time scales blur into one another. Even so, multiple time scale analysis provides useful insight into the dynamics of these complex systems. Moreover, computational methods based upon geometric singular perturbation theory can be further refined to give still more useful insights.

In mapping slow currents to an effective leak current, we treat the effective leak conductance and reversal potential as new slow variables. The time scale of the effective leak reversal potential is affected not only by the activation and inactivation rates of the slow currents, but also by the slow currents' reversal potentials. Widely differing reversal potentials may result in a fast effective leak reversal potential, even if the gating variables of the included currents are all slow. The mapping to the effective leak current works best when the slow currents have similar reversal potentials.

The mapping of slow currents into an effective leak current gives additional information that can be used to determine whether bursting might be possible in a model. The figures of section 4.3 contain gray regions that delineate possible values for the conductance and reversal potential of the effective leak current of the fast subsystems derived from a larger model. This region is determined solely by the slow currents. The extreme left point of this region is precisely the conductance and reversal potential of the true passive leak current. The lower boundary moving to the right of this point is determined by adding into the equations one slow current at a time (that is increasing its conductance from zero to its maximum value), in the order from the current with the lowest reversal potential to the one with the largest, until we reach the extreme right point where all slow currents have been added in. The upper boundary is computed similarly but taking the currents in the opposite order. Superposition of this gray region upon the bifurcation diagram of the fast subsystem restricts attention to bifurcations that might be accessible as transitions between attractors of the fast subsystem. Forcing a trajectory to cross these bifurcation curves in particular places requires slow and leak currents that vary appropriately on the slow time scale. In relating the behavior of two different models with the same fast components, comparison of the plots of the confining regions of the two sets of slow currents helps determine whether the models have similar bursting behavior. Of course, the location of the confining region is just a start, since where the trajectory goes inside the confining region depends on the specific dynamics of the slow currents.

Acknowledgments

This work was partially supported by the National Science Foundation.

References

[1] E. Benoit, J. L Callot, F. Diener, and M. Diener, Chasse au canards. *Collect. Math.* **31**, 37–119, (1981).
[2] N. M. Berezetskaya, V. N. Kharkyanen, and N. I. Kononenko, Mathematical model of pacemaker activity in bursting neurons of snail, *helix pomatia. J. Theor. Biol.* **183**, 207–218, (1996).
[3] R. Bertram, M. Butte, T. Kiemel, and A. Sherman, Topological and phenomenological classification of bursting oscillations, *Bull. Math. Biol.* **57**(3), 413–39, (1995).
[4] R. J. Butera Jr, J. W. Clark, C. C. Canavier, D. A. Baxter, and J. H. Byrne, Analysis of the effects of modulatory agents on a modeled bursting neuron: Dynamic interactions between voltage and calcium dependent systems, *J. Comp. Neurosci.* **2**, 19–44, (1995).
[5] R. J. Butera Jr, J. Rinzel, and J. C. Smith, Models of respiratory rhythm generation in the pre-Bötzinger complex. I. Bursting pacemaker neurons, *J Neurophysiol.* **82**, 382–97, (1999).
[6] G. S. Cymbalyuk and R. L. Calabrese, Oscillatory behaviors in pharmacologically isolated heart interneurons from the medicinal leech, *Neurocomput.* **32**, 97–104, (2000).
[7] G. S. Cymbalyuk and R. L. Calabrese, A model of slow plateau-like oscillations based upon the fast Na^+ current in a window mode, *Neurocomput.* **38**, 159–166, (2001).
[8] G. S. Cymbalyuk, Q. Gaudry, M. A. Masino, and R. L. Calabrese Bursting in leech heart interneurons: Cell-autonomous and network-based mechanisms, *J. Neurosci.* **22**, 10580–10592, (2002).
[9] F. Dumortier and R. Roussarie, Canard cycles and center manifolds, *Mem. Amer. Math. Soc.* **121**, no. 577, (1996).

[10] W. Eckhaus, Relaxation oscillations, including a standard chase on french ducks, *Lecture Notes in Mathematics* **985**, 449–494, (1983).

[11] R. FitzHugh, Impulses and physiological states in theoretical models of nerve membrane, *Biophys. J.* **1**, 445–466, (1961).

[12] J. M. Gambaudo, P. Glendinning, and C. Tresser, The gluing bifurcation I: symbolic dynamics of the closed curves, *Nonlinearity* **1**, 203–214, (1988).

[13] J. Guckenheimer, S. Gueron, and R. M. Harris-Warrick, Mapping the dynamics of a bursting neuron, *Phil. Trans. R. Soc. Lond. B* **341**, 345–359, (1993).

[14] J. Guckenheimer and P. J. Holmes, *Nonlinear Oscillations, Dynamical Systems, and Bifurcations of Vector Fields*, Springer-Verlag, New York, (1983).

[15] J. Guckenheimer and R. Oliva, Chaos in the Hodgkin-Huxley Model, *SIAM J. Appl. Dyn. Systems* **1**, 105–114, (2002).

[16] A. A. V. Hill, J. Lu, M. A. Masino, O. H. Olsen, and R. L. Calabrese, A model of a segmental oscillator in the leech heartbeat neuronal network, *J. Comput. Neurosci.* **10**, 281–302, (2001).

[17] B. Hille, *Ionic Channels of Excitable Membranes, 3rd edition* Sinauer, (2001).

[18] A. L. Hodgkin and A. F. Huxley, A quantitative description of membrane current and its applications to conduction and excitation in nerve, *J. Physiol.* (Lond.) **116**, 500–544, (1952).

[19] E. M. Izhikevich, Neural excitability, spiking and bursting. *Internat. J. Bifur. Chaos Appl. Sci. Engrg.* **10**, 1171–1266, (2000).

[20] C. Jones, Geometric singular perturbation theory, *Lecture Notes in Math.*, Springer, Berlin, **1609**, 44–118, (1995).

[21] R. H. Kramer and R. S. Zucker, Calcium-dependent inward current in *aplysia* bursting pace-maker neurones, *J. Physiol.* **362**, 107–130, (1985).

[22] F. Nadim, O. H. Olsen, E. DeSchutter, and R. L. Calabrese, Modeling the leech heartbeat elemental oscillator: I. Interactions of intrinsic and synaptic currents, *J. Comput. Neurosci.* **2**, 215–235, (1995).

[23] O. H. Olsen, F. Nadim, and R. L. Calabrese, Modeling the leech heartbeat elemental oscillator: II. Exploring the parameter space, *J. Comput. Neurosci.* **2**, 237–257, (1995).

[24] R. E. Plant, Bifurcation and resonance in a mathematical model for bursting nerve cells, *J. Math. Biol.* **11**, 15–32, (1981).

[25] J. Rinzel, A formal classification of bursting mechanisms in excitable

systems, Mathematical topics in population biology, morphogenesis and neurosciences (Kyoto, 1985), *Lecture Notes in Biomath.* **71**, 267–281, Springer, Berlin, (1987).

[26] J. Rinzel and B. Ermentrout, Analysis of neural excitability and oscillations, in *Methods of Neural Modeling : From Synapses to Networks*, C. Koch and I. Segev, eds., MIT Press, 135–169, (1989).

[27] J. Rinzel and Y. S. Lee, Dissection of a model for neuronal parabolic bursting, *J. Math. Biol.* **25**, 653–675, (1987).

[28] R. Roussarie, Bifurcation of planar vector fields and Hilbert's sixteenth problem. *Progress in Mathematics* **164**, Birkhuser Verlag, Basel, (1998).

[29] X. J. Wang, Multiple dynamical modes of thalamic relay neurons: Rhythmic bursting and intermittent phase-locking, *Neurosci.* **59**, 21–31, (1994).

CHAPTER 5

BURSTING IN 2-COMPARTMENT NEURONS: A CASE STUDY OF THE PINSKY-RINZEL MODEL

Amitabha Bose

Department of Mathematical Sciences
New Jersey Institute of Technology, Newark, NJ 07102, USA
e-mail: bose@njit.edu

Victoria Booth

Departments of Mathematics and Anesthesiology
University of Michigan, Ann Arbor, MI 48109, USA
e-mail: vbooth@umich.edu

The two-compartment Pinsky-Rinzel model of a hippocampal CA3 pyramidal neuron consists of electrically coupled soma and dendritic compartments, each with active ionic conductances. This model has been widely used in a variety of contexts, but little analysis has been performed on its bursting solutions. In this chapter, we provide a geometric framework to study the Pinsky-Rinzel model. Using a combination of analysis and simulations, we identify neuronal mechanisms responsible for certain salient features of the model such as burst initiation and somatic-dendritic ping-pong. Some of these mechanisms are then demonstrated in a conceptually simpler, two-compartment Morris-Lecar model.

5.1. Introduction

Neurons are spatially distributed, heterogeneous entities. Among other structures, a neuron has dendrites which collect inputs, a cell body called a soma where integration of these inputs occur, an axon for output of neuronal signals, and synapses where communication with other neurons occurs. Different parts of the neuron may contain different ionic channels with different gating kinetics. Due to these potential complexities, accurate modeling of electrical activity of neurons is a challenging endeavor. Three basic approaches have been considered. One is to model the neuron using partial differential equations to explicitly capture the spatial dependence [6, 15, 17]. Another is to use ordinary differential equations to model the neuron as a multi-compartment cell where the compartments are coupled via gap junctions [9, 14, 16, 19, 21]. The third approach is to treat the neuron as a single-compartment, point neuron [13, 20]. In choosing one of these approaches, one must balance the need for biological plausibility versus the need for mathematical rigor and understanding of underlying phenomena.

In this chapter, we shall focus on multi-compartment neuron models. Although these models have been used widely in computational modeling studies, little analysis of such models has appeared in the literature. Of particular interest to us is the development of analytic tools that can be used to better understand the dynamics that arise as the result of multiple compartments. Here, we will work primarily with the Pinsky-Rinzel (PR) model [16] which is a two-compartment reduction of a larger 19-compartment model developed by Traub *et al.* [19] of a hippocampal CA3 pyramidal cell. An important reason to study the PR model is that it introduced a specific modeling formalism which has been adopted by many others in more recent modeling studies. Namely, Pinsky and Rinzel lumped relevant active currents into a single "dendrite" compartment and segregated these from other currents lumped into a "soma" compartment. Although simple in concept, Pinsky and Rinzel demonstrated that this lumped, simplified model could qualitatively, and to a large degree, quantitatively describe the dynamics of the larger Traub model.

In the PR model, the interplay of active ionic currents between both compartments generates a wide variety of firing patterns ranging from tonic spiking to complex bursting. These features also contribute to the difficulty one faces in analyzing the dynamics of the model. The main purpose of this chapter is to provide a geometric framework from which one can begin analysis of the PR and other multi-compartment models.

For our analysis, we have modified the PR equations to simplify the gating kinetic equations for some of the ionic conductances. In this chapter, after briefly reviewing the modified PR model, we focus on two salient features of the model. First, we will show using phase plane analysis how to understand burst initiation in the PR model. We do so by deriving and analyzing a reduced set of equations which are valid in the silent state of the burst. By understanding the mechanism for burst onset, we are also able to understand how to control the burst frequency. We then turn our attention to the dynamics of two-compartment bursting, known as somatic-dendritic ping-pong [23], whereby the two compartments alternately depolarize one another throughout the burst. We consider how ping-pong can fail to occur and how the ping-pong pattern can change depending on the dynamics in each compartment. We conclude by applying some of the lessons learned from the PR model to a simpler two-compartment model where each compartment is modeled by the Morris-Lecar equations.

5.2. The Pinsky-Rinzel Model

5.2.1. *Equations and qualitative description of the complex burst*

The original Pinsky-Rinzel equations for the two-compartment pyramidal cell model consist of current balance equations for a soma and dendrite compartment that are connected by electrical coupling. The soma compartment contains inward sodium and outward, potassium delayed rectifier active currents. The dendrite compartment contains an inward calcium current, I_{Ca}, an outward, voltage-activated potassium current, I_{K-C}, and an outward, calcium-activated, potassium after-hyperpolarization current, I_{K-AHP}. The equations are of the form

$$\begin{aligned} Cv_s' &= I_s - \bar{g}_L[v_s - E_L] - \bar{g}_{Na}m_\infty^2(v_s)h[v_s - E_{Na}] \\ &\quad -\bar{g}_{K-DR}n[v_s - E_K] - g_{coup}[v_s - v_d]/p \\ Cv_d' &= I_d - \bar{g}_L[v_d - E_L] - \bar{g}_{Ca}s^2[v_d - E_{Ca}] - \bar{g}_{K-AHP}q[v_d - E_K] \\ &\quad -\bar{g}_{K-C}\chi(Ca)c[v_d - E_K] - g_{coup}[v_d - v_s]/[1-p] \end{aligned} \tag{1}$$

The variables v_s and v_d represent the somatic and dendritic membrane voltages in mV, respectively. Ca represents calcium concentration. While I_{K-C} is voltage-activated, its conductance is modulated by the function $\chi(Ca) = \min(Ca/250, 1)$, a saturation function for calcium concentration. The steady state activation function $m_\infty(v_s)$ is sigmoidal and is effectively 0 when the neuron is subthreshold, and 1 when the neuron is active. Maximal conductances are given by $\bar{g}_x$ in mS/cm^2 and reversal potentials by E_x in mV ($x = L$ leak, Na sodium, Ca calcium, $K-DR$ potassium delayed rectifier, $K-AHP$ potassium after-hyperpolarization and $K-C$ voltage-activated potassium). The parameters $I_s = 0.75$ and $I_d = 0$ μA/cm^2 are applied current terms to the soma and dendrite, respectively. The parameter $p = 0.5$ measures the percentage of the total area of the soma compartment, $g_{coup} = 2.1$ mS/cm^2 is the electrical coupling conductance and $C = 3$ μF/cm^2 is the membrane capacitance. See [16] for the h, n and q gating kinetic functions, the Ca^{2+} concentration equations and for parameter values.

The gating variables h, n and q in (1) obey first order differential equations of the form

$$y' = \alpha_y(U) - (\alpha_y(U) + \beta_y(U))y \tag{2}$$

where the argument U is v_s for $y = h, n$ and Ca for $y = q$. We have modified the equations governing the gating variables s and c for I_{Ca} and I_{K-C}, respectively, to the form

$$y' = [y_\infty(v_d) - y]/\tau_y(v_d). \tag{3}$$

The steady state activation functions $s_\infty(v_d) = 1/(1 + \exp(-(v_d + 20)/8))$ and $c_\infty(v_d) = 1/(1 + \exp(-(v_d + 10)/11))$ were fit to the corresponding functions in the original model. We simplified the time constant $\tau_s(v_d)$ to a constant $\tau_s = 2.535$ msec^{-1}. The time constant $\tau_c(v_d)$ was simplified to the piecewise linear function

$$\tau_c(v_d) = (1 - H(v_d + 10))\tau_{cc} + H(v_d + 10)(\tau_{cc} + 0.2(v_d + 10)) \tag{4}$$

where $H(v)$ is the Heaviside function. This simplification retains the break at $v_d = -10$ mV that appears in the original PR model but replaces the exponentially varying behavior for $v_d < -10$ mV with a constant $\tau_{cc} = 2.5$ msec^{-1}. The slope of $\tau_c(v_d)$ for $v_d > -10$ mV approximates the exponential behavior in the original model. The nullclines for all gating variables are sigmoidally shaped.

The modified PR model generates a complex burst essentially identical to the original model (Fig. 5.1). The burst is initiated by a sodium spike in the soma compartment. This spike back-propagates and depolarizes the dendrite compartment, activating the s, c and Ca variables. Calcium influx into the dendrite sustains dendritic depolarization which, in turn, provides sufficient depolarization through the electrical coupling to the soma to generate subsequent spikes. These subsequent spikes further depolarize the dendrite such that a partial dendritic calcium spike is induced. As a result, the soma is overdriven and the sodium spiking mechanism is shut down (depolarization block). Eventually, the burst ends when the calcium spike is shut off by I_{K-C} which builds up during the burst. The interburst length in this parameter regime, approximately 554 msec, is primarily governed by the slow decay of the potassium after-hyperpolarization gating variable q.

In Fig. 5.1, where we have projected the solution trajectory in the v_s-n and v_d-q phase planes, the direction of flow is counter-clockwise. Note

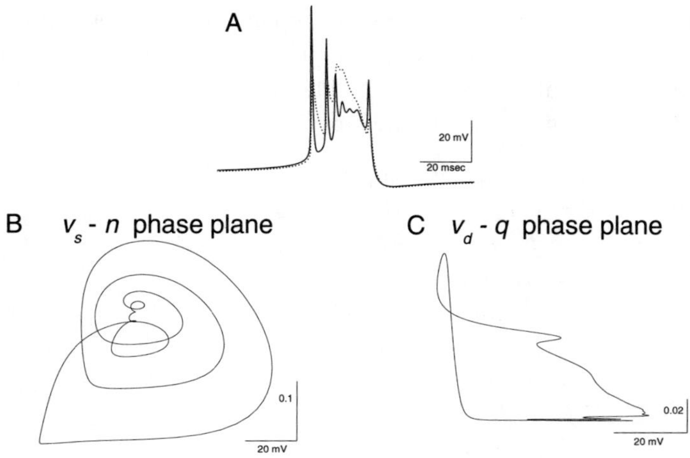

Fig. 5.1. Complex burst of the modified PR model. A: Somatic (solid curve) and dendritic (dotted curve) voltage trajectories. B,C: Burst trajectory projected onto the $v_s - n$ (B) and $v_d - q$ (C) phase planes.

that the trajectories in these phase planes intersect themselves, since these are projections of a higher dimensional flow onto two-dimensional phase planes. Phase plane analysis, as such, is not technically valid over all parts of the neuron's trajectory. However, as we will show below, it is possible to derive a set of simplified equations which govern subthreshold behavior of the neuron for which phase plane analysis is possible.

The PR model can also exhibit a wide variety of other firing patterns depending on parameter choices. These include tonic spiking in one or both compartments, mixed mode oscillations and aperiodic behavior. See [16] for more details.

One of the primary difficulties in analyzing the PR model is identifying which variables evolve on what time scales and over what parts of the cell's trajectory. The variables n and Ca decay slowly compared to all the other variables except for q which decays the most slowly. To analyze bursting, we will work with a set of slightly modified equations where we use a small parameter ϵ to demarcate fast and slow time scales. To derive them, we have broken the burst trajectory into four distinct regimes. The first is the jump up when somatic and dendritic voltages depolarize quickly at the leading edge of the burst. This occurs when $V_d^\star < v_d < v_\theta$ and $v_d' > 0$, where v_θ is some prescribed value and $V_d^\star$ will be described in detail in section 5.3.1. The second regime is the active state of the burst where $v_d > v_\theta$. The third regime is the jump down when voltages repolarize at the end of the burst. In this state, $V_d^\star < v_d < v_\theta$, but $v_d' < 0$. The final regime is the silent state or interburst interval where $v_d < V_d^\star$. The modified equations that provide for this dissection of the burst trajectory are:

$$\begin{aligned} v_s' &= F(v_s, n, h) - g_{coup}[v_s - v_d] \\ n' &= \epsilon[n_\infty(v_s) - n]/\tau_n(v_s, v_s') \\ v_d' &= f(v_d, q, Ca, s, c) - g_{coup}[v_d - v_s] \\ q' &= \epsilon\alpha(kCa - q)/\tau_q(v_d, v_d') \\ Ca' &= \epsilon[-\mu\bar{g}_{Ca}s^2[v_d - E_{Ca}] - bCa]/\tau_{Ca}(v_d, v_d') \\ s' &= [s_\infty(v_d) - s]/\tau_s \\ c' &= [c_\infty(v_d) - c]/\tau_c \\ h &= H(V_s^\star - v_s) \end{aligned} \tag{5}$$

The steady state activation functions n_∞, s_∞ and c_∞ are increasing sigmoidal functions which take values between 0 and 1, but whose values are assumed to be 0 when the neuron is silent. The value V_s^* will be defined in section 5.3.1 below.

The following time constants take on the following values in the different states of the burst:

$$\tau_n(v_s, v_s') = \begin{cases} 1 & v_s > V_s^\star, \quad v_s' > 0 \\ \epsilon & v_s > V_s^\star, \quad v_s' < 0 \\ 1/\gamma & v_s < V_s^\star, \end{cases} \tag{6}$$

$$\tau_q(v_d, v_d') = \begin{cases} 1 \text{ during jump up, active state and silent state} \\ \epsilon \text{ during jump down,} \end{cases} \tag{7}$$

$$\tau_{Ca}(v_d, v_d') = \begin{cases} 1 \text{ during jump up and silent state} \\ \epsilon \text{ during active state and jump down} \end{cases} \tag{8}$$

The parameters α, ϵ, γ, μ, k, b, τ_s and τ_c are positive. The functions $F(v_s, n, h)$ and $f(v_d, q, Ca, s, c)$ denote ionic and applied currents on the right hand sides of the v_s' and v_d' equations found in (1).

The above equations, while somewhat unwieldy, are in standard form to employ techniques of geometric singular perturbation theory. In particular, we can define relevant sets of reduced equations which will be the primary equations of interest. These equations are obtained by setting $\epsilon = 0$ in the above equations or in a rescaled version of them. Solutions of the reduced equations can then be pieced together to form a so-called singular solution. Using results of [12], for example, one can then prove that an actual solution to the ϵ small problem lies $O(\epsilon)$ close to the reduced solution. To this end, we shall work only with reduced equations.

5.3. Dynamics of the Pinsky-Rinzel Model

In this section, we describe two important aspects of the PR model, burst initiation and somatic-dendritic ping-pong. These phenomena will be discussed geometrically using phase plane analysis. We also computationally explore these issues where the effects of changing certain parameters can be addressed and illustrated.

5.3.1. *Burst initiation*

With respect to burst initiation, an issue often addressed is how bursting oscillations arise as applied current to the neuron is increased. This has led to the classification of neurons as being Type I (those that are capable of arbitrarily low frequency oscillations) or Type II (those whose frequency is bounded from below) [18]. Here, we ask a different question. Once the neuron is in the bursting regime, what is the mechanism that allows the neuron to leave the silent state, i.e. what mechanism is responsible for the onset of each burst?

To understand how firing is initiated, we derive a set of reduced equations to describe dynamics in the silent state of the neuron when $v_d < V_d^\star$. These equations are obtained from (5) when time is rescaled with the new variable $\tau = \epsilon t$ and then ϵ is set to 0:

$$\begin{aligned}
0 &= F(v_s, n, 1) - g_{coup}[v_s - v_d] \\
\dot{n} &= -\gamma n \\
0 &= f(v_d, q, Ca, s, c) - g_{coup}[v_d - v_s] \\
\dot{q} &= \alpha[kCa - q] \\
\dot{Ca} &= -bCa \\
0 &= s \\
0 &= c.
\end{aligned} \tag{9}$$

In (9), differentiation is with respect to τ. We note that c and s act as parameters in the v_d equation, and that $s = 0$ reduces the Ca equation to a simple equation of exponential decay. There are three rate constants of interest in (9); α, γ and b. Of these, α is chosen to be substantially smaller than γ and b. Therefore, it is instructive to simplify (9) by assuming $n = 0$

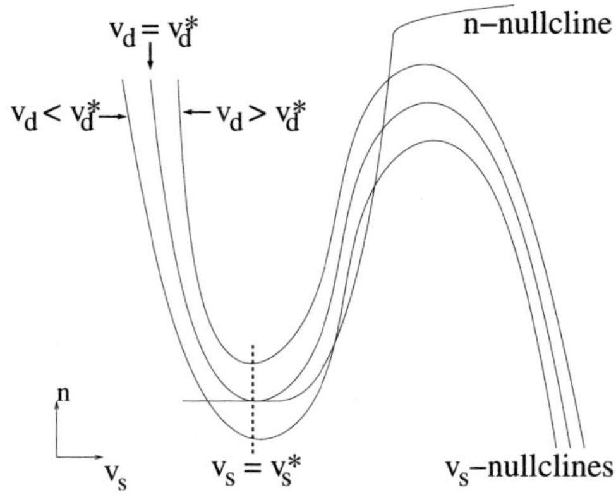

Fig. 5.2. The effect of v_d on the v_s-nullcline. A saddle-node bifurcation occurs when v_d increases through $V_d^\star$ thereby removing the two fixed points on the middle and left branch of the v_s-nullcline.

and $Ca = 0$ in the silent phase. Thus equations (9) become

$$\begin{aligned} 0 &= F(v_s, 0, 1) - g_{coup}[v_s - v_d] \\ 0 &= n \\ 0 &= f(v_d, q, 0, 0, 0) - g_{coup}[v_d - v_s] \\ \dot{q} &= -\alpha q, \end{aligned} \tag{10}$$

with the algebraic equations for $Ca = s = c = 0$. The n-nullcline is the horizontal line $n = 0$. If $g_{coup} = 0$, the v_s nullcline of (9) would simply correspond to $F(v_s, n, 1) = 0$ which is a cubic shaped curve in the $v_s - n$ phase plane. It would not intersect the n-nullcline. However, when $g_{coup} \neq 0$, the electrical coupling shifts this nullcline up or down depending on whether the quantity $I_{coup} \doteq g_{coup}(v_d - v_s)$ is positive or negative, respectively. If I_{coup} is sufficiently negative, the resulting cubic nullcline will intersect the n-nullcline, creating a fixed point in the $v_s - n$ subsystem. The existence of this fixed point prohibits the somatic trajectory from leaving the silent state. The quantity I_{coup} is continually changing during the silent state, however, since v_s and v_d are continually changing. Thus in the silent state the v_s nullcline is a two-dimensional surface consisting of the left branches of raised and lowered cubics. There is a unique value $I_{coup}^* = g_{coup}(V_d^\star - V_s^\star)$ at which the fixed point disappears and a saddle-node bifurcation occurs (see Fig. 5.2).

This bifurcation occurs when the minimum of the v_s-nullcline is tangent to the n-nullcline. The value $V_s^\star$ satisfies

$$\partial F(V_s^\star, 0, 1)/\partial v_s - g_{coup} = 0, \tag{11}$$

while $V_d^\star$ satisfies

$$F(V_s^\star, 0, 1) - g_{coup}(V_s^\star - V_d^\star) = 0. \tag{12}$$

When $v_d < V_d^\star$, because of the fast v_s and n dynamics, equation (10) shows that v_s is always in a neighborhood of $V_s^\star$. Thus the condition that $I_{coup} = I_{coup}^*$ for a saddle-node bifurcation to occur, effectively reduces to $v_d = V_d^\star$. In turn, this yields a simple conclusion: if $v_d < V_d^\star$, there exists a fixed point of the fast $v_s - n$ subsystem and the v_s trajectory lies at this fixed point. If $v_d > V_d^\star$, there is no fixed point on the left branches of the v_s nullcline and equations (9) and (10) are no longer valid. However, equations (5) and (6) then show that because of the fast v_s dynamics, the trajectory will leave a neighborhood of the left branches. Thus $V_d^\star$ provides a natural threshold for burst initiation. In short, if the trajectory is in the silent state, a burst will be initiated only when v_d increases through $V_d^\star$.

Pinsky and Rinzel [16] discuss that a burst is initiated when the variable q passes below a particular threshold. Equation (10) would appear to support this conclusion since q is the only dynamic variable in the silent state. However, we note that the values of $V_s^\star$ and $V_d^\star$ calculated from equations (11) and (12) are independent of q. While a value of q can be calculated at the moment of burst initiation, this value, in general, may change depending on the context. To elaborate, let us calculate the value of q at the bifurcation point using equation (10) for the v_d nullcline. When $g_{coup} = 0$, the graph of the v_d nullcline is a simple one-dimensional curve satisfying $f(v_d, q, 0, 0, 0) = 0$. When g_{coup} is non-zero, the v_d nullcline sweeps out a two-dimensional surface. In the silent state, however, v_s is always in a neighborhood of $V_s^\star$, so the v_d-nullcline is basically one-dimensional. At the bifurcation point, we find that $q = q_{bif}$ must satisfy $f(V_d^\star, q_{bif}, 0, 0, 0) - g_{coup}[V_d^\star - V_s^\star] = 0$. Using equation (1), we find that the value of q_{bif} satisfies

$$q_{bif} = \frac{-\bar{g}_L[V_d^\star - E_L] - g_{coup}[V_d^\star - V_s^\star]}{\bar{g}_{K-AHP}[V_d^\star - E_K]}. \tag{13}$$

For the set of parameters in Fig. 5.1, $q_{bif} = 0.155$. Note, however, that q_{bif} is inversely dependent on $\bar{g}_{K-AHP}$ indicating that a smaller value of $\bar{g}_{K-AHP}$ would allow q_{bif} to be larger. Figure 5.3 shows this situation. Here we show burst trajectories projected onto the $v_s - n$ and $v_d - q$ phase planes for $\bar{g}_{K-AHP} = 0.8$ mS/cm^2 as in Fig. 5.1 and for $\bar{g}_{K-AHP} = 0.6$ mS/cm^2. The time traces of the soma and dendrite voltages for the lower value of $\bar{g}_{K-AHP}$ are almost identical to those of Fig. 5.1, but now the

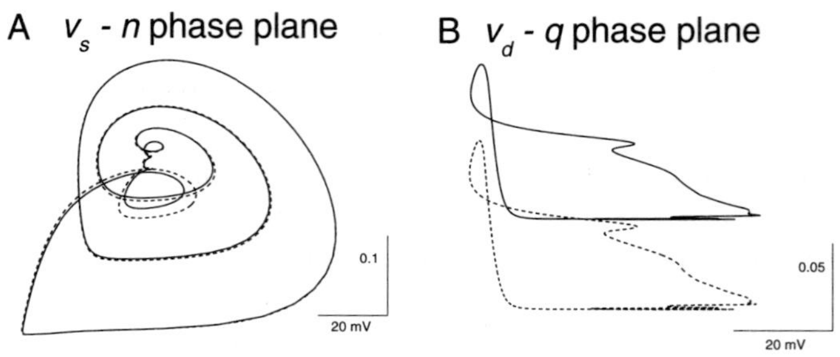

Fig. 5.3. Burst trajectories in the $v_s - n$ (A) and $v_d - q$ (B) phase planes for $\bar{g}_{K-AHP} =$ 0.8 mS/cm^2 (dashed curve, default value) and 0.6 mS/cm^2 (solid curve).

value $q_{bif} = 0.207$ at burst initiation. Lower $\bar{g}_{K-AHP}$ also increases burst frequency because not as much $I_{K-AHP} = \bar{g}_{K-AHP}q[v_d - E_K]$ is activated and it has less of a hyperpolarizing effect on the v_d trajectory. As a result, v_d only spends a small amount of time below $V_d^\star$ and the interburst interval is shortened. Note that independent of the value of $\bar{g}_{K-AHP}$, the burst is initiated when v_d passes through $V_d^\star$ which in this case is around -52 mv. (see Fig. 5.3).

The value of q_{bif} can be made smaller at burst initiation when dendritic inhibition is applied during the interburst interval. Suppose that a term $-I_{syn} = -\bar{g}_{syn}s_{inh}[v_d - E_{inh}]$ were added to the right side of the v_d' equation in (1), (9) or (10). s_{inh} is a synaptic gating variable which, at the moment of a pre-synaptic spike (or burst), is reset to one and then decays like $\exp(-\kappa t)$ for some decay rate κ. As described in [1], inhibition causes the v_d nullcline to shift down in $v_d - q$ phase space and the v_d trajectory to hyperpolarize. Suppose that the neuron is in its silent state, and the time $t = 0$ is defined such that $v_d(0^-) = V_d^\star$. Next suppose that at $t = -t_{inh}$, for some small positive value t_{inh}, the dendrite receives an inhibitory input. This causes the value of v_d to decrease further away from $V_d^\star$, thus delaying burst onset (see Fig. 3B of [1]). The burst will initiate at a time t_1 only after $s_{inh} = \exp(-\kappa t_1)$ becomes sufficiently small. The time t_1 is dependent on the decay rate of inhibition. During the time interval $[0, t_1]$, q continues to decay independently of v_d according to the dynamics $q' = -\alpha q$ and thus can become smaller at burst onset (see Fig. 3B of [1] where $q_{bif} = 0.138$ for the uninhibited case and $q_{bif} = 0.12$ for the inhibited case). The analytic value of q_{bif} can be determined on a case-by-case basis and depends on the precise timing of the inhibition to the dendrites.

Although q does not set the threshold for burst onset, it can play a role in determining the interburst duration. Indeed for large values of $\bar{g}_{K-AHP}$, the decay constant α of the q variable strongly affects the interburst length. When $\bar{g}_{K-AHP}$ is too small, the v_d trajectory is barely pushed below $V_d^\star$, so the parameter α is less important in setting the interburst duration.

5.3.2. *Somatic-dendritic ping-pong*

One way to quantify ping-pong is to measure how the somatic firing pattern changes as the result of back-propagating spikes. In and of itself, the existence of the dendritic compartment is not sufficient to substantially change the somatic firing pattern. Rather an appropriate balance of the strength and timing of interactions of these two compartments is needed. Here we will be interested in a few different questions. What are some necessary conditions for ping-pong to exist? When does ping-pong fail to exist? When ping-pong occurs, how is the somatic burst profile modulated?

A ping-pong burst generically refers to the ability of back-propagating spikes from the soma to exploit active properties of the dendritic compartment and thereby depolarize it. The depolarization of the dendrites subsequently causes depolarizing current to be re-injected to the soma and the process is given the chance to repeat. If it does, the soma and dendrite alternately depolarize one another a number of times before either outward current puts an end to the match or I_{coup} becomes too small.

Because of the electrotonic coupling between soma and dendrite, activity in one of the compartments instantly affects the other. Therefore ping-pong very much depends on the rates at which the individual compartments depolarize and hyperpolarize. Consider the parameters associated with the somatic compartment to be fixed. At the burst onset, the soma exhibits a sodium spike that then depolarizes the dendrite. The soma spike decays quickly. If the dendrite repolarizes too quickly, then it cannot return depolarization to the soma. Alternatively, if the dendrite does not repolarize quickly enough, then it can keep the soma depolarized too long, potentially overdriving the somatic spike generator. For ping-pong to occur, one compartment must be in a position in phase space to depolarize the other, and the other compartment must be in a position in phase space to be able to respond to the depolarizing current.

We now derive a necessary condition for the cycle-by-cycle existence of ping-pong. Suppose the soma has spiked at time $t = 0$ and is now repolarizing, i.e. $v_s' < 0$. In order for the soma to depolarize again, there must exist a value $\hat{v}_1 > V_s^\star$ and a time t_1 such that $v_s(t_1) = \hat{v}_1$, $v_s'(t_1) = 0$ and $v_s''(t_1) > 0$. Using equation (5), we find that a necessary condition for ping-pong is $F(\hat{v}_1, n(t_1), 1) - g_{coup}[\hat{v}_1 - v_d(t_1)] \geq 0$ or

$$v_d(t_1) \geq \hat{v}_1 - \frac{F(\hat{v}_1, n(t_1), 1)}{g_{coup}}. \tag{14}$$

If, at a later time, the dendrite is repolarizing ($v_d' < 0$) then a necessary condition for ping-pong to continue is for there to exist $\hat{v}_2 > V_d^\star$ and a time t_2 such that $v_d(t_2) = \hat{v}_2$, $v_d'(t_2) = 0$ and $v_d''(t_2) > 0$. Again using (5), this translates to

$$v_s(t_2) \geq \hat{v}_2 - \frac{f(\hat{v}_2, q, Ca, s, c)|_{t=t_2}}{g_{coup}}. \tag{15}$$

A finite sequence of such values $(\hat{v}_i, t_i)$ can be generated. Each entry in the sequence would indicate the continuation of ping-pong for another cycle.

Equations (14) and (15) are instructive in several ways. First, they show that if g_{coup} is too small, then ping-pong is unlikely to occur. Note $F(\hat{v}_1, n(t_1), 1)$ and $f(\hat{v}_2, q, Ca, s, c)|_{t=t_2}$ are both negative implying that for small g_{coup}, $v_s(t_1)$ and $v_d(t_2)$, which are bounded from above, would need to be very large. Second, if g_{coup} is too large, then equations (14) and (15) cannot be satisfied. A large value of g_{coup} tends to make the v_s and v_d trajectories lie close together both in phase space and in time, thereby making $v_s - v_d$ small for any time t. Finally, although equations (14) and (15) do not pinpoint the values of $\hat{v}_1$ and $\hat{v}_2$ nor the times t_1 and t_2, together they provide some insights into the rates of de- and repolarization of the soma and dendrite needed to sustain ping-pong. For example, if equation (14) is satisfied, then for equation (15) to hold, the dendrite compartment cannot hyperpolarize too quickly, while the soma must depolarize sufficiently fast. Thus when applied current to either or both of the compartments is too large, thereby increasing these rates, ping-pong will fail to exist.

These ideas can be illustrated by varying the activation rate of the dendritic inward current I_{Ca}. This is controlled by the gating variable s and its associated time constant τ_s. In Fig. 5.4, we show two separate simulations in which we have changed τ_s to 10 (A) and 0.1 (B) msec^{-1}. In both cases, ping-pong fails. In the former (A), it fails because the activation rate is very slow and I_{Ca} is hardly activated. The dendrite is not depolarized beyond its response to the coupling current which deactivates very quickly. Thus the dendritic compartment repolarizes too quickly. The interburst length, approximately 30 msec, is still controlled by q, but q does not build up much.

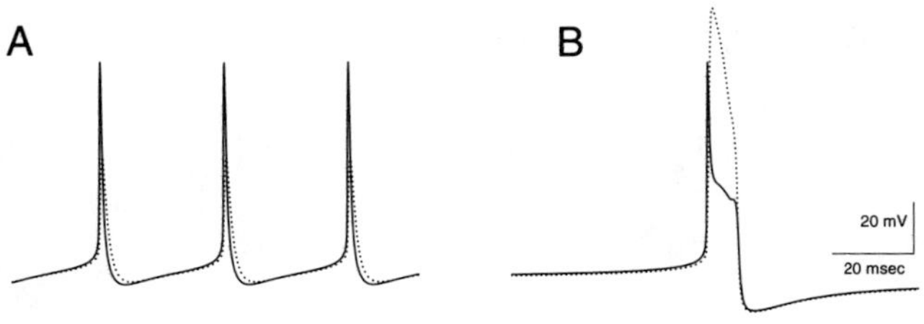

Fig. 5.4. Failure of ping-pong bursting in the modified PR model. A: Activation time constant τ_s for dendritic inward calcium current is increased to 10 msec^{-1} and dendrite repolarizes too quickly for ping-pong to occur. B: τ_s is decreased to 0.1 msec^{-1} and large dendritic spike is immediately initiated that overdrives soma. The dendrite remains depolarized too long to initiate ping-pong.

As a result, v_d spends little time below $V_d^\star$ and the frequency is relatively high. In the latter case (B), the calcium current activates very quickly and causes the v_d trajectory to stay in the active state for a relatively long time. This, in turn, drives the v_s trajectory far above its spiking threshold. When the v_d trajectory ultimately repolarizes due to I_{K-C}, the v_s trajectory does so nearly simultaneously as well. Thus neither compartment is in a position to depolarize the other and ping-pong fails. Here q builds up quite a bit, so the interburst length, approximately 512 msec, is comparable to that of the complex burst.

In both of the above cases, ping-pong fails because one of the two compartments completely dominates the activity of the other. In the former (Fig. 5.4(A)), the activity in the dendrites is slaved to that of the soma, and in the latter (B) the situation is reversed. This suggests that in order for ping-pong to work a proper balance in strength and timing of interaction between compartments needs to exist. Variations in this balance can lead to variations in the ping-pong pattern in which one compartment may have the upper hand during all or part of the burst.

In the PR complex burst (Fig. 5.1), the burst starts out with a true ping-pong between soma and dendrite. The initial somatic spike depolarizes the dendrite and partially activates I_{Ca} so that dendritic depolarization induces another soma spike. After the second spike, however, I_{Ca} activates more fully and the dendrite starts to dominate. The partial Ca^{2+} spike drives the soma into spike block, but as the dendrite repolarizes the soma is in a

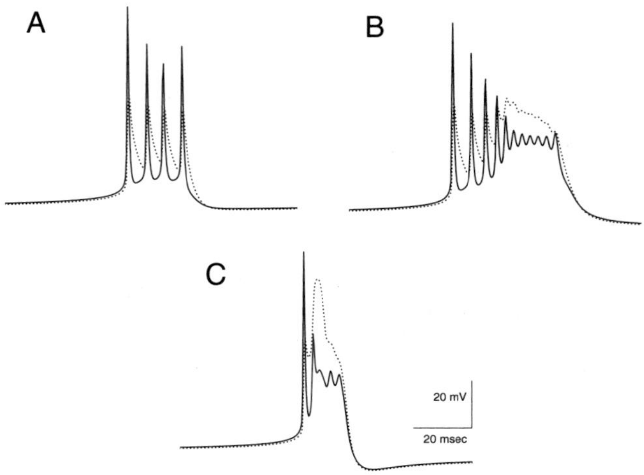

Fig. 5.5. Variations of ping-pong bursting in the modified PR model obtained by varying activation rates of dendritic calcium I_{Ca} and voltage-activated potassium I_{K-C}. Activation time constant τ_s of I_{Ca} set to 2.55 (A), 2.535 (B) and 2 (C) msec^{-1}. Parameter τ_{cc} of activation time constant $\tau_c(v_d)$ for I_{K-C} set to 0.8 (A),(B) and 3 (C) msec^{-1}.

position to rejoin the game with a final small spike.

Keeping the soma parameters fixed, we can obtain variations on the ping-pong pattern by varying the activation time constants of I_{Ca} and I_{K-C}. For example, by slowing down the activation of the calcium current ($\tau_s = 2.55$ msec^{-1}) and speeding up the activation of I_{K-C} ($\tau_{cc} = 0.8$ msec^{-1}), true ping-pong bursting is obtained (Fig. 5.5(A)). In this case, the soma and dendrite alternately depolarize one another over four spikes. The interburst interval, approximately 165 msec, is shorter than in complex bursting since the low average dendritic depolarization doesn't allow much Ca^{2+} and, hence, q accumulation.

When the calcium activation rate is increased back to the same value as for complex bursting ($\tau_s = 2.535$) $\text{msec}^{-1}$and the I_{K-C} rate remains high ($\tau_{cc} = 0.8$ msec^{-1}), the soma and dendrite ping-pong over the first three spikes of the burst (Fig. 5.5(B)). Then a partial Ca^{2+} spike is generated and the dendrite dominates the game to the end of the burst. Here, the interburst interval, approximately 713 msec, is longer than in the basic complex burst because of the longer active state of the burst.

A dendrite-dominated burst occurs when the I_{Ca} activation rate is increased further ($\tau_s = 2$) and the I_{K-C} activation rate is decreased ($\tau_{cc} = 3$ msec^{-1}) (Fig. 5.5(C)). A larger Ca^{2+} spike is initiated immediately following the leading soma spike and it drives all further somatic activity. The interburst interval is long, approximately 689 msec, because the large Ca^{2+} spike increases Ca^{2+} and q accumulation.

Dendritic depolarization can also be modulated by external sources such as synaptic inhibition. In [1] (Fig. 6), we showed how different strengths of GABA-A mediated inhibition arriving at the dendrites just after burst initiation produces different types of firing patterns as well as different frequency bursting. Inhibition of moderate strength creates a balance between soma and dendrite which can allow ping-pong to exist over several cycles. Strong dendritic inhibition yields results similar to when $\tau_s = 10$ (Fig. 5.4(A)). Thus the effect of dendritic inhibition is very similar to the effect of changing the time constant τ_s for calcium influx.

5.4. Morris-Lecar Two-Compartment Models

Ping-pong bursting can be studied more easily using a two-compartment model cell where each compartment is governed by the Morris-Lecar equations [13]. The equations of interest are:

$$\begin{aligned}
cv_s' &= I_s - g_{Ca}m_\infty(v_s)[v_s - E_{Ca}] - g_k w_s[v_s - E_K] \\
&\quad -g_l[v_s - E_L] - g_{coup}[v_s - v_d] \\
w_s' &= \phi[w_{s_\infty}(v_s) - w_s]/\tau_{w_s}(v_s) \\
cv_d' &= I_d - g_{Ca}m_\infty(v_d)[v_d - E_{Ca}] - g_k w_d[v_d - E_K] \\
&\quad -g_l[v_d - E_L] - g_{coup}[v_d - v_s] \\
w_d' &= \phi[w_{d_\infty}(v_d) - w_d]/\tau_{w_d}(v_d),
\end{aligned} \tag{16}$$

where $c = 20$, $g_{Ca} = 4$, $g_k = 8$, $g_l = 2$, $E_{Ca} = 120$, $E_K = -84$, $E_L = -60$, $I_s = 40$, $I_d = 42$ and $\phi = 0.23$. The functions $m_\infty(v) = (1 + \tanh((v - v_1)/v_2))/2$, $w_{s_\infty}(v_s) = (1+\tanh((v_s - v_3)/v_4))/2$, $w_{d_\infty}(v_d) = (1+\tanh((v_d - v_5)/v_6))/2$, $\tau_{w_s}(v_s) = \tau_{lo,w_s} + [\tau_{hi,w_s} - \tau_{lo,w_s}]t_\infty(v_s)$, $\tau_{w_d}(v_d) = \tau_{lo,w_d} + [\tau_{hi,w_d} - \tau_{lo,w_d}]t_\infty(v_d)$ and $t_\infty(v) = (1 + \tanh((v - v7)/v8))/2$, where $v_1 = -1.2$, $v_2 = 18$, $v_3 = 12$, $v_4 = 17.4$, $v_5 = -8$, $v_6 = 10$, $v_7 = 12$ $v_8 = 17.4$, $\tau_{lo,w_s} = 30$, $\tau_{hi,w_s} = 10$, $\tau_{lo,w_d} = 100$ and $\tau_{hi,w_d} = 1000$.

For this set of parameters, when the compartments are isolated, $g_{coup} = 0$, the soma compartment fires single spikes with period 1907 units (Fig. 5.6(A)) and the dendrite compartment fires wide spikes with period 3355 (Fig. 5.6(B)). With sufficiently large g_{coup}, bursting is obtained and

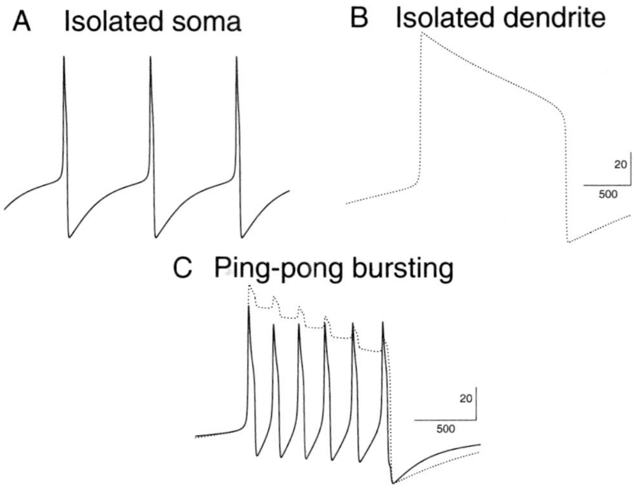

Fig. 5.6. Ping-pong bursting in the two-compartment Morris-Lecar model. Spiking trajectories in the soma (A) and dendrite (B) compartments when the compartments are uncoupled. Moderate strength coupling ($g_{coup} = 1$) results in ping-pong bursting (C, solid curve: somatic voltage, dotted curve: dendritic voltage).

the burst is initiated when the v_s- and w_s-nullclines are tangent, thereby causing a saddle-node bifurcation as in the PR model. When $g_{coup} = 1$, the soma fires a burst of spikes as a result of its interaction with the dendrite compartment. The burst is initiated by a somatic spike that then activates the dendritic spike. The dendrite dominates the ping-pong dynamics, driving the subsequent somatic spikes. Here, the dendritic depolarization does not drive the soma into spike block, as can occur in the PR model. The burst width is shorter than the isolated dendritic spike since the repolarization of each somatic spike acts to slightly repolarize dendritic voltage. The burst period is 2906 units which is shorter than the isolated dendrite period, but longer than the isolated soma period. This makes sense since the burst is now being initiated by the soma trajectory as it passes through the saddle-node bifurcation as v_d passes through the threshold value $V_d^\star$. Here $V_d^\star$ is less than the value at which the isolated dendrite compartment would have become active. When $g_{coup} = 0.05$, the coupling is too weak for the dendrite to drive a burst of somatic spikes. With $g_{coup} = 10$, the coupling is too strong and both compartments have large burst envelopes,

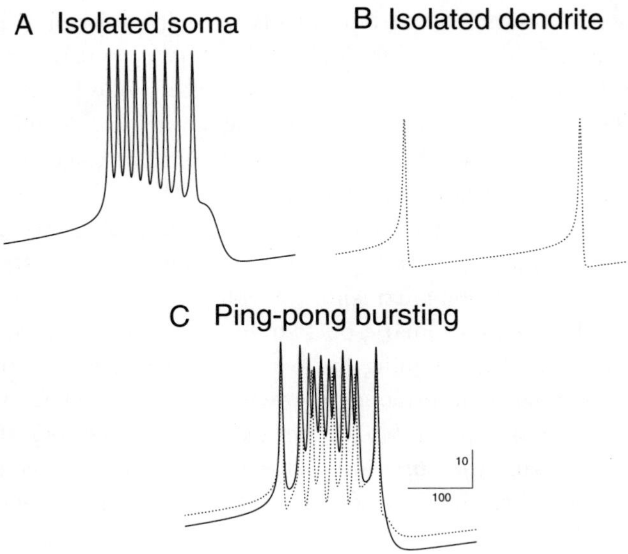

Fig. 5.7. Another example of ping-pong bursting in the two-compartment Morris-Lecar model. Isolated soma compartment displays bursting (A) and isolated dendrite repetitively spikes (B). Ping-pong bursting is obtained with moderate strength coupling $g_{coup} = 0.7$ (C, solid curve: somatic voltage, dotted curve: dendritic voltage).

but no spiking behavior (simulations not shown). The advantage of using this simplified system is that it is easy to identify which parameters affect different parts of the burst oscillation. For example, τ_{lo,w_d} and τ_{hi,w_d} control the interburst duration and burst width, respectively.

Another example of ping-pong bursting can be obtained in the Morris-Lecar two-compartment model (see Fig. 5.7) if we modify the above equations using a trick found in chapter 7.5 of Ermentrout's XPP book [5]. He shows that when the applied current of the basic Morris-Lecar equations satisfies a certain differential equation, the resulting solution exhibits a typical bursting pattern. We modified the above equations (16) to make I_s and I_d obey the following differential equation:

$$I'_x = \epsilon[v_0 - v_x], \quad x = s, d, \tag{17}$$

with $v_0 = -26$ and $\epsilon = 0.001$. We also replaced the expressions for τ_{w_s} and τ_{w_d} with a common $\tau(v) = 1/\cosh((v - v_7)/(2v_8))$ where $v_7 = 12$ and

$v_8 = 17.4$, and changed the parameters $v_5 = 7$, $v_6 = 17.4$. With these parameters, when the compartments are isolated, $g_{coup} = 0$, the soma compartment exhibits typical bursting (Fig. 5.7(A)), while the dendrite compartment fires tonically (Fig. 5.7(B)). With $g_{coup} = 0.7$, bursting is obtained and the burst is initiated through a saddle-node bifurcation of the soma compartment. The compartments engage in ping-pong, alternately depolarizing one another (Fig. 5.7(C)). The solution is not exactly periodic, but the basic phenomenon is consistent with what is seen in the PR model. The burst in this case ends at a homoclinic bifurcation when the average somatic and dendritic voltages dip below v_0. With stronger coupling, $g_{coup} = 10$, the compartments tonically spike at a frequency higher than that of the isolated somatic burst frequency. With $g_{coup} = 0.01$, there is no ping-pong as the coupling current is too weak. For certain choices of parameters, ping-pong prolongs the length of the burst far beyond the homoclinic bifurcation point. This is because the average somatic and dendritic voltages during the burst are higher in the presence of coupling than without. Interested readers can see Fig. 7.9 of [5] for further elaboration.

5.5. Discussion

The Pinsky-Rinzel two-compartment model of a CA3 pyramidal cell has attracted wide interest in the neuroscience community. In part, this is due to its success in duplicating and explaining the dynamics of the larger 19-compartment model developed by Traub *et al.* [19]. Another reason is that it was one of the first models to show how active properties of the dendrites can affect the dynamics of the soma through the phenomenon of back-propagation of action potentials.

The PR model, and slight variations of it, have been used to address the dynamics of neocortical chattering neurons [23], the effect of different dendritic morphology on firing patterns [11], bistability in hippocampal pyramidal cell networks [7], rate, temporal and calcium coding [1, 22], and patterns of burst synchrony [2]. Despite its wide usage, the PR model has been analyzed in limited cases [1, 8] and has not been the subject of a rigorous mathematical treatment. In this chapter, we have begun the work of placing the PR model in a mathematical/geometrical framework suitable for analysis. By focusing on burst initiation and the effects of back-propagation, we have provided some circumstances where the full PR equations (1) can be replaced by lower dimensional reduced equations for, at least, part of the cell's trajectory. In turn, this has allowed us to understand the mechanisms that are responsible for certain observed behaviors of the model. It also has allowed us to use this understanding to construct simpler models that exhibit effects of back propagation, but are much more transparent than the PR model.

With respect to burst initiation, we showed how changes in the coupling strength I_{coup} induce a saddle-node bifurcation in the fast v_s-n subsystem. This observation allowed us to understand through the reduced equations (10) how the length of the interburst is determined. Moreover, the analysis reveals that in any conductance-based two-compartment model, the strength of I_{coup} can affect the existence of fixed points in the silent state as well as the manner in which they disappear. For example, the phenomenon of ghost bursting, described by Doiron *et al.* [4, 10] (and see also chapter 6 of this book), can be understood in the context of our analysis. Tonic firing in that model arises through a saddle-node bifurcation of fixed points as applied current I_s to the soma compartment increases through a value called I_{s_1}. For $I_s < I_{s_1}$, from our point of view, this means that the v_s and v_d trajectories are trapped at a fixed point, $(\bar{v}_s, \bar{v}_d)$ for which $\bar{v}_d < V_d^\star$. As I_s increases, $\bar{v}_d$ increases (due to current flow through the gap junction) while $V_d^\star$ decreases (a smaller value of v_d is needed to create the bifurcation since I_s is larger), until at I_{s_1}, $\bar{v}_d(I_{s_1}) = V_d^\star(I_{s_1})$. Thus when oscillations arise for I_s slightly larger than I_{s_1}, the fixed point $\bar{v}_d$ is only slightly larger in value than $V_d^\star$. Thus the time it takes for the v_d trajectory to cross $V_d^\star$ can become arbitrarily large since it is passing near a "ghost" of a fixed point. Thus the burst frequency can become arbitrarily small. This is what Doiron *et al.* describe as "reinjection near the ghost of a saddle-node point". The transition in their model from tonic firing to more complicated firing at $I_s = I_{s_2}$ appears to reflect the fact that the rates of de- and hyperpolarization of the soma compartment depend on I_s. For $I_s < I_{s_2}$, back propagation fails to affect somatic spiking and thus the solution is a period 1 orbit (tonic firing). For $I_s > I_{s_2}$, back propagation has an effect on the soma trajectory, affecting where it resides in phase space, making the solution quasiperiodic. For larger values of I_s the solution again becomes tonic spiking, which is consistent with what we find using equations (14)-(15).

In general, we can relate the onset of oscillations arising through a saddle-node bifurcation as a result of a change in applied current to our work by understanding what affects $V_d^\star$ and what causes v_d to increase through this value. Alternatively, if the applied current in a model is fixed such that oscillations exist, one finds that the burst is initiated as I_{coup} changes strength. When the voltage of one compartment is stuck near a fixed point, I_{coup} acts like an applied current to that compartment. Increases in I_{coup} due to increases in the other compartment's voltage can then have the effect of causing a bifurcation in the number of fixed points in the other compartment.

Our analysis also suggests a few necessary conditions for back-propagation to have an effect on the firing dynamics of the soma. First, in the active state of the neurons, the amplitude of coupling current I_{coup} must be sufficiently large. Thus compartments that are nearly homogeneous are unlikely to display ping-pong. Homogeneity can be achieved either by assigning similar intrinsic properties to each compartment, or by making g_{coup} large which would have the effect of making $|v_s - v_d|$ small. Compartments that are weakly coupled (g_{coup} small) are also not likely to display ping-pong. A second condition that appears to be necessary for these effects is that one of the compartments contains a depolarizing current which decays on a slower time scale in the active state. This property gives ping-pong the chance to begin. In the PR neuron, this role is played by the calcium current in the dendrites. The third condition, and the hardest to quantify, is that the rates of depolarization and hyperpolarization of the two compartments need to be properly balanced. These rates are affected not only by intrinsic properties of the compartments, but also by the coupling conductance g_{coup} and potential external synaptic inputs. Thus when I_s or I_d is too large, ping-pong is not likely since the rates of de- and hyperpolarization are too large. In another example, in the standard PR model, the reversal potential of potassium is chosen to be $E_K = -75$ mV. With this value, and $\tau_s = 2.535$, the model exhibits a complex burst. If E_K is lowered to -84 mV, bursting gives way to tonic spiking. The lower reversal potential of potassium increases the rate of hyperpolarization of the soma and dendrite, negating the effect of back-propagation. By understanding this basic concept, it is straightforward to restore the complex burst, and there are many different ways to do so. For example, changing the reversal potential of calcium from 80 to 112 mV yields ping-pong bursting with 3-spike bursts and a slightly higher increase ($E_{Ca} = 112.5$ mV) recovers the complex burst, even with $E_K = -84$ mV. In these cases, the dendrite does not hyperpolarize as quickly, and can initiate ping-pong. See also the work of Hahn and Durand [7] who discuss other effects of changing E_K in the PR model.

In this chapter, we have laid the geometric groundwork to allow for further analysis of two-compartment neuron models. There are many open problems to be considered. While we have provided some necessary conditions for the existence of ping-pong, we are still far from analytically describing the phenomenon. Providing sufficient conditions, together with a geometric description of its existence, remains an open and challenging problem. Another open problem is to understand burst initiation in circumstances where the dynamics of the soma compartment in the silent state are not so fast. In this case, the slow manifolds associated with the silent state of each of the compartments will both be two-dimensional and the simple condition $v_d = V_d^\star$ for burst initiation would need to be replaced with $v_d = V_d^\star(v_s)$. Analysis of multi-compartment models connected by synaptic excitation or inhibition is also needed. For example in a network of PR neurons coupled by excitation, the perfectly synchronous burst solution is unstable. An analytic proof of such for a one-compartment Morris-Lecar type neuron exists [3], where a nearly synchronous solution is shown to be stable. A proof for the full or modified PR equations would be welcome.

Acknowledgments

This work was supported, in part, by the National Science Foundation (DMS - 0315862 (AB, VB) and ADVANCE DBI - 0340687 (VB)).

References

[1] V. Booth and A. Bose, Neural mechanisms for generating rate and temporal codes in model CA3 pyramidal cells, *J. Neurophysiol.* **85**, 2432–2445, (2001).

[2] V. Booth and A. Bose, Burst synchrony patterns in hippocampal pyramidal cell model networks, *Network: Comput. Neur. Syst.* **13**, 157–177, (2002).

[3] A. Bose, N. Kopell, and D. Terman, Almost-synchronous solutions for mutually coupled excitatory neurons, *Physica D* **140**, 69–94, (2000).

[4] B. Doiron, C. Laing, A. Longtin, and L. Maler, Ghostbursting: A novel burst mechanism, *J. Comput. Neurosci.* **12**, 5–15, (2002).

[5] G. B. Ermentrout, Simulating, Analyzing and Animating Dynamical Systems: A Guide to XPPAUT for Researchers and Students, Philadelphia: SIAM (2002)

[6] R. FitzHugh, Impulses and physiological states in theoretical models of nerve membranes, *Biophys. J.* **1**, 445–466, (1961).

[7] P. Hahn and D. Durand, Bistability dynamics in simulations of neural activity in high-extracellular-potassium conditions, *J. Comput. Neurosci.* **11**, 5–18, (2001).

[8] A. Kepecs and X. J. Wang, Analysis of complex bursting in cortical pyramidal neuron models, *Neurocomput.* **32**, 181–187, (2000).

[9] C. Laing and A. Longtin, A two-variable model of somatic-dendritic interactions in a bursting neuron, *Bull. Math. Bio.* **64**, 829–860, (2002).

[10] C. Laing, B. Doiron, A. Longtin, L. Noonan, R. Taylor, and L. Maler, Type I burst excitability, *J. Comput. Neurosci.* **14**, 329–342, (2003).

[11] Z. Mainen and T. Sejnowski, Influence of dendritic structure on firing pattern in model neocortical neurons, *Nature* **382**, 363–366, (1996).

[12] E. Mishchenko and N. Rozov, Differential Equations with Small Parameters and Relaxation Oscillators, New York: Plenum Press (1980).

[13] C. Morris and H. Lecar, Voltage oscillations in the barnacle giant muscle fiber, *Biophys. J.* **35**, 193–213, (1981).

[14] F. Nadim, Y. Manor, M. Nusbaum, and E. Marder, Frequency Regulation of a Slow Rhythm by a Fast Periodic Input, *J. Neurosci.* **18**, 5053–5067, (1998).

[15] J. Nagumo, S. Arimoto, and S. Yoshizawa, An active impulse transmission line simulating nerve axons, *Proc. IRL* **50**, 2061–2070, (1960).

[16] P. Pinsky and J. Rinzel, Intrinsic and network rhythmogenesis in a reduced Traub model of CA3 neurons, *J. Comput. Neurosci.* **1**, 39–60, (1994).

[17] W. Rall, Core conductor theory and cable properties in neurons, In: Handbook of Physiology **1**, 39-97, American Physiological Society, Bethesda, MD. (1977)

[18] J. Rinzel and G. B. Ermentrout, Analysis of neural excitability and oscillations, In: C. Koch, I Segev eds. Methods in Neuronal Modeling, MIT Press, Cambridge, MA 251-291 (1989).

[19] R. Traub, R. Wong, R. Miles, and H. Michelson, A model of a CA-3 hippocampal pyramidal neuron incorporating voltage-clamp data on intrinsic conductances, *J. Neurophsyiol.* **66**, 635–649, (1991).

[20] C. van Vanvreeswijk, L. Abbott, and G. Ermentrout, When inhibition, not excitation synchronizes neural firing *J. Comput. Neurosci.* **1**, 313–321, (1994).

[21] G. Wallenstein and M. Hasselmo, Gabaergic modulation of hippocampal population activity: Sequence learning, place field development, and the phase precession effect, *J. Neurophsyiol.* **78**, 393–408, (1997).

[22] X. J. Wang, Calcium coding and adaptive temporal computation in cortical pyramidal neurons, *J. Neurophysiol.* **79**, 1549–1566, (1998).

[23] X. J. Wang, Fast bursting and short-term synaptic plasticity: a model of neocortical chattering neurons, *Neurosci.* **89**, 347–362, (1999).

CHAPTER 6

GHOSTBURSTING: THE ROLE OF ACTIVE DENDRITES IN ELECTROSENSORY PROCESSING

Carlo R. Laing

Institute of Information and Mathematical Sciences, Massey University, Private Bag 102-904 NSMC, Auckland, New Zealand
e-mail: c.r.laing@massey.ac.nz

Brent Doiron

Department of Physics, University of Ottawa, 150 Louis Pasteur, Ottawa, ON, Canada, K1N 6N5
e-mail: bdoiron@cns.nyu.edu[a]

We give an overview of "ghostbursting", a novel type of bursting observed in sensory processing neurons of weakly electric fish. We discuss the steps taken to understand the bursting mechanism, including experimental manipulations and the development of multi-compartmental and minimal neuron models. Using dynamical systems theory, we emphasise the main differences between this type of bursting and other previous models. We finally review results showing how electrosensory neurons can process different components of dynamic stimuli in parallel with both bursts and isolated spikes.

6.1. Introduction

Weakly electric fish are nocturnal fresh water animals that thrive in South America and Africa. Over 60 million years they have developed a unique sensory modality — an electrosense. These fish have an electric organ that generates a weak, quasi-sinusoidal electric field. Prey, the fish's environment, and even communication calls from con-specifics modulate the amplitude of this field. The electrosensory system of the fish detects and processes

[a]Current address: Center for Neural Science, 4 Washington Place, New York, NY 10003.

these modulations to give a neural reconstruction of their environment [17]. The ability to use naturalistic dynamic inputs, and the existence of well-charted neural feedback pathways and well-characterized single neurons, have recently made weakly electric fish a popular animal in the study of neurocomputational dynamics and processing [21, 39].

Electrosensory inputs are faithfully coded by electroreceptors that densely cover the surface of the animal's body [30]. These receptors project to a dense layer of pyramidal cells in the electrosensory lateral line lobe (ELL) of the fish brain. These cells are the principal output cells within the ELL and they are devoted to the processing of a variety of sensory inputs. The single cell dynamics of these cells exhibit a form of burst discharge termed "ghostbursting" [5, 7, 27, 38]. Bursting behaviour is found in a multitude of sensory cells [21]; however, the ELL and ghostbursting offer distinct advantages for the study of bursting and sensory coding. ELL pyramidal cells are only one synapse from the outside world — an outside world that is simply describable in terms of electric field modulations rather than complex visual or olfactory scenes. Feedback from higher brain centers is segregated and is known to contextually modulate pyramidal cell spiking behaviour [4, 6]. Finally, the burst discharge is dependent on active dendritic processes [38] which offers several methods for modulation of burst behaviour [8, 31].

In this chapter we review a host of experimental, computational, and theoretical results of ELL pyramidal cell burst discharge. We first present the core burst mechanism and relate it to experimental and computational results. Next we present several reduced mathematical descriptions of the burst mechanism occurring in ELL pyramidal cells, which are useful for gaining an understanding of the mechanism from the point of view of dynamical systems theory. A comparison between ghostbursting and more classical burst mechanisms will show that ghostbursting has some unique properties. The final section of this review outlines recent results detailing how ELL pyramidal cells use their burst mechanism to differentially code low and high frequency inputs.

6.2. Bursting Mechanism

In the early 1990s, R. W. Turner and L. Maler observed a novel form of burst discharge from ELL pyramidal cells in brain slices of the electric fish *Apteronotus leptorhynchus* [38]. These observations were of a repetitive and high frequency burst discharge in response to a constant current injection;

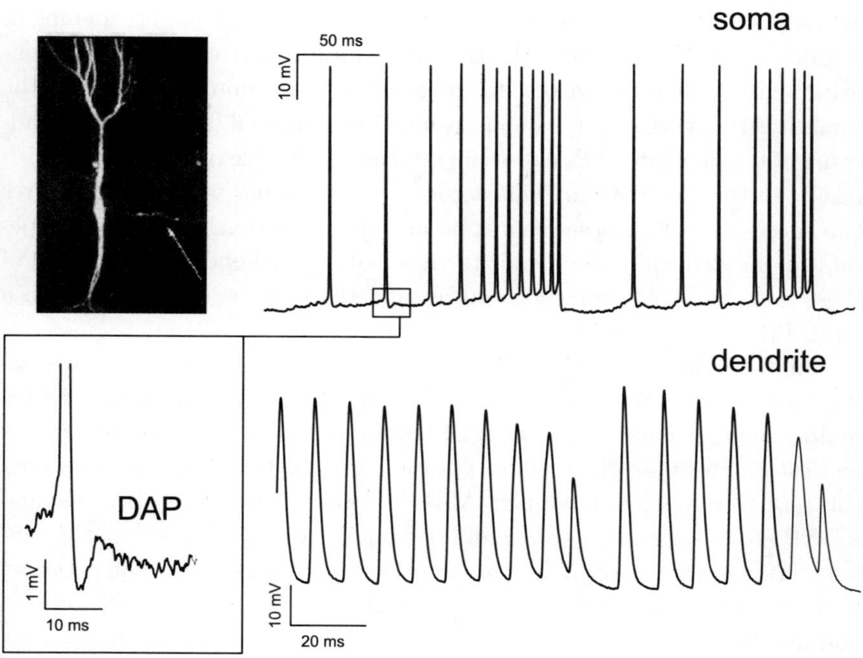

Fig. 6.1. Ghostbursting in ELL pyramidal cells. Somatic and dendritic membrane potentials recorded from an *in vitro* ELL slice preparation. A constant depolarizing input current was applied to elicit the action potential trains shown in both the somatic and dendritic spike sequences. The expanded portion of the somatic potential shows the depolarizing after-potential (DAP) that occurs shortly after a somatic action potential. The dendritic potential clearly shows the failure of action potential backpropagation after a high frequency somatic spike discharge. This dendritic failure causes a large hyperpolarization at the soma, signalling a burst termination. Note that the somatic and dendritic potentials should not be directly compared since they are recorded from different cells. Data provided by Anne-Marie Oswald. At top left is a confocal image of a Lucifer-yellow filled ELL basilar pyramidal cell.

see Fig. 6.1 for an example recording. The bursts were observed to have a monotonic increase in instantaneous frequency through the burst (i.e. the time between successive action potentials monotonically decreases during a burst). This study was also one of the first to determine that there were active sodium channels in the neuron's dendrite, and that their presence was necessary for bursting to occur. Burst mechanisms dependent on active dendritic processes are now quite familiar occurring in varied forms and in diverse systems [21, 40].

Further experimental work [27, 39] determined that the acceleration of action potentials (APs) during a burst was due to a gradual broadening of the dendritic APs. Because the somatic APs are narrower than the dendritic, current flows from the dendrite to the soma immediately after the somatic AP, giving rise to a depolarising after potential (DAP). The broadening of the dendritic APs causes an increase in the size of the DAPs, which results in the acceleration. This acceleration continues until the soma fires two successive APs whose separation in time is less than the refractory period of the dendrite. The dendrite then fails to respond to the second of these APs, the DAP does not appear, and the burst is terminated with a large after-hyperpolarization.

The experimentally-determined aspects of the bursting were successfully modelled by Doiron *et al.* [7], who constructed and studied a detailed multi-compartmental model of an ELL pyramidal cell. Using measurements and estimates of ion channel densities and parameters, these authors used this model to reproduce realistic APs, different AP refractory periods, and a DAP at the soma. However, it did not reproduce bursting without the introduction of cumulative inactivation of dendritic potassium. The necessity for this assumption will be clear once the ghostburster system is introduced and analysed.

The biophysically-based compartmental model successfully reproduced the bursting seen *in vitro* but, being very detailed, was slow to simulate. Also, it was not clear which aspects of the model were essential for bursting to occur, although it was clear that some components were necessary. Because of this, the authors developed a much simpler model [5]. This simpler model was produced by lumping all of the compartments representing the neuron's dendrite together (there were over 300 compartments representing the dendrite in the model of Doiron *et al.* [7]), and by not including ion channels whose dynamics were not thought to be essential for bursting. The result was a model comprising two compartments (the soma and the dendrite) coupled by a resistance, and described by the following six differential equations:

$$C\frac{dV_s}{dt} = I - g_{Na,s}[m_{\infty,s}(V_s)]^2(1-n_s)(V_s - V_{Na}) \\ -g_{dr,s}n_s^2(V_s - V_K) - g_L(V_s - V_L) - \frac{g_c}{\kappa}(V_s - V_d) \tag{1}$$

$$\frac{dn_s}{dt} = \frac{n_{\infty,s}(V_s) - n_s}{0.39} \tag{2}$$

$$C\frac{dV_d}{dt} = -g_{Na,d}[m_{\infty,d}(V_d)]^2 h_d(V_d - V_{Na}) - g_{dr,d}n_d^2 p_d(V_d - V_K)$$
$$-g_L(V_d - V_L) - \frac{g_c}{1-\kappa}(V_d - V_s) \quad (3)$$
$$\frac{dh_d}{dt} = h_{\infty,d}(V_d) - h_d \quad (4)$$
$$\frac{dn_d}{dt} = \frac{n_{\infty,d}(V_d) - n_d}{0.9} \quad (5)$$
$$\frac{dp_d}{dt} = \frac{p_{\infty,d}(V_d) - p_d}{\tau_p} \quad (6)$$

Subscripts s and d refer to somatic and dendritic variables, respectively. Equations (1) and (3) are current balance equations for the soma and dendrite of the neuron, respectively, and the other equations govern the ion channel dynamics. The variables m and h are activation and inactivation of Na^+, respectively, and n and p are activation and inactivation of K^+, respectively. Parameter values are $C = 1\mu F/cm^2$, $\tau_p = 5$, $g_{Na,s} = 55$, $V_{Na} = 40$, $g_{dr,s} = 20$, $V_K = -88.5$, $g_L = 0.18$, $V_L = -70$, $g_c = 1$, $\kappa = 0.4$, $g_{Na,d} = 5$, $g_{dr,d} = 15$, where voltages are measured in mV, time in ms, and conductances in mS/cm^2. I is the somatic input current, g_c is the coupling conductance, and κ is the ratio of the somatic area to the total area of the cell. Other functions are $m_{\infty,s}(V) = 1/[1 + \exp(-(V+40)/3)]$, $n_{\infty,s}(V) = 1/[1+\exp(-(V+40)/3)]$, $m_{\infty,d}(V) = 1/[1+\exp(-(V+40)/5)]$, $h_{\infty,d}(V) = 1/[1+\exp((V+52)/5)]$, $n_{\infty,d}(V) = 1/[1+\exp(-(V+40)/5)]$, $p_{\infty,d}(V) = 1/[1+\exp((V+65)/6)]$. These functions and parameter values are the same as those used in the multi-compartmental model previously discussed [7]. Note that the time constant for h_d is 1 ms, so p_d is the slowest variable by a factor of 5.

Behaviour of the ghostburster model (1)-(6) is shown in Fig. 6.2; for comparative purposes bursts from both experimental data and the large multi-compartmental model are also shown.

We will now describe the bursting in detail, referring to the model (1)-(6) and its behaviour as seen in Fig. 6.2(B). The presence of both sodium and potassium channels in the soma and the dendrite make both capable of generating action potentials and somatic DAPs as discussed above. During a burst the variable representing the cumulative inactivation of dendritic potassium, p_d, slowly decreases. This directly causes the dendritic APs to broaden, as it is associated with the flow of repolarizing potassium ions. This causes the DAPs to slowly grow in magnitude, which in turn accelerates the rate of production of APs in the soma. This acceleration occurs

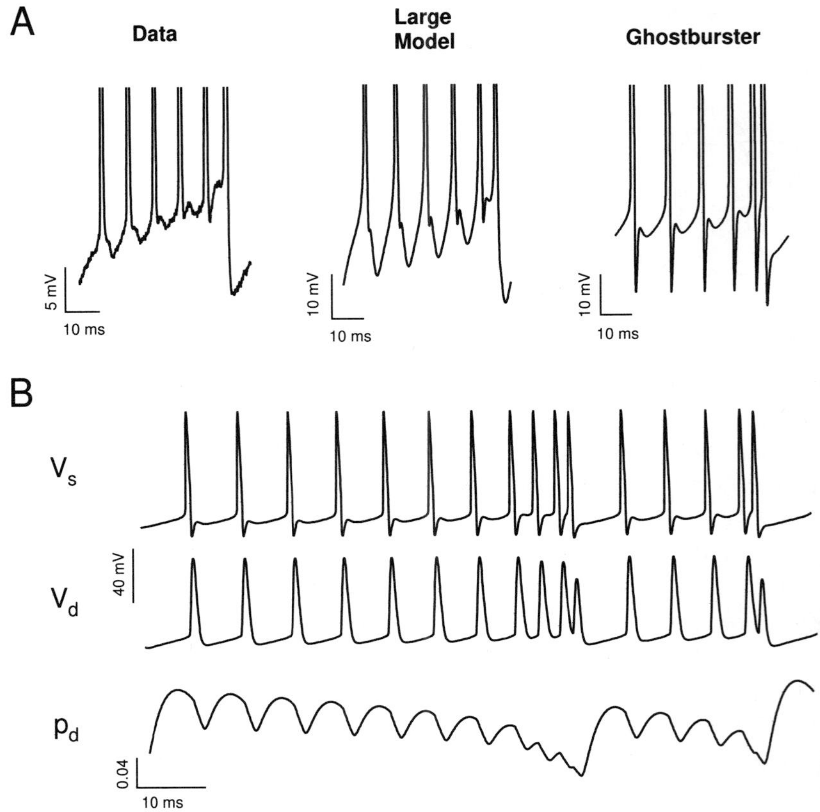

Fig. 6.2. Ghostbursting in data and models. **A.** Typical somatic bursts in experimentally-observed data (left), the large compartmental model [7] (middle), and the model (1)-(6) for $I = 9$ (right). The bursts all terminate with a fast "doublet" event. The gradual potentiation of DAPs is visible during the evolution of a burst. **B.** Simulations of (1)-(6) with $I = 9$. Top: V_s (somatic voltage). Middle: V_d (dendritic voltage). Bottom: p_d (inactivation of dendritic potassium). Note the rapid reset of p_d in between bursts.

until the soma fires two APs (a "doublet") that are so close together that the dendrite can respond to only the first of this pair, as the second occurs within the refractory period of the dendrite. This failure of the dendrite to respond to the second AP in the doublet (seen as a drop in AP amplitude in the middle panel of Fig. 6.2(B)) eliminates the current that would normally flow from the dendrite to the soma, and thus the DAP. There is then a relatively long wait until the soma fires again, of its own accord. During this gap (the "inter-burst interval") p_d recovers to its value near the start of a burst and the process starts again. While there is no direct experimental evidence for a p_d-like variable in ELL pyramidal cells, it was included in the models as the most plausible mechanism for causing the slowly broadening dendritic APs during a burst. Frequency-dependent spike broadening resulting from potassium inactivation has been shown in several invertebrate systems [1, 29].

Now that a reduced two-compartment description of ELL pyramidal cell behaviour is available, a more mathematical understanding of ELL burst discharge is possible. This will allow for a better comparison between ghostbursting and other more traditional types of bursting. This is the focus of the next section.

6.3. Ghostburster Dynamics

A bifurcation analysis of the full system (1)-(6) using the injected current I as a parameter was presented in Doiron *et al.* [5], and a similar diagram is shown in Fig. 6.3. For small enough I, the system is quiescent. As I is increased, there is a saddle-node bifurcation of fixed points on an invariant circle, leading to periodic firing. This bifurcation is seen in a number of other model neurons [10, 35]. As the current is increased further, there is a saddle-node bifurcation of limit cycles, and the system starts bursting. The bifurcation diagram suggests that for some values of I, this bursting is *chaotic* [16]. This chaotic nature was shown by Doiron *et al.* [5], where the most positive Lyapunov exponent of (1)-(6) was calculated as a function of I. Intervals of I for which this exponent was positive were found, indicating that the dynamics were chaotic. Note that the chaotic nature implies that no two bursts will be identical. This is clearly seen in Fig. 6.2(B).

A standard way of analysing bursting systems [18, 20, 35] is to notice that for many of them there is a separation of timescales, so that the system can be written

$$\frac{dx}{dt} = f(x, y) \tag{7}$$

$$\tau\frac{dy}{dt} = g(x, y) \tag{8}$$

where $1 \ll \tau$ and f and g are of similar magnitude. The analysis proceeds by treating y in (7) as a constant, and performing a bifurcation analysis of the "fast" subsystem (7) with y as the bifurcation parameter, yielding,

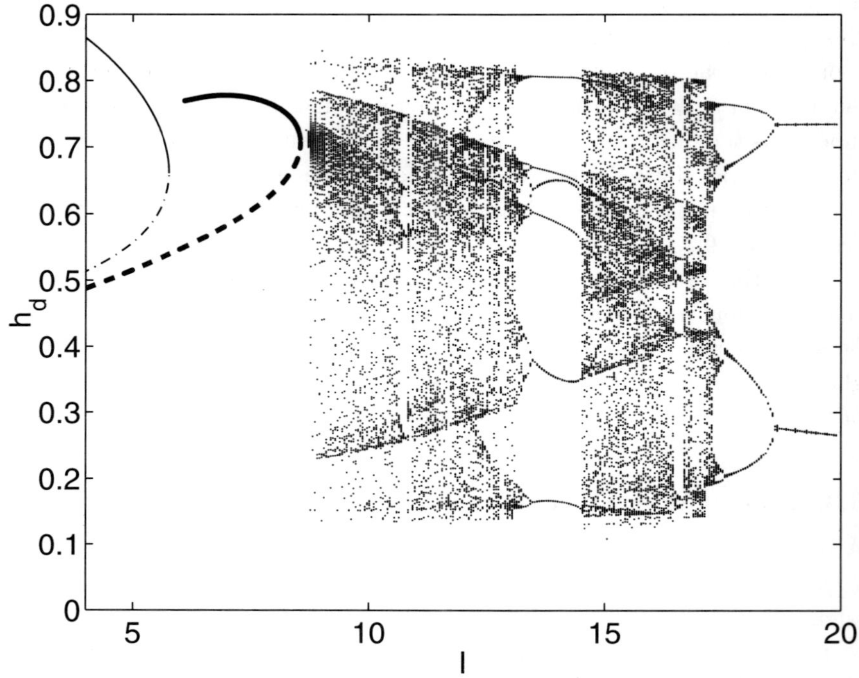

Fig. 6.3. Bifurcation diagram for (1)-(6) as a function of I. The value of h_d for the stable and unstable fixed points is shown with the thin solid and dash-dotted lines, respectively. The maximum of h_d over one period for the stable and unstable periodic orbits is shown by the thick solid and dashed lines, respectively. During bursting, the maximum values of h_d during a period of 500 ms are shown (after transients).

typically, bistability between a periodic oscillation in x and a stable steady state, over a range of values of y. Now considering the full system (7)-(8), imagine that $g(x, y)$ is such that when x is oscillating, y slowly increases (say) until it reaches a value for which there is a bifurcation destroying the periodic oscillation (for example, a homoclinic bifurcation). The system then jumps to the branch of fixed points, on which y slowly decreases (say). This continues until another bifurcation destroys the fixed point (for example, a saddle-node bifurcation of fixed points), at which point the system jumps back to the branch of periodic oscillations, and the cycle starts again. Thus the system as a whole slowly alternates between periodic firing and quiescence, i.e. it bursts [35].

Another possibility is that the fast subsystem (7) is not bistable for any value of y, but does have bifurcations of fixed points and periodic orbits. If y is at least two-dimensional, y could undergo slow oscillations that cause (7) to repeatedly cycle through regions in which there were alternately oscillations and fixed points, thus giving bursts of oscillations separated by quiescent periods [35]. By understanding the bifurcations that (7) undergoes as y is varied, qualitative aspects of the bursting can be determined. Indeed, by combining pairs of bifurcations in different ways, a large number of theoretically-possible bursters can be enumerated [18].

This type of analysis was also carried out for the system (1)-(6), even though the separation of timescales is not so clear, with p_d being the slowest variable by a factor of only 5 (see Eq. (6)). Treating p_d as a parameter, the "fast" subsystem (1)-(5) undergoes a bifurcation from periodic firing with one oscillation of V_d per period to periodic firing with two oscillations of V_d per period as p_d is decreased, as shown in Fig. 6.4. The top panel in this Figure provides a "skeleton" upon which the bursting of the full system can be superimposed.

To determine the dynamics on this skeleton, we need to know the dynamics of p_d. From (6) we see that p_d is driven by V_d only, and so the p_d nullcline (where $dp_d/dt = 0$) will be a curve in the $p_d - V_d$ plane. This is plotted in Fig. 6.5, along with the curves from the top panel of Fig. 6.4 and a single burst of the full system (1)-(6). We see that during the first part of the burst, p_d slowly decreases — this is due to the trajectory spending most of its time in the region where $dp_d/dt < 0$. The burst ends when p_d decreases below the value at which there is a bifurcation in the fast subsystem ($p_d \approx 0.102$), a fast "doublet" is fired, and V_d drops below the p_d nullcline. p_d is then reinjected to higher values, crosses the nullcline again, and another burst starts.

Finally, by choosing parameter values carefully it is possible to use the two saddle-node bifurcations shown in Fig. 6.3 to set the timescales of bursting. This effect is shown in Fig. 6.6 where the slow passage associated with both the saddle-node bifurcations of fixed points and limit cycles dictate the inter-burst and burst timescales respectively. The slow passage through a region of phase space where a saddle-node bifurcation occurs is often referred to as sensing the ghost of the bifurcation [37]; it is this effect that gives the bursting mechanism its name. (Also, the common name for the weakly electric fish *Apteronotus leptorhynchus* is the "brown *ghost* knife fish".)

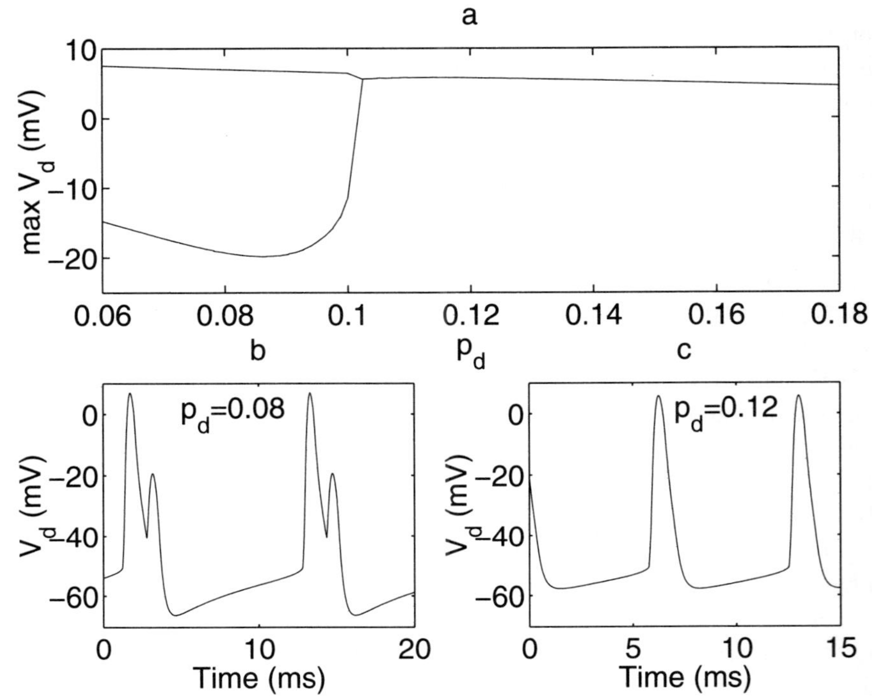

Fig. 6.4. Bifurcation analysis of the fast subsystem (1)-(5) for $I = 9$. There is a bifurcation from period-one firing to period-two firing as p_d is decreased. a: Maxima of V_d during periodic firing as a function of p_d. b: V_d as a function of time for $p_d = 0.08$. c: V_d as a function of time for $p_d = 0.12$.

6.4. Unique Features

In this section we contrast the ghostburster with other models of bursting, pointing out some unique features. As mentioned in Sec. 6.2, many bursting systems are analysed by splitting them into "fast" and "slow" subsystems [18, 35]. For many of these systems, the fast subsystem is bistable for some values of the (one-dimensional) slow variable (for example, the square-wave or elliptic bursters [20, 35]). Upon splitting the model (1)-(6) like this, with p_d as the slow variable, we do not find bistability for any value of p_d. Indeed, we do not even find stable fixed points for any relevant value of p_d, only a family of periodic orbits. In contrast, some other bursting models do not have bistability in their fast subsystem, but have a slow subspace with two or more dimensions (for example, the parabolic burster [20, 35]). The

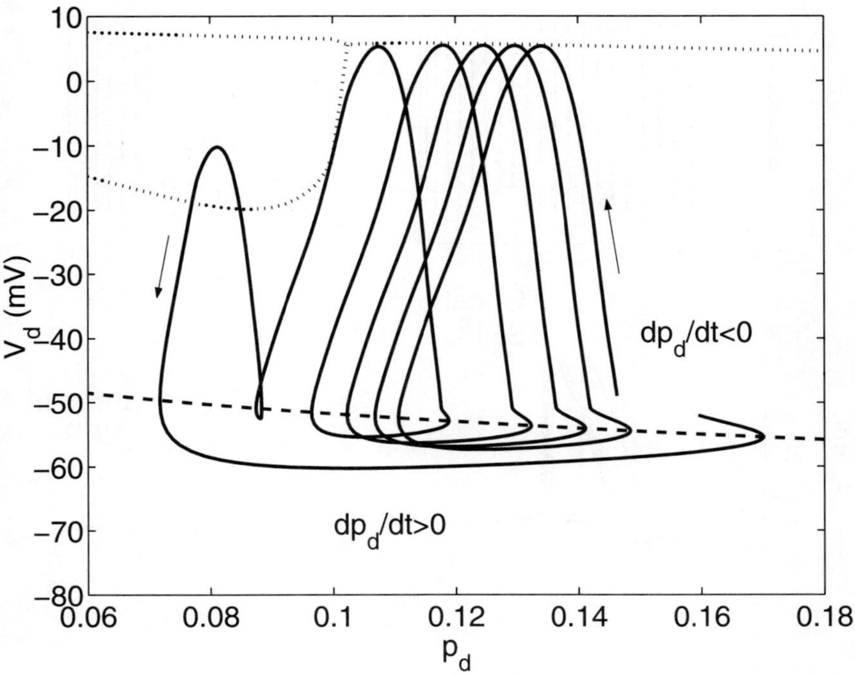

Fig. 6.5. A single burst (solid line) superimposed on the skeleton shown in the top panel of Fig. 6.4 (dotted). The p_d nullcline is shown dashed (above this, $dp_d/dt < 0$, and below it $dp_d/dt > 0$). Arrows show the direction through the burst.

ghostburster is not of this type either, as we have only one slow variable, p_d.

Another difference between the ghostburster and any other bursters of which we are aware is the presence of a period-one to period-two bifurcation in the fast subsystem (see Fig. 6.4). This transition involves a rapid change in the appearance of the periodic orbit over a small interval of p_d values, and is a result of the threshold nature of action potential (AP) production. To the right of the bifurcation in Fig. 6.4, the DAP that appears at the soma is not large enough to trigger another AP, but to the left it is, resulting in two APs in quick succession. It is this "doublet", and the failure of the dendrite to respond to the second of the APs, that allows p_d to recover and another burst to commence. The exact nature of this bifurcation has not been determined, but it may be related to the formation of a canard [15].

A further difference is in the way the system responds when the slowest timescale in the system, τ_p, is increased. For other bursters such as the

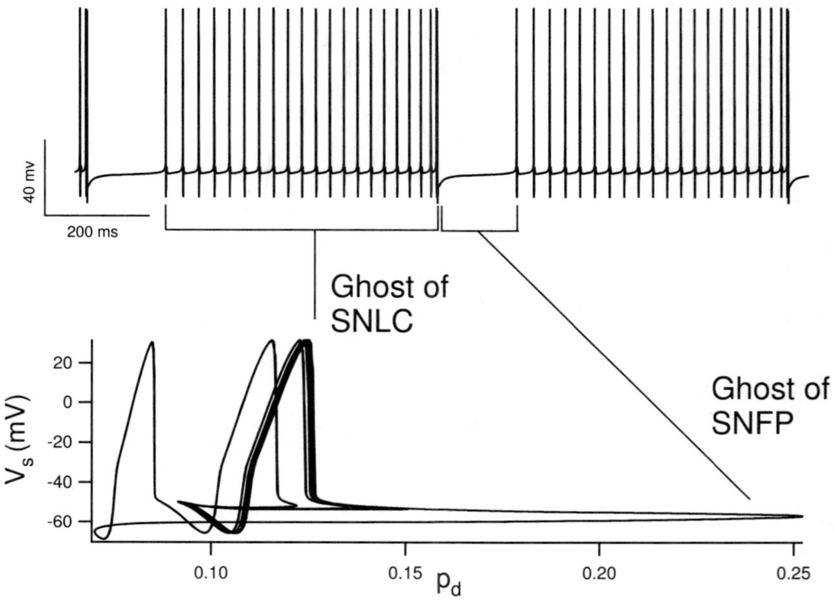

Fig. 6.6. A demonstration of the effects of the saddle-node bifurcations on the dynamics. Simulations of the system (1)-(6) with $I = 5.748$ and $g_{Dr,d} = 12.14$. These values put the system near both the saddle-node bifurcation of fixed points (SNFP) and of limit cycles (SNLC) shown in Fig. 6.3. Top: Time series of V_s; note the clear bursting pattern. Bottom: Phase trajectory as projected in the (V_s, p_d) axis. In phase space the burst discharge occurs with the slow passage through the ghost of the SNLC, where the firing is almost periodic. The inter-burst interval is determined by another slow passage, this time through the ghost of the SNFP.

square-wave, parabolic and elliptic [35], increasing the timescale of the slow process(es) leads to the durations of both the active (spiking) and quiescent phases of the bursting being increased. This continues as the slow timescale is made arbitrarily large. However, for the ghostburster there are qualitative changes as τ_p is increased. As this timescale is increased, recognisable bursts become longer, but the interburst intervals do not. Instead, between bursts there are a number of doublets that occur as p_d slowly increases to its value at the start of the burst, as shown in Fig. 6.7 (top). This is because the interburst interval is not actually caused by the fast subsystem tracking a branch of stable fixed points, as happens in many other bursters [18]. Fig. 6.7, bottom, shows the effect of further increasing I on the behaviour shown in the top panel; we have a slow modulation of dou-

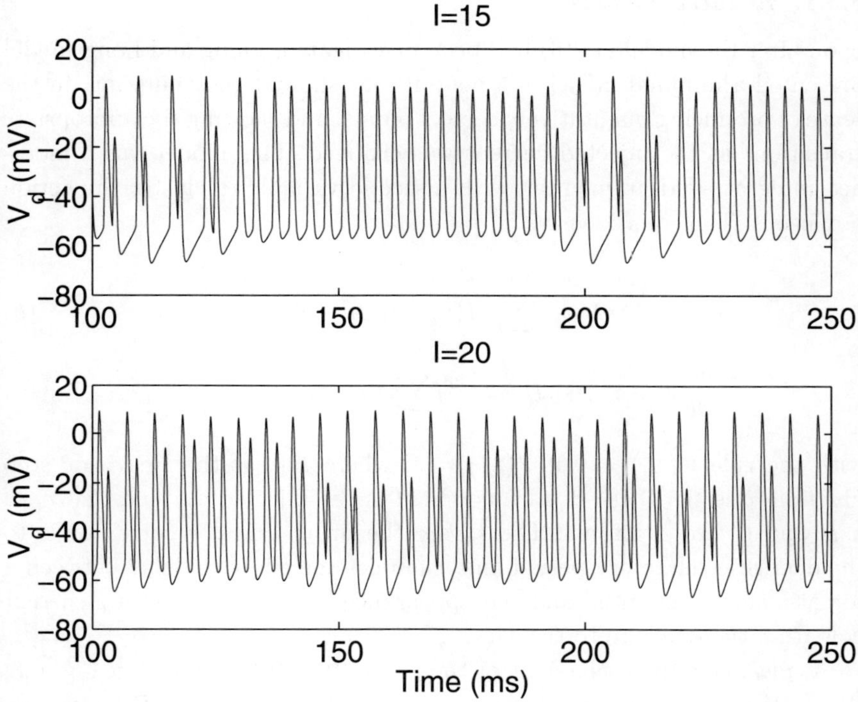

Fig. 6.7. The effects of increasing the slowest timescale, τ_p. V_d as a function of time for $\tau_p = 55$ms and $I = 15$ (top) and $I = 20$ (bottom).

blets, with dendritic failure to a greater or lesser extent. Decreasing I leads to periodic firing, while increasing τ_p further just increases the number of doublets between bursts (not shown). There is also a lower limit on the value of τ_p (approximately 2 ms), below which the system does not burst for any values of I (data not shown). Thus, τ_p must lie in a finite interval for ghostbursting to occur.

It is for these reasons that ghostbursting can be regarded as "novel".

6.5. Extensions and Other Work

Various aspects of the ghostbursting described above have been investigated further [22–26, 31]. We now describe some of this work in more detail.

6.5.1. *Reduced models*

Soon after the model (1)-(6) had been investigated, Laing and Longtin [25] presented a minimal model of a neuron that showed ghostbursting, in the sense of producing qualitatively correct bursts, and showing the appropriate transitions as the injected current was changed. This model was a modified integrate-and-fire neuron, with a second variable to cluster the action potentials. The equations are

$$\frac{dV}{dt} = I - V + c\sum_n H(t_n - t_{n-1} - r)\delta(t - t_n - \sigma) \tag{9}$$

$$\frac{dc}{dt} = -c/\tau + (B + Cc^2)\sum_n \delta(t - t_n) \tag{10}$$

with the rule $V(t_n^+) = 0$ if $V(t_n^-) = 1$, where $H(\cdot)$ is the Heaviside step function, δ is the Dirac delta function, I is the injected current, and r, σ, τ, B and C are constants. The t_n are the firing times, r corresponds to the dendritic refractory period and σ mimics the effective delay between a somatic action potential and the appearance of a DAP caused by current flow from the dendrite to the soma.

Typical bursting behaviour of the model (9)-(10) is shown in Fig. 6.8. We see that c is incremented at each action potential: $c \mapsto c + B + Cc^2$, and decays exponentially to zero otherwise, with a time constant τ. Also, at a fixed delay (σ) after most action potentials, V is incremented by the current value of c. If two successive action potentials are too close in time (less than r apart), V does not get incremented after the second of those two APs, and there is a gap until the next burst starts. If I is gradually decreased, the bursts get longer, and then the system starts behaving periodically, in agreement with the other models (not shown).

Because (9)-(10) is piecewise linear, we can explicitly integrate from one firing time to the next, obtaining a firing time map

$$\Delta_{n+1} = \begin{cases} \sigma & \text{if } \Delta_n > r \text{ and } I + s_n > 1 \\ \sigma + \ln\left[s_n/(1 - I)\right] & \text{if } \Delta_n > r \text{ and } I + s_n < 1 \\ \ln\left[I/(I - 1)\right] & \text{if } \Delta_n < r \end{cases} \tag{11}$$

$$c_{n+1} = c_n e^{-\Delta_{n+1}/\tau} + B + C\left[c_n e^{-\Delta_{n+1}/\tau}\right]^2 \tag{12}$$

where $\Delta_n = t_n - t_{n-1}$, $c_n = c(t_n^+)$, and $s_n = c_n e^{-\sigma/\tau} - Ie^{-\sigma}$.

This exact map avoids the introduction of errors through numerical integration and allows one to quickly generate a sequence of firing times. It is

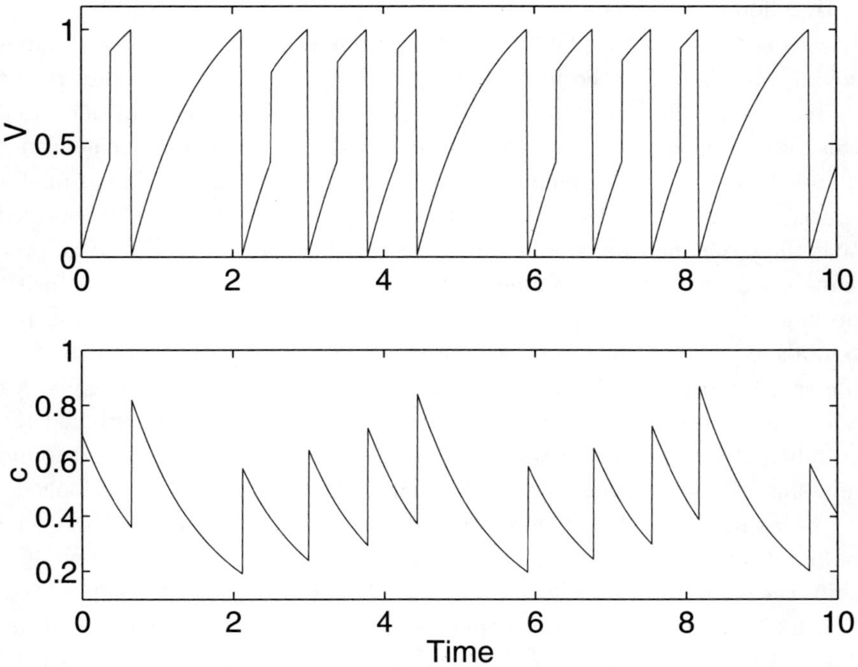

Fig. 6.8. Voltage (V, top) and c (bottom) as functions of time for the minimal model (9)-(10). Two complete bursts are shown. Parameter values are $\sigma = 0.4, \tau = 1, r = 0.7, B = 0.35, C = 0.9, I = 1.3$.

also easy to use this map to see how changing parameters will change the behaviour of the system (9)-(10) through, for example, bifurcations of specific types of solution [25]. Although bursting in maps has been previously studied [36], we believe this to be the first map from one firing time to the next that shows bursting.

6.5.2. *Periodic forcing*

The pyramidal cell under study receives input from electroreceptors on the skin of the fish [30]. These detect the electric field around the fish. For a freely-swimming animal, the electric field and thus the input to the pyramidal cells will be time-dependent. A natural way to study the effects of time-dependent input on a pyramidal cell is to study periodic input. This periodic input could come from at least two sources: the periodic electric organ discharge itself, or the "beat" frequency that occurs when two fish with different frequencies meet.

Laing and Longtin [25] studied the minimal model (9)-(10) with sinusoidal modulation of the input current I. Because of the simplicity of the system, a map for firing times could again be derived. These authors used this map to show how resonance (Arnol'd) tongues — in which the neuron is "mode locked" to the forcing frequency — could be traced out in parameter space. They also investigated the effects of noise on such a map and showed that the model neuron could display *stochastic resonance* [14], in which the signal-to-noise ratio is maximised at a moderate value of noise intensity, provided that bursts were used as the "signal", rather than all action potentials. Subsequently, Laing and Coombes [22] studied the model (9)-(10) under arbitrary periodic forcing, analysing general $p : q$ mode locking, for which the neuron fires p times during q forcing periods. They studied the stability of these types of solutions by linearising about them, and found non-smooth bifurcations in the flow that had been previously overlooked.

Laing and Longtin [26] also studied the model (1)-(6) under sinusoidal modulation of the input current I. They found that the modulation could shift the value of I corresponding to the periodic/burst transition (see Fig. 6.3) in either direction, depending on the frequency of modulation. They also found stochastic resonance, provided that bursts be used as the signal rather than action potentials, in agreement with previous results [25].

6.5.3. *Burst excitability*

The concept of "burst excitability" was first introduced by Laing and Longtin [25] and then studied in detail by Laing *et al.* [24] Burst excitability is a generalisation of "normal" excitability, seen in neural and other systems [20, 35]. The usual notion of excitability is that a system is at rest and there exists a threshold such that if a perturbation pushes the system past the threshold, it undergoes a large stereotypical excursion in phase space before returning to rest. If the perturbation is not large enough to push the system past threshold, it returns directly to the rest state.

Such excitability occurs in neural systems for which the bifurcation from quiescence to periodic firing as the injected current is increased is a saddle-node-on-a-circle bifurcation [10]. The essential ingredients here are the saddle-node bifurcation, and the existence of a "global reinjection" mechanism that takes the trajectory (once it has passed the threshold) through a large excursion in phase space and returns it to the stable fixed point. These ingredients also exist for the ghostburster near the bifurcation from periodic firing to bursting. There is a saddle-node bifurcation (of periodic orbits) and a global reinjection mechanism in the form of the decrease of p_d during a burst and then its rapid increase between bursts. Thus there should be excitable behaviour near the bifurcation from periodic firing to bursting, but with the quiescent fixed point and action potential (for normal excitability) replaced by periodic firing and a burst, respectively [24].

This type of burst excitability is shown in Fig. 6.9. Here, I was stepped from 8.3 to either 10.5 (thin line) or 11 (bold line) during the interval $300 < t < 310$. (Note that for $I = 8.3$, the system is firing periodically.) The smaller step failed to induce a burst (i.e. did not push the system past threshold) and the system returned directly to its previous state, namely periodic firing. The slightly larger step did induce a burst, as seen from the slow decrease and then rapid increase in p_d. Note that most of the burst occurred after I had returned to its original value, another signature of the excitable nature of the system.

This type of burst excitability was also shown to occur in the minimal model [25] (9)-(10) and Laing *et al.* [24] showed that it occurred in the more realistic multi-compartmental model [7]. These authors also discussed the possible relevance of burst excitability to communication between weakly electric fish, and derived a scaling relationship between the size and duration of a stimulus that is needed to produce a burst in the ghostburster (or any other similar excitable system). Several authors have proposed that bursts rather than action potentials could be the fundamental units of neural communication [19, 28], and the ghostburster is an example of a neuron which robustly produces bursts in response to physiologically-realistic perturbations in input.

6.5.4. *Differential modulation of burst discharge*

The multi-compartmental model [7] and a modification of the minimal model presented in Sec. 6.5.1 were used by Noonan *et al.* [31] to reproduce and understand the different effects that somatic and dendritic potassium channels have on burst length. As explained above, the different widths of the somatic and dendritic action potentials (APs), and the slow increase in the width of the dendritic APs during a burst, are an essential part of the bursting mechanism. In both the soma and the dendrite, the flow of potassium ions is responsible for the repolarization of APs. By blocking potassium channels in the neuron's dendrite, dendritic APs become wider, enhancing the size of the DAPs that appear at the soma. This causes bursts

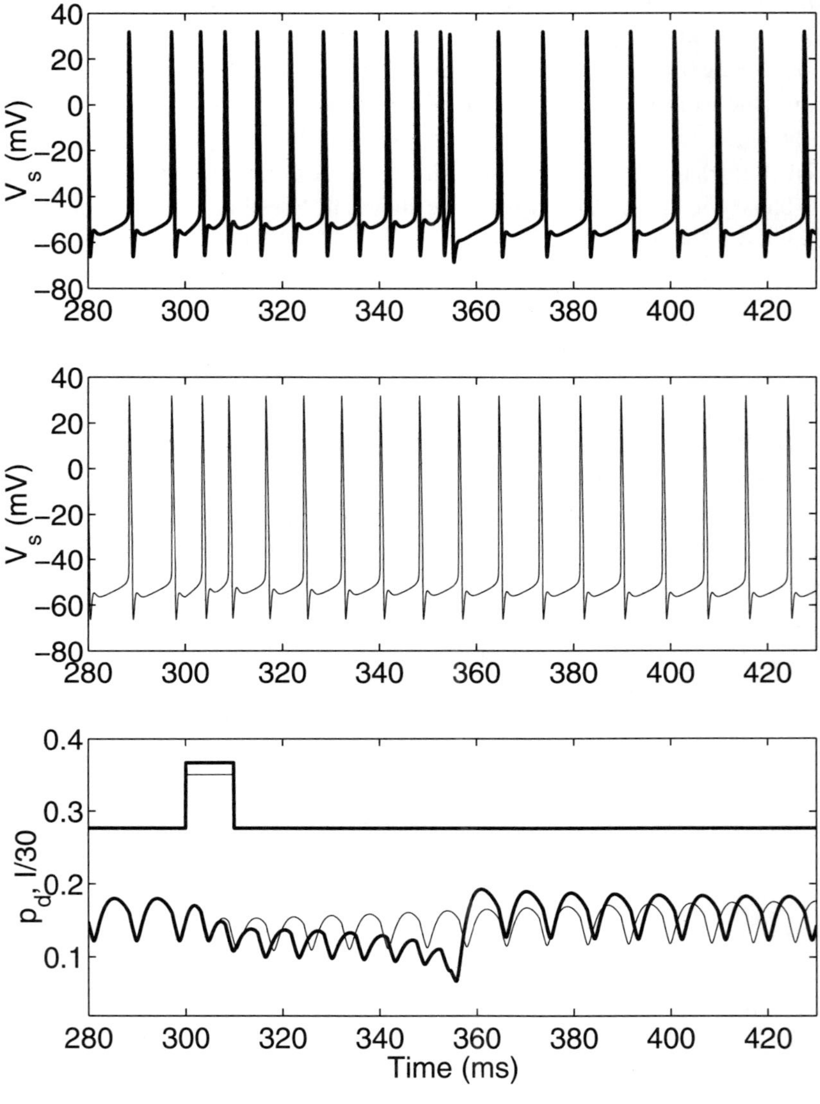

Fig. 6.9. Burst excitability in (1)-(6). Two different current pulses (shown in bottom panel, 1/30 their actual size) were applied. The larger one (bold) induced a burst (top panel, where the somatic voltage is plotted), while the smaller one (thin line) did not (middle panel, showing somatic voltage). Top and middle panels: V_s as a function of time. Bottom panel: p_d and $I/30$. See text for more detail.

to become shorter (if the neuron is already bursting) or can cause the neuron to start bursting (if it is below, but near, the periodic/burst bifurcation).

Conversely, if potassium channels at the soma are blocked, somatic APs become wider, thus lessening the size of the DAPs. This causes bursts to become longer (if the neuron is already bursting) or stop altogether, leaving the neuron firing periodically. The advantage of using such a simple model as (9)-(10) to study an effect like this is that the behaviour of interest could be seen by simply following a curve of saddle-node bifurcations of fixed points in the parameter plane [31].

6.6. Parallel Processing with Bursts and Isolated Spikes

The original experimental characterization of ELL pyramidal cell burst discharge was in response to static depolarizing inputs [27, 38, 39]. As described above, there have been successful theoretical efforts in characterising the response of the ghostburster system to periodic inputs as well as to instantaneous step depolarizations. However, weakly electric fish thrive in a sensory environment with very rich temporal structure. Prey inputs and natural scenes, such as the electric image of the fish's own tail, are typically composed of only low frequency components (0-10 Hz). This is in contrast to intra-specific communication calls that are broadband in their spectral content (0-200 Hz). An often-used simplification of natural scenes is to model its temporal structure as Gaussian band-limited noise. It should be mentioned that this simplification is not always appropriate, most notably in the auditory system [34]. Nevertheless, this strategy has been successfully employed on numerous occasions in *in vivo* electric fish studies [3, 4, 13]. A study of how the *in vitro* ghostburster system processes stochastic inputs has only recently been undertaken [9, 32]. This section will briefly describe the main findings of these studies.

6.6.1. *Ghostbusting the ghostburster*

In Oswald *et al.* [32] broadband Gaussian stimuli (0-60 Hz) were applied to ELL pyramidal cells in a slice preparation. The spike trains observed were quite distinct from those observed in response to static depolarizations. Notably, the random stimuli elicited a mixture of both isolated spike discharge and bursting, with bursts often consisting of only two spikes and without the characteristic large after-hyperpolarizing potential at burst termination. The difference between autonomous and driven burst discharges is presumably that the high-frequency components in the stimulus — specifically, rapid hyperpolarizations — prematurely terminate burst discharges before a full burst is completed. This assumption can be used to greatly simplify the mathematical modelling of the burst mechanism.

The ghostbursting mechanism described in Sec. 6.2 involves three main components: 1) a dendritic dependent DAP at the soma, 2) a potentiation of the DAP over a burst event, and 3) a longer refractory period of the dendritic action potential as compared to the somatic action potential. The relatively slow timescale of the dendritic potassium inactivation allows for significant DAP potentiation, typically only over bursts of many spikes; this is evident in both Figs. 6.1 and 6.2. Somewhat less apparent from the modelling presented in this review is that the dendritic refractory period is not a fixed quantity, but increases as more spikes occur during a burst. This was demonstrated experimentally by Noonan *et al.* [31]. In this paper the authors forced the neuron to discharge periodically with inter-spike intervals between 5 and 7 ms and observed that dendritic spike failures occurred only after multiple (approximately 5) dendritic spikes, indicating that earlier spikes acted to dynamically increase the dendritic refractory period.

The lack of many-spike bursts in response to broadband Gaussian stimuli permits an approximation of ELL burst dynamics that contains only DAPs and ignores burst mechanism components 2) and 3). Motivated by past leaky integrate-and-fire modelling of ghostbursting [25, 31] the following description was postulated [9, 9, 33]

$$\frac{dV}{dt} = -V + \gamma x(t-\sigma) + I_{stim}(t) \tag{13}$$

$$\frac{dx}{dt} = y \tag{14}$$

$$\frac{dy}{dt} = -\alpha^2 x - 2\alpha y + \alpha^2 \sum_n \delta(t-t_n) \tag{15}$$

with the rule that once V reaches 1 from below, V is reset to 0 and held there for a time τ_r before being allowed to continue evolving under (13). Time is measured in units of the membrane time constant. The firing times, $\{t_n\}$, are defined to be the times at which V reaches 1.

The dynamics of (13)-(15) is quite simple in comparison to those of the full conductance-based ghostbursting system (1)-(6) or even those of the reduced model (9)-(10). Equation (13) is a standard leaky integrate-and-fire description of spiking dynamics with a refractory period τ_r. The solution of the subsystem (x, y) with the initial conditions $x(0) = 0$ and

$y(0) = \alpha^2$ is the so-called alpha function: $x(t) = \alpha^2 t e^{-\alpha t}$. Every time $V(t)$ spikes, there is a time delay σ, after which an alpha function of intensity γ drives the membrane dynamics; this models the dendritic DAP's influence on somatic spike generation. In contrast with (9)-(10), the DAP dynamics are linear without the possibility of potentiation or refractory dynamics. When $I_{stim}(t) = I$, independent of time, the system (13)-(15) gives simple tonic discharge for all values of I. Thus (13)-(15) is not an autonomous burster, unlike many of the models reviewed in this book. There is no saddle-node bifurcation of limit cycles or chaos for any value of I. We have thus removed (or "busted") the "ghosting" behaviour so crucial for our understanding of burst response to static inputs. However, when $I_{stim}(t)$ is a stochastic process with Gaussian spectra between 0-60 Hz, the dynamics of (13)-(15) reproduces the experimentally-measured first and second order statistics of both the spike train and ISI sequence, as well as the linear signal processing of a broadband input stimulus.

Figure 6.10(A) shows numerical simulations of (13)-(15) when driven with broadband Gaussian input. Note the presence of both isolated spikes and bursts of two spikes. Both the dendritic DAP, $x(t)$, and the stimulus, $I_{stim}(t)$, are also shown. Figure 6.10(B) shows bimodal inter-spike interval (ISI) histograms of pyramidal cell spike train data. The model shows similar behaviour with active dendrites ($\gamma > 0$) but unimodal ISI histograms when the dendrite is passive ($\gamma = 0$). To measure action potential patterning we compute the spike train autocorrelation [12] defined as

$$A(\tau) = \frac{\langle s(t)s(t+\tau)\rangle}{\langle s(t)^2\rangle}. \tag{16}$$

where $s(t) = \sum_n \delta(t - t_n)$ and $\langle\cdot\rangle$ is an average over time. $A(\tau)$ is the mean corrected probability of observing a spike τ time units after (or $-\tau$ time units before) another spike. "Mean corrected" implies that when $A(\tau) = 0$ the statistics of $s(t)$ should be interpreted as having the equivalent statistical structure as a simple Poisson process with the same firing rate.

$A(\tau)$ is shown for both the model and the data in Fig. 6.10(C). After an interval of reduced probability of spiking again, due to refractoriness, there is an interval of enhanced probability of firing a spike at approximately 5–7ms after the previous spike. The probability of firing again then decays rapidly back to Poisson statistics within 10ms of the previous spike. The passive dendrite model ($\gamma = 0$) shows that this increased probability is due to the DAP current promoting spike discharge after a spike, but only for a short period. The combination of both the bimodal ISI distributions as well as the distinct non-Poissonian spike statistics as observed from $A(\tau)$ allow us to describe the stochastic behaviour of (13)-(15) as bursting. Similar statistics were used to characterize the burst discharge of *in vivo* ELL pyramidal cells [2].

6.6.2. *Spike train processing*

To investigate the processing done by pyramidal cells, we introduce the coherence $C(f)$ between the input stimulus S and the spike train response R:

$$C(f) = \frac{P_{SR}(f)^2}{P_{SS}(f)P_{RR}(f)}. \tag{17}$$

$P_{SR}(f)$ is the cross spectrum between S and R, $P_{SS}(f)$ is the power spectrum of S and $P_{RR}(f)$ is the power spectrum of R. Quite simply, $C(f)$ is the frequency-dependent linear correlation between S and R; it is a number between 0 and 1 with 0 representing no correlation and 1 representing perfect correlation at a given frequency f. The coherence between the full spike train and the stimulus for both the data and the model system (13)-(15) is relatively broadband (slightly lowpass), as shown in Fig 6.11(B). This is similar to *in vivo* results when the stimulus is applied to a small fraction of the total receptive field [3].

In order to better understand pyramidal cell coding, Oswald *et al.* [32] partitioned the full spike train into two component trains: an isolated-spikes train and a burst train. This partitioning is schematically shown in Fig. 6.11(A) and briefly described here. Every spike in a spike train defines two ISIs: the ISI that it begins and the one that it terminates. An ISI threshold corresponding to the local minimum of the ISI probability distribution is set. If both ISIs that a given spike defines are greater than this threshold, then that spike is considered an isolated spike. In a complementary sense, if one or both of the ISIs are less than the threshold then that spike is involved in a burst. The burst train is further simplified by removing all but the first spike in a burst; the results presented are not sensitive to this reduction.

Interestingly, the coherence between the burst train and the stimulus is low-pass while the coherence between the isolated-spikes train and the stimulus is high-pass (sometimes band-pass). This occurs in a statistically-significant fashion in experiments, in the reduced model (13)-(15), and in a modified version of the full ghostburster system (1)-(6). (See Fig. 6.11(B) and Oswald *et al.* [32] for results not shown.) Thus, this separation of the

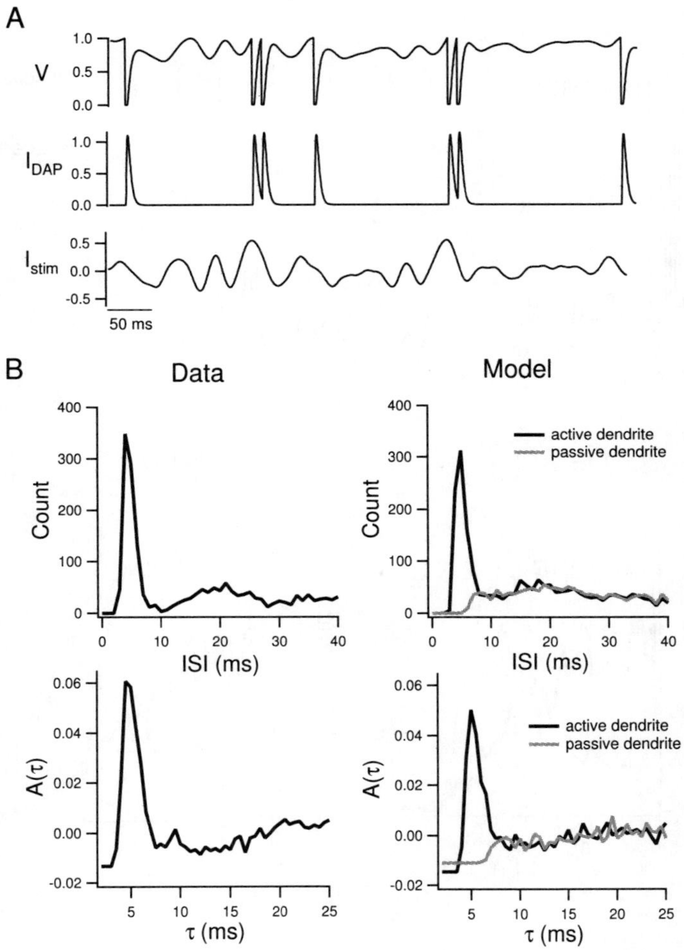

Fig. 6.10. Stochastic burst discharge in electrosensory pyramidal cells. **A** Time series of $V(t)$ (top) and $x(t)$ (middle) when driven with I_{stim} (shown in the bottom panel). Note the lack of refractory period in the dendritic response $x(t)$. **B** ISI histograms (top) and spike train autocorrelation (bottom) for both slice experiment data and the model (13)-(15), computed from 100 seconds of spiking activity. The model results show simulations when the dendrite is active ($\gamma = 1.2$), and when the dendrite is passive ($\gamma = 0$). Other model parameters are $\sigma = 0.2, \tau_r = 0.2, \alpha = 12.5, \langle I_{stim} \rangle = 0.88$, and $\sqrt{\langle I_{stim}^2 \rangle - \langle I_{stim} \rangle^2} = 0.185$. The membrane time constant was taken to be 5 ms. The experimental methodology is as described in Oswald *et al.* [32]. Data provided by Anne-Marie Oswald.

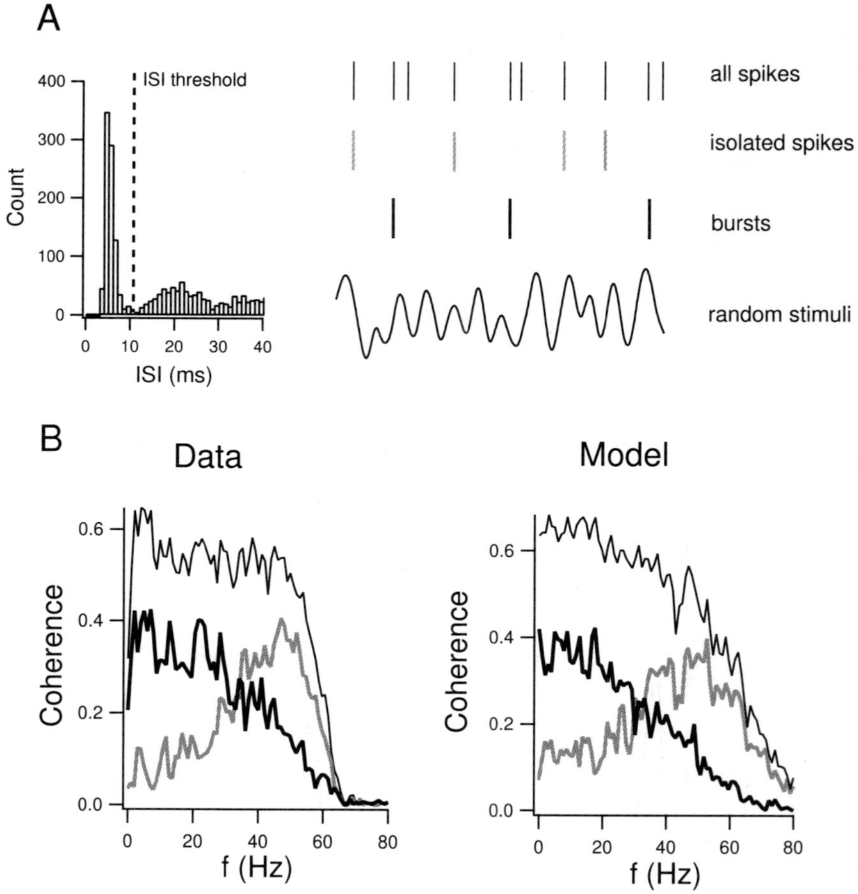

Fig. 6.11. Parallel processing of dynamic stimuli by bursts and isolated spikes. **A** An ISI threshold of 10ms is used to partition the spike train into isolated spikes (for which both neighbouring ISIs are greater than 10ms) and bursts (spikes for which an ISI is less than 10ms). The time at which a burst occurs is taken to be the time at which the first spike in the burst occurs. **B** The coherence between the full spike train (thin black line), isolated spike train (gray line) and burst train (thick black line), and the stimulus (Gaussian noise with power between 0-60 Hz). The details for both the data and the model are identical to those for Fig. 6.10. Data provided by Anne-Marie Oswald.

spike train reveals the potential for the pyramidal cell to selectively code for both low-frequency components via bursts and high-frequency components via isolated spikes. Furthermore, this coding occurs in parallel since the full spike train simultaneously carries both bursts and isolated spikes (providing that the stimulus is dynamic).

The usefulness of this parallel coding by bursts and isolated spikes of a broadband signal presupposes that the decoding mechanisms of higher brain centers are sensitive to this sort of encoding. ELL pyramidal cell output is decoded in the torus semicircularis (TS) of the midbrain. Fortune and Rose [11] have shown that different TS cells have distinct tuning properties with respect to external *in vivo* inputs: specifically, some show low-pass characteristics while others have a high-pass nature. Oswald *et al.* [32] suggested that their low-/high-pass nature was synaptically mediated to respond selectively to either bursts or isolated spikes from ELL pyramidal cells. However, much more work must be done to decisively conclude this point.

6.7. Summary

We have given an overview of a recently-characterised form of neural bursting, known as "ghostbursting", that occurs in pyramidal cells of weakly electric fish. We have described the various stages involved in its analysis, from experimental observations and the construction of a multi-compartmental model to the analysis of simple caricatures involving two or three differential equations. In the process of analysis we have found a number of features of ghostbursting that do not appear in any previous bursting models. We have also discussed the possible "use" made of the bursting dynamics by the electric fish, in terms of the processing of electrosensory signals, and found that these neurons seem to be capable of transmitting at least two parallel streams of information, encoded in the timing of bursts and isolated spikes.

Acknowledgements

We would like to thank our many ghostbursting collaborators whose ideas have helped to shape the results presented here: André Longtin, Leonard Maler, Ray Turner and students, Anne-Marie Oswald, and Maurice Chacron. We particularly thank Anne-Marie Oswald for providing data for several of the figures and André Longtin for carefully reading the manuscript. B.D. was supported by NSERC (Canada) during the writing of this chapter.

References

[1] R. Aldrich, P. Getting, and S. Thomson, Mechanism of frequency-dependent broadening of molluscan neuron soma spikes, *J. Physiol. (Lond)* **291**, 531–544, (1979).

[2] J. Bastian and J. Nguyenkim, Dendritic modulation of burst-like firing in sensory neurons, *J. Neurophysiol.* **85**, 10–22, (2001).

[3] M. J. Chacron, B. Doiron, L. Maler, A. Longtin, and J. Bastian, Non-classical receptive field mediates switch in a sensory neuron's frequency tuning, *Nature* **423**, 77–81, (2003).

[4] B. Doiron, M. J. Chacron, L. Maler, A. Longtin, and J. Bastian, Inhibitory feedback required for network oscillatory responses to communication but not prey stimuli, *Nature* **421**, 539–543, (2003).

[5] B. Doiron, C. Laing, A. Longtin, and L. Maler, Ghostbursting: a novel neuronal burst mechanism, *J. Comput. Neurosci.* **12**, 5–25, (2002).

[6] B. Doiron, B. Lindner, A. Longtin, L. Maler, and J. Bastian, Oscillatory activity in electrosensory neurons increases with the spatial correlation of the stochastic input stimulus, *Phys. Rev. Lett.* **93**, 048101(4), (2004).

[7] B. Doiron, A. Longtin, R. W. Turner, and L. Maler, Model of gamma frequency burst discharge generated by conditional backpropagation, *J. Neurophysiol.* **86**, 1523–1545, (2001).

[8] B. Doiron, L. Noonan, N. Lemon, and R. W. Turner, Persistent Na^+ current modifies burst discharge by regulating conditional backpropagation of dendritic spikes, *J. Neurophysiol.* **89**, 324–337, (2003).

[9] B. Doiron, *Electrosensory Dynamics: Dendrites and Delays*, PhD Thesis, Univeristy of Ottawa, (2005).

[10] B. Ermentrout, Type I membranes, phase resetting curves, and synchrony, *Neural Comput.* **8**, 979–1001, (1996).

[11] E. Fortune and G. Rose, Passive and active membrane properties contribute to the temporal filtering properties of midbrain neurons in vivo, *J. Neurosci.* **17**, 3815–3825, (1997).

[12] F. Gabbiani and C. Koch, Principles of spike train analysis, in *Methods in Neuronal Modeling: From Ions to Networks*, Ed. C. Koch and I. Segev, MIT Press, Cambridge, MA, (1998).

[13] F. Gabbiani, W. Metzner, R. Wessel, and C. Koch, ¿From stimulus encoding to feature extraction in weakly electric fish, *Nature* **384**, 564–567, (1996).

[14] L. Gammaitoni, P. Hänggi, P. Jung, and F. Marchesoni, Stochastic

resonance, *Rev. Mod. Phys.* **70**, 223–287, (1998).

[15] J. Guckenheimer, K. Hoffman, and W. Weckesser, Numerical computation of canards, *Int. J. Bifurcat. Chaos* **10**, 2669–2687, (2000).

[16] J. Guckenheimer and P. Holmes. *Nonlinear Oscillations, Dynamical Systems, and Bifurcations of Vector Fields*, Springer-Verlag, New York, (1983).

[17] W. Heilengenberg, *Neural Nets in Electric Fish*, MIT Press,Cambridge, MA, (1991).

[18] E. M. Izhikevich, Neural excitability, spiking, and bursting, *Int. J. Bifurcat. Chaos* **10**, 1171–1266, (2000).

[19] E. M. Izhikevich, N. S. Desai, E. C. Walcott, and F. C. Hoppensteadt, Bursts as a unit of neural information: selective communication via resonance, *Trends Neurosci.* **26**, 161–167, (2003).

[20] J. Keener and J. Sneyd. *Mathematical Physiology*, Springer-Verlag, New York, (1998).

[21] R. Krahe and F. Gabbiani, Burst firing in sensory systems, *Nat. Rev. Neurosci.* **5**, 13–23, (2004).

[22] C. R. Laing and S. Coombes, Mode locking in a periodically forced "ghostbursting" neuron model, *Int. J. Bifurcat. Chaos* **15**, (2005).

[23] C. R. Laing, B. Doiron, A. Longtin, and L. Maler, Ghostbursting: the effects of dendrites on spike patterns, *Neurocomputing*, **44-46**, 127–132 (2002).

[24] C. R. Laing, B. Doiron, A. Longtin, L. Noonan, R. W. Turner, and L. Maler, Type I burst excitability, *J. Comput. Neurosci.* **14**, 329–342, (2003).

[25] C. R. Laing and A. Longtin, A two-variable model of somatic-dendritic interactions in a bursting neuron, *Bull. Math. Biol.* **64**, 829–860, (2002).

[26] C. R. Laing and A. Longtin, Periodic forcing of a model sensory neuron, *Phys. Rev. E*, **67**, 051928(7), (2003).

[27] N. Lemon and R. W. Turner, Conditional spike backpropagation generates burst discharge in a sensory neuron, *J. Neurophysiol.* **84**, 1519–1530, (2000).

[28] J. E. Lisman, Bursts as a unit of neural information: making unreliable synapses reliable, *Trends Neurosci.* **20**, 38–43, (1997).

[29] M. Ma and J. Koester, Consequences and mechanisms of spike broadening of R20 cells in Aplysia-Californica, *J. Neurosci.* **15** 6720–6734, (1995).

[30] M. E. Nelson, Z. Xu, and J. R. Payne, Characterization and modeling

of P-type electrosensory afferent responses to amplitude modulations in a wave-type electric fish, *J. Comp. Physiol. A* **181**, 532–544, (1997).

[31] L. Noonan, B. Doiron, C. R. Laing, A. Longtin, and R W. Turner, A dynamic dendritic refractory period regulates burst discharge in the electrosensory lobe of weakly electric fish, *J. Neurosci.* **23**, 1524–1534, (2003).

[32] A-M. M. Oswald, M. J. Chacron, B. Doiron, J. Bastian, and L. Maler, Parallel processing of sensory input by bursts and isolated spikes, *J. Neurosci* **24**, 4351–4362, (2004).

[33] A-M. M. Oswald, *Burst Firing in Electrosensory Processing*, PhD Thesis, Univeristy of Ottawa, (2005).

[34] F. Rieke, D. A. Bodnar, and W. Bialek, Naturalistic stimuli increase the rate and efficiency of information transmission by primary auditory afferents, *Proc. R. Soc. Lond. B* **262**, 259–265, (1995).

[35] J. Rinzel and G. B. Ermentrout, Analysis of neural excitability and oscillations, in *Methods in Neuronal Modeling: ¿From Ions to Networks,* Ed. C. Koch and I. Segev, MIT Press, Cambridge MA, (1998).

[36] N. F. Rulkov, Regularization of synchronized chaotic bursts, *Phys. Rev. Lett.* **86**, 183–186, (2001).

[37] S. H. Strogatz, *Nonlinear Dynamics and Chaos with Applications to Physics, Biology, Chemistry, and Engineering*, Addison-Wesley, Reading, MA., (1994).

[38] R. W. Turner, L. Maler, T. Deerinck, S. R. Levinson, and M. H. Ellisman, TTX-sensitive dendritic sodium channels underlie oscillatory discharge in a vertebrate sensory neuron, *J. Neurosci.* **14**, 6453–6471, (1994).

[39] R. W. Turner and L. Maler, Oscillatory and burst discharge in the apteronotid electrosensory lateral line lobe, *J. Exp. Biol.*, **202**, 1255–1265, (1999).

[40] X. J. Wang, Fast burst firing and short-term synaptic plasticity: a model of neocortical chattering neurons, *Neuroscience* **89**, 347–362, (1999).

PART II:
BURSTING AT THE NETWORK LEVEL

CHAPTER 7

ANALYSIS OF CIRCUITS CONTAINING BURSTING NEURONS USING PHASE RESETTING CURVES

Carmen Canavier

Department of Psychology, University of New Orleans
2000 Lakeshore Dr., New Orleans, La, USA, 70471
e-mail: ccanavie@uno.edu

Closed circuits composed of bursting neurons were analysed using the phase resetting observed in a postsynaptic neuron in response to a burst in the presynaptic neuron in the open loop condition without feedback. Phase resetting before (first order) and after (second order) burst initiation was considered separately. Existence and stability criteria were derived for small networks composed of endogenously bursting neurons assuming that the effect of a perturbation is the same under open or closed loop conditions, postulating only that the resetting is complete by the time a subsequent input is received. Synaptic delays could be accomodated as long as the above postulate was satisfied. The method had excellent success in small networks of model neurons, and good success in hybrid circuits composed of one biological and one model neuron. The latter success was limited somewhat by the inherent variability in biological neurons and by changes in burst durations resulting from feedback in the closed circuit. Stability criteria were also derived for variable burst duration, and the dependence of first order resetting in a biological bursting neuron on duration was elucidated as the first step into accomodating variability in burst duration into the theoretical framework.

7.1. Introduction

The analysis of systems of coupled oscillators often begins with the assumption of limit cycle oscillators. Phase resetting theory [16, 42] further assumes that a perturbation instantaneously displaces the trajectory along the limit cycle, with a phase advance causing the trajectory to skip ahead on the limit cycle and a delay causing it to jump backwards. This has the effect of either shortening or lengthening the particular cycle in which the perturbation occurs. Phase resetting theory reduces the analysis to a single dimension, absolute phase, representing the position along the limit cycle. Often the oscillators are assumed to move around a common, identical limit cycle and the relative phase of the oscillators is assumed to change on a slower time scale than the absolute phase [12, 22–24]. This assumption, which is equivalent to weak coupling, allows the consideration of only the relative phase between oscillators, and further reduces the dimensionality. One elegant method suggested for the analysis of weakly coupled oscillators is to approximate each oscillator as a time-varying linear system such that the time-varying impulse response of the system as a function of the phase is designated the instantaneous phase resetting curve (iPRC). Then the response of the oscillator to arbitrary perturbations of finite duration can be obtained by convolution. Assuming infinite attraction, or instantaneous relaxation, to the limit cycle and a synaptic pertubation in current, which appears in the derivative of membrane potential only, simplifies the form of the iPRC [12, 19]. The effect of the coupling can be averaged over a cycle as a function of relative phase and the coupled period can be predicted by applying periodicity and stability criteria.

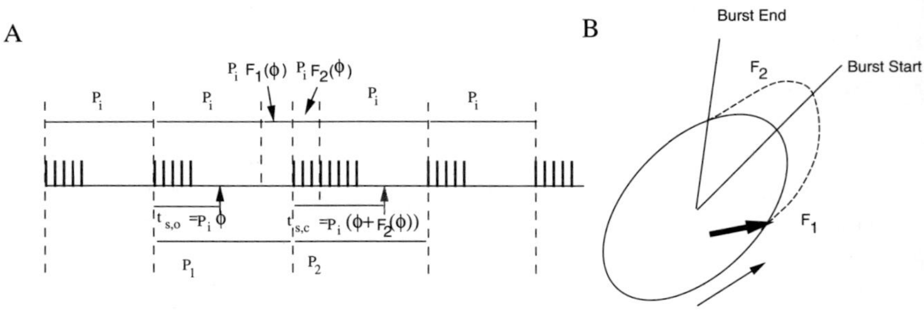

Fig. 7.1. **Importance of Second Order Phase Resetting. A.** Time Domain. The unperturbed period of the oscillator is P_i. The open and closed loop stimulus intervals are $t_{s,o} = P_i\phi$ and $t_{s,c} = P_i(F_2(\phi) + \phi)$, respectively, and the vertical arrows indicate stimuli applied at the same phase. The cycle containing the perturbation is elongated by the interval designated $P_iF_1(\phi)$. The cycle after the perturbation is also elongated, by an interval designated $F_2(\phi)$. **B**. Phase Plane. The burst start and end occur when the trajectory crosses the labeled lines, whether this motion occurs on the unperturbed limit cycle (solid curve) or on the perturbed trajectory (dashed line). The contributions of $F1$ and $F2$ occur before and after burst initiation, respectively. The direction of motion along the limit cycle is indicated by the thin arrow and the thick arrow indicates the point of application of an arbitrary input.

There are several important shortcomings of these methods as applied to neural oscillators. One is that neural oscillators usually exhibit some sort of threshold phenomenon such as a spike (action potential) or a burst. The well-known theta model [11, 18, 21] was developed as a result of the realization that spike (or burst) timing is important, but still cannot capture complexity greater than that of an integrator with an infinitely attractive limit cycle. Another complication is that pulsatile coupling frequently causes large excursions from the limit cycle such that the approximation as a time-varying linear system does not hold, nor does the assumption of an infinitely attractive limit cycle. An innovative aspect of our methodology based on phase resetting is that it can accomodate strong coupling, both in the sense that the relative phase varies on the same or faster time scale as the absolute phase and that the perturbations induced by the coupling produce significant excursions from the limit cycle. The essential innovation [7] is the generation of the PRCs using a perturbation that approximates as closely as possible the actual input that a neuron will receive in a closed loop circuit. This input is usually the conductance pulse caused by a spike or burst in the neuron that is presynaptic to the neuron under study. Phase resetting curves (PRCs) are generated in an open loop configuration as the oscillator under study is perturbed without feedback. We propose that the second order phase resetting [7] that occurs after the threshold event immediately following the perturbation must be accounted for in addition to the first order phase resetting that occurs before the threshold event.

Figure 7.1(A) shows a schematic of the two components of resetting in an open loop phase resetting protocol for a bursting neuron in the time domain, and Fig. 7.1(B) illustrates our geometric understanding of this two-pronged phase resetting. The unperturbed intrinsic period of the oscillator is P_i, and a burst containing five spikes is shown. The initiation of the burst is designated as a phase of zero, and the termination as a phase of one. A perturbation of arbitrary shape, amplitude, and duration is applied at the first arrow at a phase of ϕ corresponding to an open loop stimulus interval after the burst initiation of $t_{s,o} = P_i\phi$. The cycle containing the perturbation is in this case elongated by $P_iF_1(\phi)$, where $F_1(\phi)$ is the first order resetting due to a perturbation at a phase ϕ. The phase is decremented by $F_1(\phi)$ as a result of the input, so that it now requires a longer time to reach the burst threshold, producing a delay. A shortening would produce an advance instead. The cycle after the perturbation is also elongated in this case, by an amount designated the second order resetting, $F_2(\phi)$. The phase is again decremented, but this second reset occurs immediately after burst initiation. The time interval required after the next burst initiation until restoration of the phase ϕ at which the input was originally applied is

$P_i[F_2(\phi) + \phi]$. This is also the required interval $t_{s,c}$ (second vertical arrow) between burst initiation and a repetitively applied perturbation at the same phase used to generate the open loop PRC at an elapsed time interval of $t_{s,o}$. Thus, the application of open loop PRC data based on $t_{s,o}$ to the prediction of the phasic relationships in closed loop phase-locking requires second order PRCs in addition to first order PRCs. The use of time intervals [13] rather than phase obviates the need for phase to be well-defined, and would therefore be prefereable, but the requirement that phases be updated twice per cycle precludes the possiblity of using only time intervals and not phases in our analysis. Although the second order phase resetting is often measured with reference to the entire cycle labeled P_2, the essential constraint on our analysis is that the second order resetting be complete by the time of the next input, so that the trajectory is close enough to the limit cycle that the phase is well defined for each input. Figure 7.1(B) is a schematic representation of a limit cycle oscillator that exhibits a threshold phenomenon. An arbitrary input (thick arrow) causes a deviation from the limit cycle such that the time elapsed until the burst starts is altered by an amount $F_1(\phi)$. The burst is initiated before the return to the limit cycle and its duration is altered by an amount $F_2(\phi)$. In model bursting neurons, we have found that $F_2(\phi)$ is largely accounted for by changes in burst duration [29].

7.2. Stability Analysis for Two Coupled Oscillators

The stability analyses presented here are an extension of the work of Perkel *et al.* [32]. Our original assumptions [10] were that 1) all component neurons in the circuit are endogenous oscillators (bursting or spiking neurons), 2) there are no synaptic delays, 3) each neuron receives one perturbation (synaptic input) per cycle, as in an open loop circuit composed only of a presynaptic neuron driving a postsynaptic one, and 5) each neuron returns to its unperturbed limit cycle before the next input is received. However, assumptions 2 and 3 are not required as long as assumption 5 is met, and in section 7.7 assumption 4 is relaxed.

Figure 7.2(A) shows how the open loop phase resetting functions calculated as in Fig. 7.1(A) can be applied to a heterogenous closed loop circuit. The stimulus interval ($t_{s,k}$) is the time elapsed between the initiation of a spike (or burst) in neuron k and the receipt of an input at a phase ϕ_k such that this interval is analogous to $t_{s,c}$ in Fig. 7.1 and is given by $t_{s,k} = P_{ki}[\phi_k + F_{2k}(\phi_k)]$, where P_{ki} is the intrinsic period. The recov-

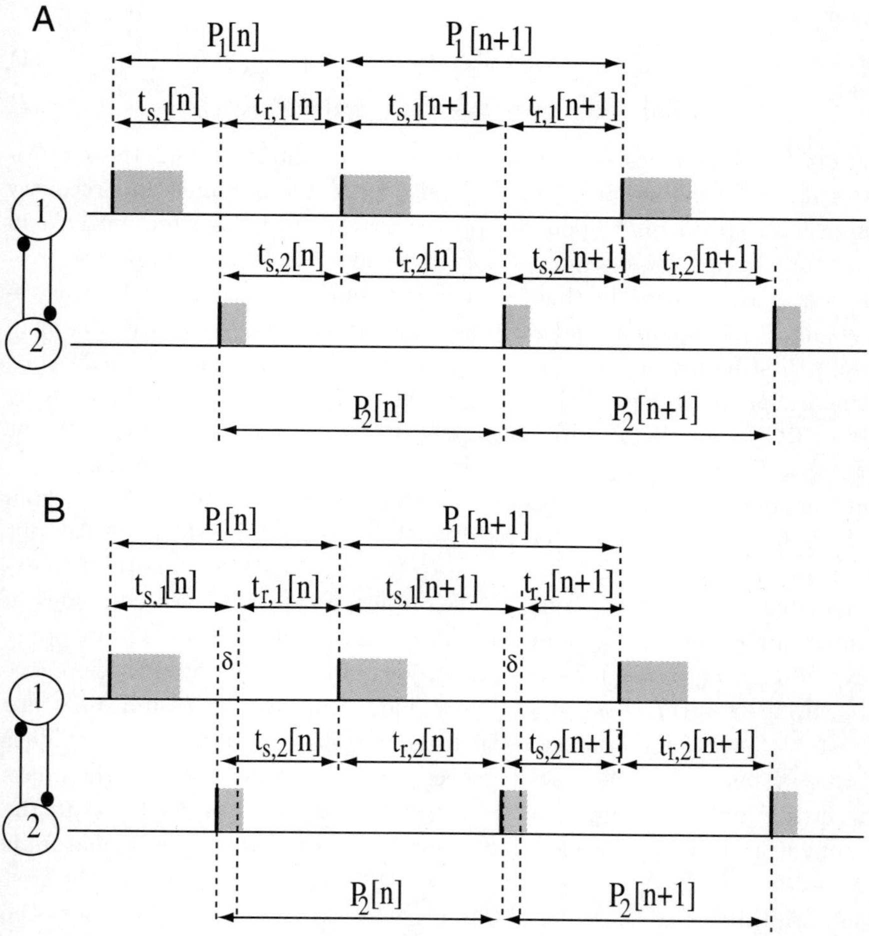

Fig. 7.2. **Stability Analysis for Two Coupled Oscillators. A.** Stimulus and recovery times in a phase-locked mode with no delays. **B.** Stimulus and recovery times in a phase-locked mode with an offset (δ) between presynaptic burst initiation in neuron 2 and postsynaptic receipt of the input in neuron 1. The gray bars indicate burst duration, which is not considered until section 7.7.

ery interval ($t_{r,k}$) is the time elapsed between the receipt of an input at a phase ϕ_k and the next spike (or burst) produced by neuron k, such that $t_{r,k} = P_{ki}[1 - \phi_k + F_{1k}(\phi_k)]$. Any 1:1 locking must satisfy the periodicity criteria that the sum of the stimulus and recovery intervals in each neuron equal the phase-locked period, and that the recovery interval in each neuron equals the stimulus interval in the other: $t_{s,1} = t_{r,2}$ and $t_{s,2} = t_{r,1}$, such that

$$P_{1i}[\phi_1^* + F_{21}(\phi_1^*))] = P_{2i}[1 - \phi_2^* + F_{12}(\phi_2^*)] \quad (1)$$

$$P_{2i}[\phi_2^* + F_{22}(\phi_2^*))] = P_{1i}[1 - \phi_1^* + F_{11}(\phi_1^*)] \quad (2)$$

where the quantities on the left are stimulus intervals and the quantities on the right are recovery intervals. Since the stimulus and recovery intervals depend only upon the phases at which inputs were received in previous cycles, expressions can be obtained [10] that describe the evolution of the system in time. If the contribution of the second order resetting F_{2k} is ignored, and a stable phase locking at (ϕ_1^*, ϕ_2^*) is assumed, the nth stimulus interval can be expressed as $t_{s,k}[n] = P_{ki}(\phi_k^* + \Delta\phi_k[n])$ where $\Delta\phi_k[n]$ is the perturbation from the steady phase locking. Linearizing the PRC about this fixed point, the nth cycle length can be expressed as $P_k[n] = P_{ki}(1 + F_{1k}(\phi_k^*) + m_{1k}\Delta\phi_k[n])$, where m_{1k} is the slope of F_{1k} at ϕ_k^*, and again ignoring $F_{2k}(\phi)$. However, each $P_k[n]$ can also be written as a sum of stimulus intervals such that $P_1[n] = P_{1i}(\phi_1^* + \Delta\phi_1[n]) + P_{2i}(\phi_2^* + \Delta\phi_2[n])$ and $P_2[n] = P_{1i}(\phi_1^* + \Delta\phi_1[n+1]) + P_{2i}(\phi_2^* + \Delta\phi_2[n])$. Setting the two expressions for each $P_k[n]$ equal to each other, a system of two equations in three unknowns can be obtained. After eliminating $\Delta\phi_2[n]$, the mapping $\Delta\phi_1[n+1] = (1 - m_{11})(1 - m_{12})\Delta\phi_1[n]$ is obtained. The perturbation goes to zero if $-1 < (m_{11} - 1)(m_{12} - 1) < 1$, indicating that the assumed pattern is stable [10]. If the analysis is then redone [27] considering F_{2k}, a higher order system results because it is necessary to consider not only the phase resetting due to the input in the current cycle, but also that due to the input in the previous cycle. The result for two heterogenous oscillators is $\lambda^2 - [(m_{11} - 1)(m_{12} - 1) - m_{21} - m_{22}]\lambda + m_{21}m_{22} = 0$ where the first subscript indicates the order of the phase resetting, and λ is the root of the characteristic equation of the linearized system about the point of phase-locking. In order for the phase-locking to be stable, the absolute value of λ must be less than one. If the second order terms $m_{2,k}$ are set to zero, the previous result is recovered.

Interestingly, the stability results are not changed by the presence of small synaptic delays, as shown in Fig. 7.2(B). One possible offset is illustrated here that is representative of a synaptic delay. The existence criterion can be obtained by rewriting the relationship of the offset interval and the stimulus and recovery times to each other and the period to correspond to the algebraic relationships illustrated in the figure. Instead of $t_{s,2} = t_{r,1}$ and $t_{s,1} = t_{r,2}$ as in Fig. 7.2(A), in Fig. 7.2(B) $t_{s,2} = t_{r,1} + \delta$, where δ is the offset, and $t_{s,1} = t_{r,2}$ is unchanged. The phase-locked period P_1 at steady state is now $t_{s,1} + t_{r,1} + \delta$ rather than $t_{s,1} + t_{r,1}$ as before. The rewrite can also be accomplished in an analogous manner for the postsynaptic receipt of a input that precedes presynaptic burst initiation, as might be the case in graded synaptic transmission.

7.3. Analysis of a Circuit of Two Model Neurons

In the application of PRC theory to a ring circuit of N oscillators, each oscillator is assumed to independently follow its own limit cycle, with the only effect of the coupling being to reset the phase of the postsynaptic oscillator along the limit cycle at the time of a burst in the presynaptic oscillator. The hallmark of a pattern, or mode, is that the phasic relationships between pre and postsynaptic oscillators are constant. Therefore, in a space composed of the $(N-1)$ relative phases of the oscillators, a pattern is simply a fixed point. The coordinates of these points can be determined by finding the points that satisfy the existence criteria. In a model system of identical, identically coupled neurons, the relative phases (with respect to a reference oscillator) in a mode that satisfies the existence criteria can be calculated by arbitrarily setting one to zero ($\theta_1 = 0$) and adding the normalized stimulus times around the ring to obtain the others: $\theta_n = \sum_{i=2}^{n}[\phi_i + F_2(\phi_i)]$. The analysis can easily be rewritten to include the effect of heterogeneity (see section 7.6). Given an intrinisic frequency and an initial phase for each oscillator in a ring, iterative tabulation of the phase resetting can predict all future behavior of the system under our assumptions; this process is referred to as circuit emulation. The phase of an oscillator is advanced along the limit cycle with the passage of time, but may also be instantaneously reset by being moved forward (advanced) or backward (delayed) along the limit cycle as a result of an input perturbation: $\dot{\theta}_i(t) = f - \delta(t - t_{n,i-i})F_1(\theta_i(t_{n,i-1})) - \delta(t - t_{n,i})F_2(\theta_i(t_{n-1,i-1}))$ where $F_1(\phi)$ constitutes the PRC curve for the effect on the first burst, $F_2(\phi)$ the effect on the second burst, f is the intrinsic frequency, t_n is the time of the most recent spike in the indexed oscillator, t_{n-1} is the time of the previous one, and $i-1$ is the index of the presynaptic oscillator. In other words, at the time an oscillator receives an input, its phase is instantaneously reset by the tabulated effect of an input on the next burst ($F_1(\phi)$), then, at the time this same oscillator fires its next burst, it is again instantaneously reset, but this time by the tabulated effect of the previous input on the second burst ($F_2(\phi)$).

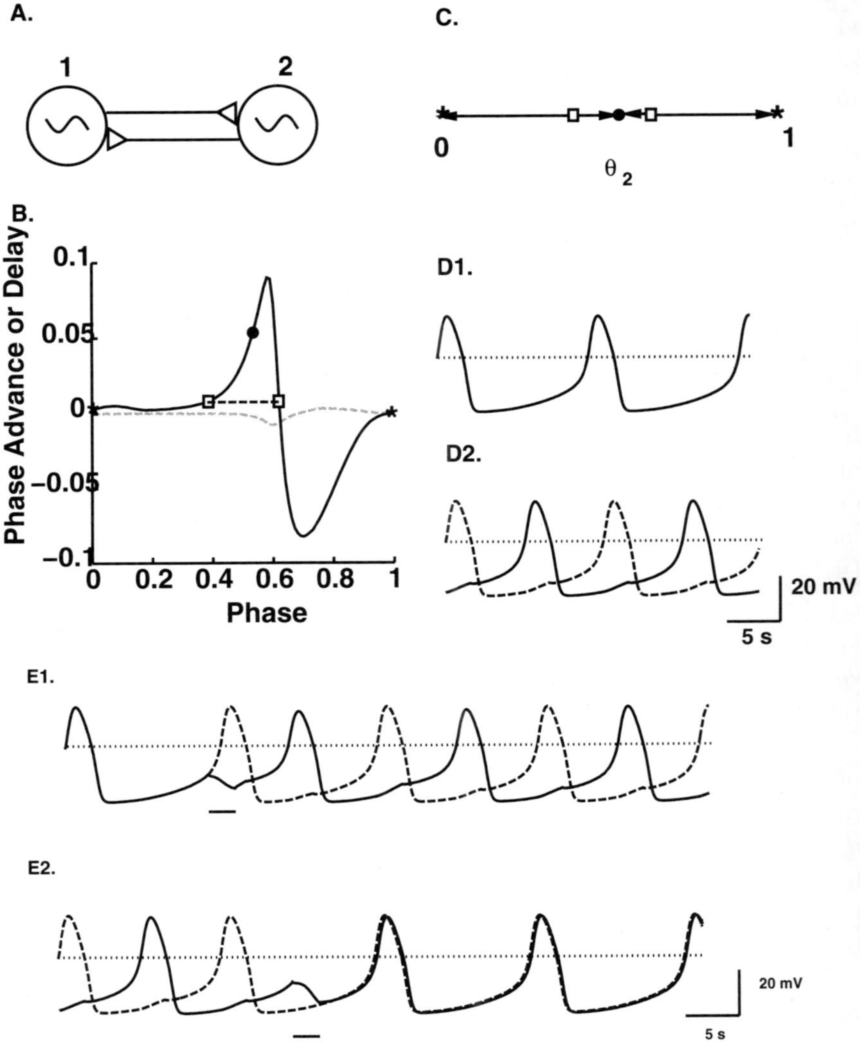

Fig. 7.3. **Ring of Two Oscillators Can Produce Two Stable Modes. A.** Circuit Diagram. **B.** Phase Response Curve. This PRC used a single presynaptic burst as the perturbation. The solid line shows $F(\phi)$, and the dotted line shows the contribution of $F_2(\phi)$. **C.** Emulator Phase Diagram. **D.** This circuit is capable of exhibiting a synchronous mode (**D1**) or an alternating mode (**D2**). The dotted line in both **D1** and **D2** as well as **E1** and **E2** indicates the threshold for the beginning of a burst. **E. E1** Transition from synchronous to alternating **E2** Transition from alternating to synchronous.
Adapted from Canavier *et al.* [6].

For this example and for the one for a ring of three model neurons in the next section, the model of Butera *et al.* [5] was used with the parameters set as in Figs. 5A and 6A of that study, except as noted in Canavier *et al.* [6]. This model is a four variable reduction of a model of a bursting neuron [8] that does not explicitly model spikes, but instead has a state variable that represents spiking frequency. For the purposes of this chapter, the model neuron can be considered to be spiking when the membrane potential exceeds a certain threshold. Fig. 7.3(A) shows two reciprocally connected identical oscillators with identical excitatory connections. The PRC shown in Fig. 7.3(B) predicts a stable synchronous mode with intervals equal to 0, as indicated by the asterisks as well as a stable alternating mode with intervals equal to $0.52P_i$, as indicated by the filled circle. In addition, a mode characterized by alternating intervals of $0.39P_i$ and $0.62P_i$, as indicated by the open squares, is predicted to be unstable. In the 1-D space of the emulator shown in Fig. 7.3(C) using the same symbols, the boundaries between the two stable modes are indicated on a line with the arrows indicating the direction of the flow, where 1 is equivalent to 0, and the unstable alternating mode forms the boundaries of the basins of attraction of the two stable modes. Using a transient switch signal, transitions between the synchronous and alternating modes could be induced by applying the stimulus at a phase of about 0.9 when the phase of the oscillator indicated by the dashed lines was reset by about 0.5 in order to produce a speedy transition (see Fig. 7.3(E)).

7.4. Stability Analysis for a Three Neuron Ring Circuit

The case for $N = 2$, where N is the number of oscillators in the ring, is the only one for which a closed form solution can be obtained in terms of the slopes of the PRCs (m_{ik}). For the case of $N > 2$, the system can not be reduced to a single state variable, but requires $N - 1$ coupled equations, if, for simplicity, second order resetting is ignored. In this section, the oscillators are assumed to be identical and identically connected. For circuits with more than two neurons, the firing order no longer has just a single possiblity other than synchrony: in the case of three neurons shown schematically in Fig. 7.4, the firing of neuron 2 can follow either neuron 1 (clockwise around the ring, panel (A)) or neuron 3 (counterclockwise, panel (B)). In the first case, the steady state stimulus intervals as defined above sum to the phase-locked period P_e, whereas in the second they sum to $2P_e$. Since all oscillators are phase locked at the same frequency, the sum of these

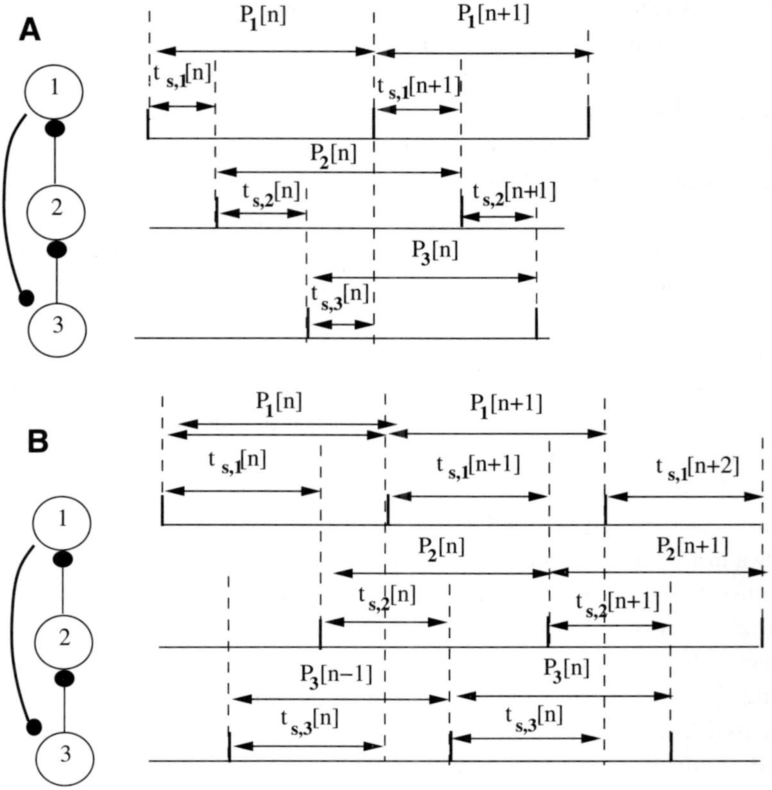

Fig. 7.4. **Ring of Three Oscillators Can Produce Different Firing Patterns.**

firing interval for a ring of N oscillators must be an integral multiple of P_e. The integral multiplier is designated j, takes a value from 1 to $N-1$, and uniquely characterizes the firing pattern. As in the previous sections, one can assume a stable phase locking, at $(\phi_1^*, \phi_2^*, \phi_3^*)$ and linearize about this fixed point of a discrete mapping of the phase. Note that for the firing mode in panel (A), each of the cycle periods can be expressed as a sum of three consecutive stimulus intervals, for example, $P_1[n] = t_{s,1}[n] + t_{s,2}[n] + t_{s,3}[n]$. The period can then be expressed both as having a linearized dependence on the phase of the input received in that cycle and, in the mode shown in Panel (A), as a sum of the stimulus intervals, where $t_{s,k} = P_i\phi_k$:

$$P_1[n] = P_i[1 + F_1(\phi_1^*) + m_{11}\Delta\phi_1[n]] = P_i\phi_1[n] + \phi_2[n] + \phi_3[n] \quad (3)$$

where $\phi_k[n] = \phi_k^*[n] + \Delta\phi_k$ and $\Delta\phi_k$ is the perturbation in phase from the assumed steady value. The assumed steady phase-locked period is equal to either $P_i[1 + F_1(\phi_k^*)]$ or $P_i(\phi_1^* + \phi_2^* + \phi_3^*)$. Similar equations can be written for the cycle periods of the other two neurons, and the steady state components on both sides cancel out to obtain a system of three equations can be written in terms of the perturbation in phase:

$$\Delta\phi_1[n] + \Delta\phi_2[n] + \Delta\phi_3[n] = m_{11}\Delta\phi_1[n] \quad (4)$$

$$\Delta\phi_2[n] + \Delta\phi_3[n] + \Delta\phi_1[n+1] = m_{12}\Delta\phi_2[n] \quad (5)$$

$$\Delta\phi_3[n] + \Delta\phi_1[n+1] + \Delta\phi_2[n+1] = m_{13}\Delta\phi_3[n] \quad (6)$$

The left hand side of each equation above gives the sum of the perturbations in each stimulus time, and the right hand side gives the linearized deviation in phase resetting from the steady state value in each cycle period due to the pertubation in stimulus time. The variable $\Delta\phi_3[n]$ can be eliminated by substitution using Eq. 4. This results in the following system:

$$\Delta\phi_1[n+1] = (1 - m_{11})\Delta\phi_1[n] + m_{12}\Delta\phi_2[n] \quad (7)$$

$$\Delta\phi_2[n+1] = m_3(m_{11} - 1)\Delta\phi_1[n] + (1 - m_{12} - m_{13})\Delta\phi_2[n] \quad (8)$$

The stability of this system can then be determined according to linear systems theory, which state that if the eigenvalues of the state matrix all have absolute value less than 1, the oscillatory mode associated with the linearized state matrix is stable.

The simplest way to set up the state matrix is to begin with the algebraic relationships of the form $t_{s,1}[n] + P_2[n] = P_1[n] + t_{s,1}[n+1]$ for each $t_{s,k}[n]$ (see Fig. 7.4). Eliminating the steady steady components gives the system:

$$\Delta\phi_1[n] + m_{12}\Delta\phi_2[n] = m_{11}\Delta\phi_1[n] + \phi_1[n+1] \quad (9)$$

$$\Delta\phi_2[n] + m_{13}\Delta\phi_3[n] = m_{12}\Delta\phi_1[n] + \phi_2[n+1] \quad (10)$$

$$\Delta\phi_3[n] + m_{11}\Delta\phi_3[n+2] = m_{13}\Delta\phi_3[n] + \phi_3[n+1] \quad (11)$$

A different approach is required in order to substitute for $\Delta\phi_3[n]$ in the first two equations, but this approach generalizes well [10] to higher values of N and j. In constrast to Panel (A) in Fig. 7.4, in Panel (B), j is equal to two rather than one such that two successive cycle lengths (rather than just one) can then be expressed as a sum of the stimulus intervals, such that:

$$\begin{aligned} P_1[n] + P_1[n+1] &= t_{s,1}[n] + t_{s,2}[n] + t_{s,3}[n] \\ &= P_i(\phi_1[n] + \phi_2[n] + \phi_3[n]) \end{aligned} \quad (12)$$

Each cycle can also be expressed as having a linearized dependence on the perturbation in phase from the assumed steady state of the inputs received in those cycles such that:

$$P_1[n] + P_1[n+1] = P_i[2 + 2F_1(\phi_1^*) + m_{11}(\Delta\phi_1[n] + \Delta\phi_1[n+1])] \quad (13)$$

Setting the above two expressions for $P_1[n] + P_1[n+1]$ equal to each other and eliminating steady components on either side gives:

$$\Delta\phi_1[n] + \Delta\phi_2[n] + \Delta\phi_3[n] = m_{11}\Delta\phi_1[n] + \Delta\phi_1[n+1] \quad (14)$$

This can easily be rewritten to allow substitution into Eqs. 9 and 10 above. Because the assumed firing pattern is different than in Panel (A), a different state matrix results:

$$\Delta\phi_1[n+1] = (1 - m_{11})\Delta\phi_1[n] + m_{12}\Delta\phi_2[n] \quad (15)$$

$$\Delta\phi_2[n+1] = m_{13}(1 - m_{11})^2\Delta\phi_1[n] + (1 - m_{12} - m_{13} + m_{11}m_{12}m_{13})\Delta\phi_2[n] \quad (16)$$

These equations result in a different characteristic equation, hence different eigenvalues than for the mode shown in Panel (A), given the same set of m_{1k}. This method has been generalized for any N, and appropriate j [10]. The stability criteria for $N = 3$ that include the contribution of second order resetting and allow for heterogeneity are derived in Oprisan and Canavier [28]. A different but equivalent derivation of the existence criteria is given in Luo *et al* [25].

Note the dependence of the stability criteria on firing order. In order to derive a criterion for the stability of synchrony, all possible firing modes that may occur upon a perturbation from synchrony must be anticipated, and all such perturbations must decay as indicated by eigenvalues with an absolute value less than one. In the case of synchrony, the likelihood that the slope of the PRC is different as a phase of zero is approached from the left or right is high [17], therefore in order guarantee stability at synchrony, one needs to confirm that the synchronous solution is robust to a perturbation giving rise to any possible firing order, in either direction using the left (m_{ik}^-) and right (m_{ik}^+) slopes as appropriate for the assumed convergence to synchrony.

7.5. Analysis of a Circuit of Three Model Neurons

The power of this method is illustrated by an example [6] in which it is applied to a system composed of three oscillators coupled in a ring via excitatory synapses (Fig. 7.5(A)), in order to produce the three distinct patterns

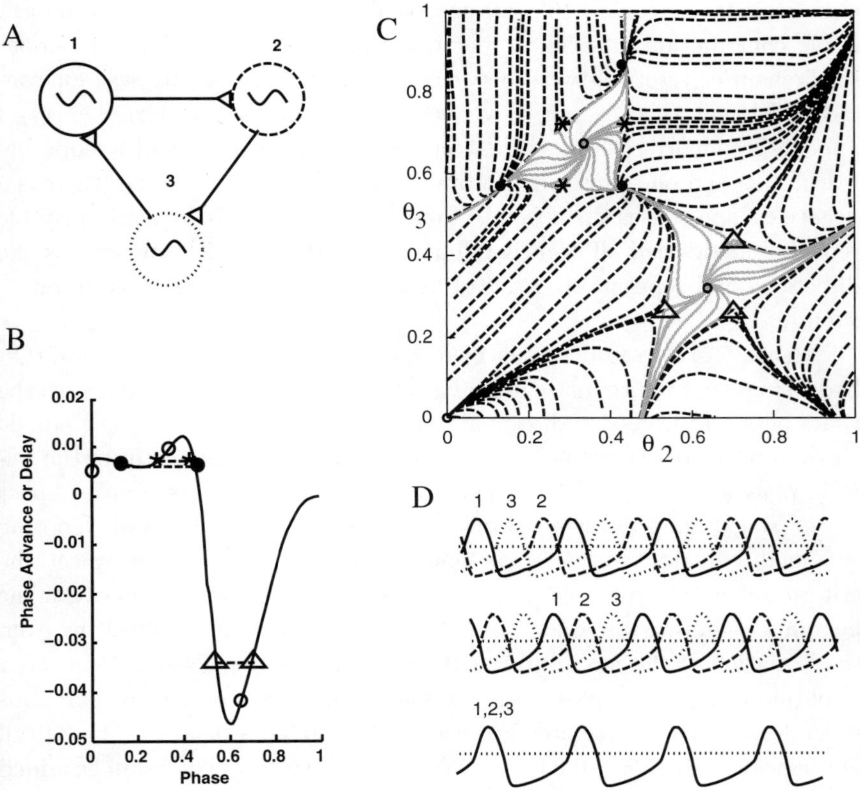

Fig. 7.5. **Ring of Three Oscillators Can Produce Three Stable Modes. A.** Three neuron circuit. **B.** Phase Response Curve. The counterclockwise (1,3,2) mode was predicted by the open circle at a phase of 0.337 in the phase response curve at the left and by the attractor (open circle at (0.34,0.67)). predicted in the θ_2/θ_3 plane at the right (see arrows). The clockwise (1,2,3) mode was predicted by the open circle at a phase of 0.638 on the PRC and by the attractor at (0.64,0.32). The synchronous mode was predicted by the open circle at a phase of zero on the PRC and by the attractor at (0,0) on the right. The boundaries for the attractive basins of the three modes are given by one unstable mode (filled circles) and two saddles (asterisks and open triangles). **C.** Emulator Phase Plane Portrait. Same symbols as in B. **D.** Three modes: top, counterclockwise, middle clockwise, bottom, synchrony. Adapted from Canavier *et al.* [6].

shown in Fig. 7.5(D). As in the example using two neurons, the model of Butera *et al.* [5] was used. The open loop PRC shown in Fig. 7.5(B) was used to predict all the periodic modes that fit the existence criteria given above. The criteria developed in the previous section apply except in the case of synchrony, so the stability of synchronous modes was determined using the rule of thumb that stable attractive modes have a small positive slope on the PRC at each values of ϕ. The form of the state matrix and characteristic equations [10] were such that in every case that we examined, if the contribution of second order resetting was ignored and if all slopes for first order resetting were between zero and one, stability was guaranteed. Although this was not proven for the general case, the term $(1-m_{1k})$ appears frequently in the expressions for the eigenvalues, and a slope between zero and one causes its absolute value to be less than one whereas a negative slope causes the absolute value to exceed one. In general, unstable repelling modes had all negative slopes, and saddles, which attract in some directions and repel in others, had at least one positive and one negative value.

All of the stable modes, identified by open circles in Fig. 7.5(B) and (C), had a single ϕ, or normalized stimulus interval, associated with them, so the times between successive threshold crossings were identical, and each mode corresponded to a single point in the phase plane constructed from the relative phases (see Fig. 7.5(C)). Synchronous, counterclockwise (with respect to the ring), and clockwise modes were predicted and observed. Ignoring the small contribution of $F_2(\phi)$, one can see that these modes meet the criteria by adding the succesive normalized stimulus intervals between the beginning of a burst in a neuron and the receipt on an input resulting from the initiation of the next burst in the neuron presynaptic to it to in order to obtain integer multiples of the normalized entrained period: synchronous $(0+0+0=0(1+0))$, counterclockwise $(0.337+0.337+0.337=1(1+0.01))$, and clockwise $(0.638+0.638+0.638=2(1-0.043))$. The number added to one in the parentheses is the normalized predicted first order resetting. Note that each of the three stable modes has a different integer value of j. In addition to the three stable patterns, the analysis of the PRC predicted an unstable mode with one ϕ of 0.139 and two of 0.438, indicated by the two connected filled circles $(0.139+0.438+0.438=1(1+0.015))$. This mode is an unstable repellor because the slopes associated with both of these ϕ are negative. Finally, two saddles, corresponding to the pairs of points represented by asterisks and by open triangles, were also identified, each with one positive slope and one negative. The pairs of points that compose each saddle are also connected by a horizontal dashed line: the upper set of asterisks is at 0.285 (value of ϕ repeated twice) and 0.437, and the lower set of asterisks is at 0.532 and 0.705 (repeated twice). These also meet the criteria: $(0.285+0.285+0.437=1(1+0.007))$ and $(0.532+0.705+0.705=2(1-0.029))$. Each of these "border" modes has two distinct phases, or stimulus times associated with it, so they are asymmetric and have three rotational variants each because the value repeated only once can be associated with any of the three distinct stimulus intervals. These rotational variants are indicated by the appropriate symbols in the phase plane on the right. The curves in the phase plane at the right of Fig. 7.5 indicate the trajectories in this space that were emulated as described above, using the equation for $\dot{\theta}$ also given above, and confirmed by simulations of the full model system. The entire flow can be mapped by the trajectories emanating from the three unstable fixed points (filled circles), which are first attracted and then repelled by the six saddle points (asterisks and triangles) and ultimately end up on one of the three attractors (open circles). This map shows the basin of attraction for synchrony by the dashed black lines, whereas the other two basins of attraction are shown in gray. Transitions between modes in this multistable system could be achieved using transient perturbations from one basin to another (not shown) [6]. Similar complete analyses of circuits composed of four oscillators have been conducted [6], and the method can be applied to any unidirectional ring circuit of oscillators and completely describes the activity of the circuit under the assumption of 1:1 entrainment.

7.6. Analysis of a Two Neuron Hybrid Circuit

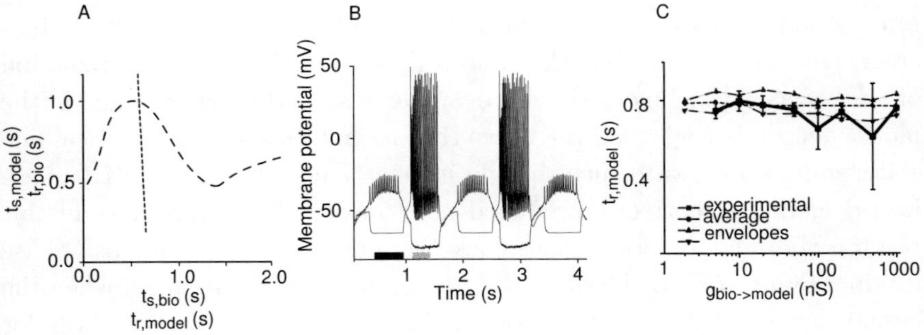

Fig. 7.6. **Prediction of Phase-locking in the Hybrid Circuit. A.** The intersection of t_s in the model neuron (short dashes, vertical line) with t_r in the biological neuron (curve, longer dashes) gives the predicted intervals in 1:1 phase-locking. **B.** Membrane potential waveforms for both the model (tall) and biological (short) neuron in the observed phase locking. The intrinsic burst duration for each neuron is shown as a bar on the x-axis. **C.** Results of predictions not only using the average PRC but also the upper and lower envelopes of the PRC compared to average experimentally observed values (thick line). Adapted from Oprisan *et al.* [29].

It is crucial to apply our methods to real neurons as well as to models because neural oscillators are not mathematical abstractions but rather living cells. In order to test the applicability of our circuit analysis to physiological neurons, a hybrid circuit of one modeled bursting neuron and one biological bursting neuron was constructed. The biological bursting "neuron" used here was actually three electrically coupled neurons in the pyloric circuit in the stomatogastric ganglion of the lobster: the AB pacemaker and two PD neurons. These three neurons were treated as a single functional oscillator, and all recordings were made from one of the PD neurons. The hybrid circuit was constructed using the Dynamic Clamp protocol [38] to implement reciprocally inhibitory computer-generated synapses. Open loop PRCs were generated for both the model and the biological neurons using a rectangular pulse in synaptic conductance with a duration equal to the free-running burst duration in its partner in the hybrid circuit. In the closed loop circuit, the synaptic conductances had a steep dependence on presynaptic membrane potential, so that the pulses in conductances were also rectangular and active when the presynaptic neuron exceeded a preset threshold. A total of 164 hybrid networks [29] were formed by varying the component neurons and the synaptic conductances. The prediction of the presence or absence of 1:1 phase locking agreed qualitatively with the experimental observations, except in three hybrid circuits in which 1:1 locking was predicted but not observed. Figure 7.6(A) shows pairs of stimulus and recovery intervals calculated for the model and biological neuron. The intersection of these curves satifies the periodicity constraints for a heterogenous two-neuron network given in Eqs. 1 and 2 and is the prediction of a 1:1 phase locked mode. In this example, if second order resetting in the model neuron is neglected, the curve that resembles a straight vertical line shifts shifted downward such that no intersection exists, and the 1:1 phase locked mode is incorrectly predicted not to exist. The significance of this result is that manipulations that block $F_2(\phi)$ are predicted to abolish phase locking. Figure 7.6(B) shows the 1:1 phase-locked mode obtained when the circuit was closed. The intersection point in part A predicted 0.773s for $t_{r,model}$ compared to an actual average value of 0.776s, (0.4% error), 0.656s for $t_{r,bio}$ versus 0.746s, (12% error), and 1.429s for the phase-locked period versus 1.522s (6% error). This reasonable agreement was obtained despite the increase in model neuron burst duration to 0.5s in the closed loop from its open loop value of 0.28s. A summary of the predictions of recovery intervals for the model is shown in Fig. 7.6(C) over a range of conductance values. The quantitative accuracy of the predictions generally fell within the variability (10%) in the experimentally observed intrinsic period and PRC.

In addition, in 9 out of the 164 hybrid circuits stable phase-locking would be incorrectly predicted to be unstable if the effects of the second order phase resetting on the stability criterion were not considered. The method was robust to offsets between the initiation of bursting in the presynaptic neuron and the activation of the synaptic coupling with the postsynaptic neuron when these offsets were incorporated in the definition of the stimulus or recovery intervals as appropriate.

A central role for neurons that are endogenous bursters in the neuromodulatory contexts of their particular CPGs [37] has been demonstrated in the heartbeat of crustacea [40], the swimming CPG of the mollusc *Clione limacina* [3], the pyloric and gastric CPGs of the crustacean stomatogastric system [20, 31, 36], the feeding CPG in molluscs [2, 3], flight in the locust [33], swimming in the lamprey [41] and respiration in neonatal rodents [39]. Therefore, the results obtained for bursting neurons may be widely applicable.

7.7. Effect of Changing Burst Durations in the Two Neuron Circuit

In the three out of a total of 164 hybrid circuits in which incorrect predictions were made, it is likely that the reason was that the burst duration was indeed variable as a result of burst truncation in the biological neuron at precisely the phases at which locking was predicted. Therefore, existence and stability criteria for the case of variable burst duration [28] were derived under the following assumptions: 1) In 1:1 locking, the phasic relationships remain constant with the additional contraint that the burst duration in each neuron is constant in the steady phase-locked mode. 2) The duration of the postsynaptic burst in the closed loop configuration can be inferred from the open loop effects of a perturbation on burst duration. The change ($G_{1k}(\phi_k, \tau)$) from the intrinsic burst duration $b_{k,i}$ observed in the open loop condition in the burst that contains the perturbation as well as the change ($G_{2k}(\phi_k, \tau)$) in the duration of the burst in the cycle after the one that contains the perturbation, where τ_j is the normalized duration of the perturbation in the presynaptic neuron, can be directly measured. These effects are additive and dissipate by the time the next input is received. 3) The sensitivity of the change in burst duration in the postsynaptic neuron in the closed loop condition to a slight change in input phase (duration) can be determined from the slope of a plot of $G_{ik}(\phi_k, \tau_j)$ versus phase (duration) with duration (phase) held constant. This produces the required partial derivatives. 4) The phase resetting curves can be determined as a function of presynaptic burst duration as well as phase: $F_{ik}(\phi_k, \tau_j)$, where i is the order and k is the kth neuron. 5) The shape of the conductance pulse either does not vary independently from duration or any variation does not affect the resultant phase resetting, such that all conductance pulses in the open and closed loop conditions that have the same duration produce the same resetting and the same change in burst duration.

The additional criterion that the normalized steady state burst duration (b_k^*) in each neuron remain constant under closed loop conditions can be written as follows:

$$b_1^* = 1 + G_{11}(\phi_1^*, (P_{2i}/P_{1i})b_2^*) + G_{12}(\phi_1^*, (P_{2i}/P_{1i})b_2^*) \tag{17}$$

$$b_2^* = 1 + G_{12}(\phi_2^*, (P_{1i}/P_{2i})b_1^*) + G_{22}(\phi_2^*, (P_{1i}/P_{2i})b_1^*) \tag{18}$$

Only pairs of (ϕ_1, ϕ_2) for which the above conditions hold need be considered. The pair of (b_1^*, b_2^*) values for each (ϕ_1, ϕ_2) pair can be determined, and the location of the fixed point can then be determined using a slight modification of the periodicity criteria given in Eqns. 1 and 2 to incorporate dependencies on burst duration:

$$P_{1i}[\phi_1^* + F_{21}(\phi_1^*, b_2^*))] = P_{2i}[1 - \phi_2^* + F_{12}(\phi_2^*, b_1^*)] \tag{19}$$

$$P_{2i}[\phi_2^* + F_{22}(\phi_2^*, b_1^*))] = P_{1i}[1 - \phi_1^* + F_{11}(\phi_1^*, b_2^*)] \tag{20}$$

where the terms on the left are the stimulus intervals and the terms on the right are the response intervals. The solution can be visualized as before, by plotting the values of t_{sk} and t_{rk} after identifying sets of $(\phi_1, \phi_2, b_1, b_2)$ that satisfy the equalities given above. The intersection point is the predicted 1:1 phase-locked mode.

Thus the revised stability criterion includes the effects of the first and second order resetting plus the dependence of the PRC on the duration of the normalized input perturbation $\tau_j[n]$, using the derivative of the PRC $h_{ik} = (\partial F_{ik}/\partial \tau)_\phi$ with respect to burst duration, as well as on the previously defined derivative with respect to phase $m_{ik} = (\partial F_{ik}/\partial \phi)_\tau$, where the subscript i refers to the order and k to the neuron. Two state variables were added to the system of linearized equations that was obtained previously because of the need to keep track of input durations as well as input phases in order to calculate the phase resetting. The derivatives of the transient change in postsynaptic burst duration curve with respect to phase and presynaptic burst duration are given by $p_{ik} = (\partial G_{ik}/\partial \phi)_\tau$ and $q_{ik} = (\partial G_{ik}/\partial \tau)_\phi$. The characteristic equation (not shown) associated with the resultant linearized system of equations was obtained as before using the Z-transform method on the linearized perturbation in the state vector, which has four dimensions $\Delta[n] = [\Delta\phi_1[n], \Delta\phi_2[n], \Delta\tau_1[n], \Delta\tau_2[n]]$. The mapping treats phase resetting based on the input phase and duration, but if the duration of the burst is changed (truncated or elongated) in the same cycle as the perturbation is received, the duration of an input may change *after* the phase resetting attributed to that input has already been calculated, hence the mapping and the stability result only strictly applies as written if the burst is not truncated ($\Delta b_{1k}(\phi_k, \tau_k) = 0$). This problem with causality could be resolved by treating a presynaptic burst as having two components, one occurring before the postsynaptic burst and one after.

In the three cases for which incorrect predictions were made in the in the hybrid circuits described above [29], stable 1:1 phase-locking was predicted but no 1:1 locking was observed. Instead, a firing pattern that was highly variable was observed. The failures were the only cases in which the biological neuron was predicted to receive an input at a phase that would truncate its burst. It is likely that the predicted modes did not satify the additional criteria given above for the burst duration to remain constant within a phase locked mode.

7.8. Phenomenology of Resetting in a Biological Bursting Neuron

In order to generalize our results to real neurons in which the burst duration and perhaps other parameters vary as a result of closing the loop, it is important to understand the phenomenology of phase resetting in bursting neurons and how it depends on such parameters. A test of our understanding of phase resetting is whether it can be predicted from just the time series of the membrane potential in an unperturbed oscillator. The AB/PD oscillator kernel described above was again used as an exemplar of an endogenously bursting biological oscillator. All recordings were made from one of the PD neurons, and the perturbations used to generate PRCs were applied to the same PD neuron using the Dynamic Clamp [38]. The perturbation was a pulse in synaptic conductance, and the synaptic current generated by such a pulse was calculated in real time by the Dynamic Clamp software based on the postsynaptic potential in the PD neuron. The first order phase resetting [30] in a biological bursting neuron was predicted by assuming that the bursting neuron could be characterized as a relaxation oscillator rather than as an integrator or resonator. A relaxation

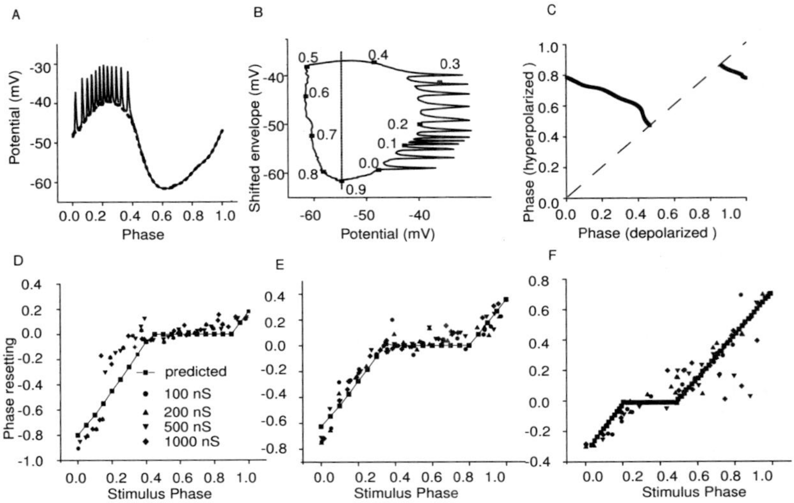

Fig. 7.7. **Phase Resetting in the PD Neuron A.** The solid line indicates the membrane potentisl, and the dashed line is the membrane envelope. **B.** The membrane potential is plotted against a delayed version of the envelope, producing a limit cycle. The vertical line separates the depolarized and hyperpolarized branches. The numbered squares indicate the temporal phase. **C.** The map between phases on the hyperpolarized and depolarized branches at a constant value of the envelope potential. **D.** Predicted phase resetting (black square) including only normal resetting for 100 msec pulses at 4 different values of synaptic conductance. **E.** Predicted phase resetting (black squares) including both normal resetting and wait time for a 250 msec pulse at four conductance values. **F.** Same as E for a 750 msec pulse. Adapted from Oprisan *et al.* [30].

oscillator has a predominant slow time scale, and its limit cycle has two distinct stable branches, here hyperpolarized, silent branch corresponding to the interburst, and a depolarized, spiking branch corresponding to the burst. The trajectory jumps between branches at the "knees" corresponding to the termination points of the stable branches. The slow variable provides the negative feedback that causes switching between branches resulting in periodic bursting. The limit cycle was reconstructed (Fig. 7.7(A) and (B)), using the membrane potential plotted versus a delayed version of the envelope of the membrane potential. The envelope is a spline fit to the potential waveform with the spikes removed, and provides the slow time scale required to the reconstruction of a relaxation oscillator. Only inhibitory perturbations were used, and all perturbations were assumed to be strong enough to induce a switch from the depolarized to the hyperpolarized branch, resulting in premature burst termination. The membrane potential was assumed to vary much more rapidly than the presumed slow variable such that the displacement caused by the perturbation applied on the depolarized branch is parallel to the x-axis in Fig. 7.7(B) and results in a transition along a horizontal line to the hyperpolarized branch. On the other hand, a short pulse applied during the interburst was assumed not to disturb the trajectory, but rather result in zero phase resetting. A map (Fig. 7.7(C)) was constructed of the phase on the depolarized branch to the phase on the hyperpolarized branch that shared a common value of the y-axis. The difference between the two phases predicts the phase advance due to a switch between branches. These assumptions resulted in predictions in reasonable agreement with the data for short pulses (100msec) (Fig. 7.7(D)). The magnitude of the conductance did not affect predictions since all pulses were assumed to be strong enough to cause a jump. For short pulses, the trajectory could be assumed to be instantaneously reset without significant error. For longer pulses, the inhibition was often still active at the time the trajectory would be predicted to jump from the hyperpolarized to the depolarized branch. Therefore, a delay was incurred because the jump could not be made until pulse offset. The "waiting" component of the phase resetting can be easily calculated, and allowed the successful prediction (Fig. 7.7(E) and (F)) of pulses as long as 750msec, which was half of the intrinsic period.

7.9. Significance

A recent line of research (for a review see [35]) also derived stability and existence criteria for synchrony and antisynchrony while making few assumptions except that the component neurons are endogenous oscillators with synaptic coupling, but the criteria developed were in terms of the equations that characterize the oscillator and synaptic dynamics. In contrast, our predictions of phase-locked modes and stability results do not assume any knowledge of the system equations, but rather use PRCs that can readily be generated experimentally to confirm the mapping between theory and reality. In addition, our methods dispense with restrictive assumptions commonly used in proofs regarding phase-locking. One such assumption is to consider only integrators rather than resonators or relaxation oscillators. Results regarding the existence and stability of phase-locked modes have been obtained for integrators with weak coupling under the assumption of a nonphysiological concave down waveform [26], for electrically coupled integrators [9] or for integrators with strong coupling [4]. Others have assumed Type I excitability (an integrator) and employed the concept of a recovery interval to derive results for synchronization with delays [13]. However, even recent work [17] that is based on our own proposed PRC methodology assumes resetting at a phase of zero is equal to zero and does not include second order resetting, and consequently does not consider the possibility that firing order does not remain constant during the convergence to synchrony. Other recent theoretical work [1] has suggested the need to incorporate second order resetting, and experimental observations [34] have shown that pyramidal neocortical spiking neurons do indeed exhibit second order resetting. The contribution of $F_2(\phi)$ is likely to be maximal when an input is delivered just prior to a spike, as may often occur during convergence to synchrony. This in turn may cause violation of a cherished assumption encountered in decades of stability of synchrony proofs [17, 24, 26], that the firing order of the oscillators is invariant.

Whereas the methods presented herein were able to incorporate short duration synaptic delays, a similar study employing phase response methods analysed the effects of long delays in feedback to a single oscillator [14, 15]. Our methodology is applicable to pulsatile coupling under the assumption that the trajectory return close to the limit cycle before the next input is received. This requirement is essential, because if the trajectory is not on the limit cycle one cannot calculate the phase in order to apply the open loop PRC. The other essential assumption is that the phase resetting produced by the synaptic inputs in the closed loop can be approximated (or inferred from) the inputs from the same sources in the open loop condition. This assumption is quite valid for spiking neurons, but bursting neurons have special problems that probably do not apply to spiking neurons in that closing the loop can change the duration and shape of the burst, which in turn changes the input received by the neurons to which it projects. For the bursting neuron studied in the previous section, the phase resetting is often but not always invariant to burst duration. In sum, the innovation presented herein of considering the second order resetting for bursting neurons may also be necessary for spiking neurons in some cases, but the problem of variable input duration is unique to bursting neurons. The methodology presented herein can be applied to many different circuit configurations, as long as the phase is well defined at the time that an input is received.

Acknowledgments

I would like to acknowledge the important contributions to the research presented in this chapter that were made by Sorinel Oprisan, Rob Butera,

Doug Baxter, Jack Byrne, Ron Dror, John Clark, Chuan Luo, Astrid Prinz, Vatsala Thirumalai, and Eve Marder. This work was partially supported by a National Science Foundation grant number 0118117 (CCC), a Whitaker Foundation Biomedical Engineering Transitional Funding grant number TF-98-033 (CCC), and two NIH grants to Doug Baxter (R01 RR11626 and P01 NS38310).

References

[1] C. Acker, N. Kopell, and J. White, Synchronization of strongly coupled excitatory neurons: relating network behavior to biophysics, *J. Computationl Neurosci.* **15**, 71–90, (2003).

[2] Y. Arshavshy, T. Deliagina, G. Orlovsky, and Y. V. Panchin, Control of feeding movements in pteropod mollusc *Clione limacina*, *Exp. Brain Res.* **78**, 387–397, (1989).

[3] Y. Arshavshy, S. Grillner, G. Orlovsky, and Y. V. Panchin. Central pattern generators and the spatiotemporal pattern of movements. In eds. J. Fagard and P. Wolff, *The Development of Timing Control*, pp. 93–115. Elsevier, Amsterdam, (1991).

[4] P. Bressloff and S. Coombes, Dynamics of strongly-coupled spiking neurons, *Neural Computation.* **12**, 91–129, (2000).

[5] R. J. Butera Jr., C. C. Canavier, D. A. Baxter, J. W. Clark, and J. H. Byrne, Analysis of the effects of modulatory agents on a model bursting neuron: Dynamic interactions between voltage and calcium-dependent systems, *J. Comp. Neurosci.* **2**, 19–44, (1995).

[6] C. C. Canavier, D. A. Baxter, J. W. Clark, and J. H. Byrne, Control of multistability in ring circuits of oscillators, *Biol. Cybernetics.* **80**, 87–102, (1999).

[7] C. C. Canavier, R. J. Butera, R. O. Dror, D. A. Baxter, J. W. Clark, and J. H. Byrne, Phase response characteristics of model neurons determine which patterns are expressed in a ring circuit model of gait generation, *Biol. Cybernetics.* **77**, 367–380, (1997).

[8] C. C. Canavier, J. W. Clark, and J. H. Byrne, Simulation of the bursting activity of neuron R15 in *Aplysia*: Role of ionic currents, calcium balance, and modulatory transmitters, *J. Neurophysiol.* **66**, 2107–2124, (1991).

[9] C. Chow and N. Kopell, Dynamics of spiking neurons with electrical coupling, *Neural Computation.* **12**, 1643–1678, (2000).

[10] R. O. Dror, C. C. Canavier, R. J. Butera, J. W. Clark, and J. H.

Byrne, A mathematical criterion based on phase response curves for the stability of a ring network of oscillators, *Biol. Cybernetics.* **80**, 25–44, (1999).

[11] G. B. Ermentrout, Type I membranes, phase resetting curves, and synchrony, *Neural Computation.* **8**, 979–1002, (1996).

[12] G. B. Ermentrout and N. Kopell, Multiple pulse interactions and averaging in systems of coupled neural oscillators, *J. Math. Biology.* **50**, 125–146, (1991).

[13] G. B. Ermentrout and N. Kopell, Fine structure of neural spiking and synchronization in the presence of conduction delays, *PNAS.* **95**, 1259–1264, (1998).

[14] J. Foss and M. J, Multistability in recurrent neural loops arising from delay, *J. Neurophysiol.* **84**, 975–985, (2000).

[15] J. Foss, F. Moss, and M. J, Noise, multistability, and delayed recurrent loops, *Physical Review E.* **55**(4), 4536–4543, (1997).

[16] L. Glass and M. C. Mackey, *From Clocks to Chaos: the Rhythms of Life.* (Princeton University Press, Princeton, N. J., 1988).

[17] P. Goel and G. B. Ermentrout, Synchrony, stability, and firing patterns in pulse-coupled oscillators, *Physica D.* **163**, 191–216, (2002).

[18] B. S. Gutkin and G. B. Ermentrout, Dynamics of membrane excitability determine interspike interval variability: A link between spike generation mechanisms and cortical spike train statistics, *Neural Computation.* **10**, 1047–1065, (1998).

[19] D. Hansel, G. Mato, and C. Meunier, Synchrony in excitatory neural networks, *Neural Computation.* **7**, 307–335, (1995).

[20] R. Harris-Warrick, E. Marder, A. Selverston, and M. Moulins, Eds., *The Stomatogastric Nervous System.* (MIT Press, Cambridge, MA, 1992).

[21] F. C. Hoppensteadt and E. Izhikevich, *Weakly Connected Neural Networks.* vol. 126, *Springer Series of Appled Mathematical Science*, (Springer-Verlag, New York, 1997).

[22] E. Izhikevich, Neural excitability, spiking, and bursting, *International Journal of Bifurcation and Chaos.* **10**(6), 1171–1266, (2000).

[23] N. Kopell and G. B. Ermentrout, Symmetry and phaselocking in chains of weakly coupled oscillators, *Communications on Pure and Applied Mathematics.* **90**, 87–109, (1988).

[24] Y. Kuramoto, *Chemical Oscillations, Waves and Turbulence.* (Springer-Verlag, Berlin, 1984).

[25] C. Luo, C. Canavier, D. Baxter, J. Byrne, and J. Clark, Multimodal

behavior in a four neuron ring circuit: mode switching., *IEEE Transactions on Biomedical Engineering.* **51**, 205–218, (2004).

[26] R. Mirollo and S. Strogatz, Synchronization of pulse-coupled biological oscillators, *SIAM Journal of Applied Mathematics.* **50**, 1645–1662, (1990).

[27] S. A. Oprisan and C. C. Canavier, Stability analysis of rings of coupled pulse-coupled oscillators: The effect of phase resetting in the second cycle after the pulse is important at synchrony and for long pulses, *Differential Equations and Dynamical Systems.* **9**, 242–259, (2001).

[28] S. A. Oprisan and C. C. Canavier, Stability criterion for a two-neuron reciprocally coupled network based on the phase and burst resetting curves, *Neurocomputing.* (in press).

[29] S. A. Oprisan, A. Prinz, and C. C. Canavier, Phase resetting and phase locking in hybrid circuits of one model and one biological neuron, *Biophys. J.* **87**, 2283–2298, (2004).

[30] S. A. Oprisan, V. Thirumalai, and C. C. Canavier, Dynamics from a time series: Can we extract a phase resetting curve from a time series?, *Biophys. J.* **84**, 2919–2928, (2003).

[31] Y. V. Panchin, Y. Arshavshy, A. Selverston, and T. Cleland, Lobster stomatogastric neurons in primary culture, *J. Neurophysiol.* **69**, 1967–1992, (1993).

[32] D. H. Perkel, J. H. Schulman, T. H. Bullock, G. P. Moore, and J. P. Segundo, Pacemaker neurons: effects of regularly spaced synaptic input, *Science.* **145**, 61–63, (1964).

[33] J. Ramirez and K. Pearson, Octopominergic modulation of interneurons in the flight system of the locust, *J. Neurophysiol.* **66**, 1522–1537, (1991).

[34] A. Reyes and E. E. Fetz, Two modes of interspike interval shortening by brief transient depolarizations in cat neocortical neurons, *J. Neurophysiol.* **69**, 1661–1672, (1993).

[35] J. E. Rubin and D. Terman. Geometric singular perturbation analysis of neuronal dynamics. In ed. B. Fiedler, *Handbook of Dynamical Systems: Toward Applications*, vol. 2. Elsevier, Amsterdam, (2002).

[36] A. Selverston and M. Moulins, Eds., *The Crustacean Stomatogastric System.* (Springer, Berlin, 1987).

[37] A. Selverston, Y. V. Panchin, Y. Arshavshy, and G. Orlovsky. Shared features of invertebrate central pattern generators. In eds. P. S. G. Stein, S. Grillner, A. I. Seleverston, and D. G. Stuart, *Neurons, Networks, and Motor Behavior*, pp. 105–117. The MIT Press, Cambridge,

Massachusetts, (1997).
[38] A. Sharp, M. O'Neil, L. Abbott, and E. Marder, The dynamic clamp: computer-generated conductances in real neurons, *J. Neurophysiol.* **69**, 992–995, (1993).
[39] J. Smith, H. Ellenberger, K. Ballanyi, D. Richter, and J. Feldman, Pre-Botzinger complex: A brainstem region that may generate respiratory rhythm in mammals, *Science.* **254**, 726–729, (1991).
[40] K. Tasaki and I. M. Cooke, Characterization of Ca current underlying burst formation in lobster cardiac ganglion motorneurons, *J. Neurophysiol.* **63**, 370–384, (1990).
[41] P. Wallen and S. Grillner, N-methyl D-aspartate receptor-induced, inherent oscillatory activity in neurons active during fictive locomotion in the lamprey, *J. Neurosci.* **7**, 2745–2755, (1987).
[42] A. T. Winfree, *The Timing of Biological Clocks.* (Scientific American Books, New York, 1987).

CHAPTER 8

BURSTING IN COUPLED CELL SYSTEMS

Martin Golubitsky
Krešimir Josić
Department of Mathematics, University of Houston
Houston TX 77204-3008, USA
e-mail: mg@uh.edu; josic@math.uh.edu

LieJune Shiau
Department of Mathematics, University of Houston–Clear Lake
Houston TX 77058, USA
e-mail: shiau@cl.uh.edu

Periodic bursting in fast-slow systems can be viewed as closed paths through the unfolding parameters of degenerate singularities. Using this approach we show that bursting in coupled systems can have interesting behavior. We focus on two identical cell systems and use the $\mathbf{Z}_2$ symmetry present in such systems to illustrate interesting bursting phenomena. In particular, we show that Hopf/Hopf mode interactions can lead to bursting between in phase and out of phase periodic solutions and symmetry-breaking Takens-Bogdanov singularities can lead to bursting that randomly chooses between two (symmetrically related) limit cycles.

8.1. Introduction

Many processes in nature are characterized by transitions between different modes of activity, such as periodic, quasiperiodic, chaotic and quiescent states. An example of an autonomous differential equation whose behavior alternates between near steady-states and trains of approximate spike-like oscillations was analyzed by Rinzel [13, 16], and such behavior has since been referred to as bursting. From a mathematical point of view, it is also natural to consider transitions between other attracting states in a similar vein, and this is the viewpoint we will adopt in this chapter.

The large number of possible states and transitions between them necessitates a coherent method of classifying different types of bursting systems. Early classifications using roman numerals assigned to the different bursters in the order of their description in the literature, or based on qualitative properties of the timeseries proved impractical. Systematic methods were soon introduced (see [2, 11], for example).

In [6, 11] a method was introduced for classifying the types of bursting that occur in models in which variables evolve on two different timescales, i.e., fast-slow systems. The classification is based on the observation that the bifurcations of the fast system that lead to bursting can be collapsed to a single local bifurcation, generally of higher codimension. The bursting is recovered as the slow variables periodically trace a closed path in the universal unfolding of this singularity. The codimension of a periodic bursting type is then defined to be the codimension of the singularity in whose unfolding it first appears. Using this definition, all of the known universal unfoldings of codimension one and two bifurcations were analyzed to classify the codimension one and two bursters.

This local approach has several advantages over global analytic and geometric methods that are also used to classify bursters. Many bifurcations that are first observed globally can be studied more easily by using the unfolding theory of degenerate singularities, since the local theory provides methods by which global phenomena can be found locally using calculus and numerical techniques. Moreover, the local theory provides a rational method of classification by codimension that indicates how complex a system needs to be in order for it to support bursters of given types.

The goal of this chapter is to illustrate how the ideas described in [6] can be extended to networks of bursting systems. To avoid technicalities, and give an accessible introduction to these ideas, we only consider networks of two coupled identical cells. The assumption that the cells are identical leads to $\mathbf{Z}_2$ symmetry in the equations of motions. The unfoldings of singularities in the presence of such symmetries can be very different from the general case and lead to new and surprising phenomena.

The chapter is organized as follows. In section 8.2, we review the theory introduced in [6], and in section 8.3 we adapt the discussion to two-cell systems. In section 8.4 we review the codimension one and two bifurcations in $\mathbf{Z}_2$-equivariant systems. Bursters associated to steady-state pitchfork bifurcations are discussed in section 8.5. Those associated with Hopf/Hopf mode interactions and Takens-Bogdanov bifurcations are discussed in sections 8.6

and 8.7. Hopf/Hopf mode interactions can lead to bursting between in phase and out of phase periodic solutions and symmetry-breaking Takens-Bogdanov bifurcations can lead to a form of chaotic dynamics where the bursting randomly chooses between two symmetrically related limit cycles and steady-states. A similar phenomenon can occur in pitchfork bifurcations, but only when noise is added to the system.

8.2. Unfolding Theory and Bursting in Fast-Slow Systems

We consider bursting that occurs in models consisting of variables that evolve on a fast and a slow timescale, and can therefore be described by equations of the form

$$\begin{aligned} x' &= f(x, y) \\ y' &= \varepsilon g(x, y), \end{aligned}$$

where $\varepsilon > 0$ is small, $x \in \mathbf{R}^n$, $y \in \mathbf{R}^k$, $f : \mathbf{R}^n \times \mathbf{R}^k \to \mathbf{R}^n$, and $g : \mathbf{R}^n \times \mathbf{R}^k \to \mathbf{R}^k$.

In periodic bursters, the slow variables y oscillate periodically, and thus provide a time-periodic forcing in the fast x' equation. In turn, the solution of the fast equation visits various invariant sets in order. The slow variables either provide this forcing effectively *without* feedback from the fast system, or *with* feedback from the fast system. In the former case, the system may be modeled as:

$$\begin{aligned} x' &= f(x, y) \\ y' &= \varepsilon g(y), \end{aligned} \tag{2}$$

with the slow component only depending on the slow variable y. A reduction to (2) can also be made in the latter case, under certain assumptions.

Assuming that the slow system varies periodically, we rewrite (2) as

$$x' = f(x, y(\varepsilon t)). \tag{3}$$

If ε is sufficiently small, the solution of (3) visits the stable invariant states of the frozen system

$$x' = f(x, y^*)$$

where $y^* = y(\varepsilon t^*)$ for some t^*, i.e., the time-periodic evolution of $y(\varepsilon t)$ forces the solution trajectory $x(t)$ to transition between these invariant sets. The transition from one invariant state to another occurs at values of y^* at which the state that is currently shadowed by the orbit of the fast system, loses stability in some type of bifurcation. As $y(\varepsilon t)$ passes such a value, the orbit of (3) leaves the vicinity of such a state and is attracted to another state which is stable for the current value of the "parameter" y. We note that for analytic systems the orbit may remain in the vicinity of an unstable state long after $y(\varepsilon t)$ passes through a bifurcation value for the frozen system. This *delayed loss of stability* is discussed in more detail in [10, 14], and references therein. Although this phenomenon does not typically persist for noisy systems, it can be observed in numerical simulations, as is demonstrated below.

A *periodic burster type* is determined by the set of stable attractors (equilibria, periodic orbits, *etc.*) that the system visits, as well as the bifurcations in which these states lose their stability. For a precise definition see [6].

To illustrate the local birth of periodic bursters, we assume that the frozen system

$$x' = f(x, 0)$$

has a singularity of codimension k at $x = 0$ and that the y variables are universal unfolding parameters for this singularity. In this context, we assume that the unfolding theorem is valid and $y(\varepsilon t)$ is a small amplitude periodic path in $\mathbf{R}^k$. Of course, our discussion only refers to an unspecified neighborhood of the origin in $\mathbf{R}^k$, so that the convention of writing the parameter space of k parameters as $\mathbf{R}^k$ is a slight abuse of notation.

Locally, near the origin, the universal unfolding defines a codimension one transition variety $\mathcal{V} \subset \mathbf{R}^k$. This variety consists of parameter values at which singularities of codimension at least one occur. These singularities include, but are not limited to, saddle-node bifurcations, Hopf bifurcations, and homoclinic trajectories.

For different values on the periodic orbit $y(\varepsilon t)$, different states may be stable, and may lose their stability as the path crosses $\mathcal{V}$. Therefore traversing a path in the unfolding of this singularity can lead to transitions between various stable states, and hence periodic bursting. Note that many different paths can lead to the same type of transitions, and can be considered *path equivalent* (for a precise definition see [6]). In fact, typically a small change in the path will preserve the bursting type observed in the fast system.

Among all of those singularities whose unfoldings contain a given bursting type, the one with smallest codimension gives an intrinsic measure of the complexity of that burster. The *codimension* of a periodic bursting type is the minimum codimension of a bifurcation point in the fast system in whose unfoldings that type of bursting occurs.

In [6] codimension one bursters (from a nondegenerate Hopf bifurcation in the fast subsystem), codimension two bursters (from the cusp singularity, degenerate Hopf bifurcation, Takens-Bogdanov bifurcation, Hopf-steady state mode interaction, and Hopf-Hopf mode interaction), and certain codimension three bursters are described from this viewpoint. Somewhat surprisingly, the systems traditionally labeled as Type III (or elliptic) bursters have codimension two, whereas the other most commonly studied bursters — those labeled as Types Ia (square-wave), Ib, II (parabolic) and IV — first occur in the unfoldings of a codimension three bifurcation [2].

The path in the unfolding of the degenerate Hopf bifurcation that leads to Type III bursting, and a typical resulting timeseries is shown in Fig. 8.1. The path through the unfolding of this codimension two bifurcation is depicted on the lower left. Suppose we start at the leftmost point on the path. For this value of the slow parameter the fast system approaches a stable fixed point at the origin. As the slow system traverses the path, this fixed point loses stability in a subcritical Hopf bifurcation, and, after a delay, the orbit of the fast system approaches the unique periodic orbit that exists in this region of parameter space. As the slow system follows the path through the unfolding from right to left, this periodic orbit loses stability in a collision with an unstable periodic orbit (the same orbit that arose in the subcritical Hopf bifurcation discussed earlier). After this bifurcation, the fast system again approaches the stable fixed point at the origin, and the process repeats.

8.3. Bursting in Two Coupled Cells

In many applications one studies the dynamics of two identical coupled cells. We further assume that each cell is a fast-slow system, and that the cells are coupled symmetrically, so that the evolution of the network is described by

$$\begin{aligned} x_1' &= f(x_1, y_1, x_2, y_2) \qquad & x_2' &= f(x_2, y_2, x_1, y_1) \\ y_1' &= \varepsilon g(x_1, y_1, x_2, y_2) \qquad & y_2' &= \varepsilon g(x_2, y_2, x_1, y_1). \end{aligned}$$

It is frequently observed in practice that the slow variables of such a system can be (approximately) synchronous, even when the fast variables are desynchronized. Suppose that each cell bursts, and that the active state is oscillatory. Moreover, assume that the average of the fast, oscillating variables x_1 and x_2 is equal, although the two are not necessarily synchronized. In this case, after averaging the fast variables over each cycle in their

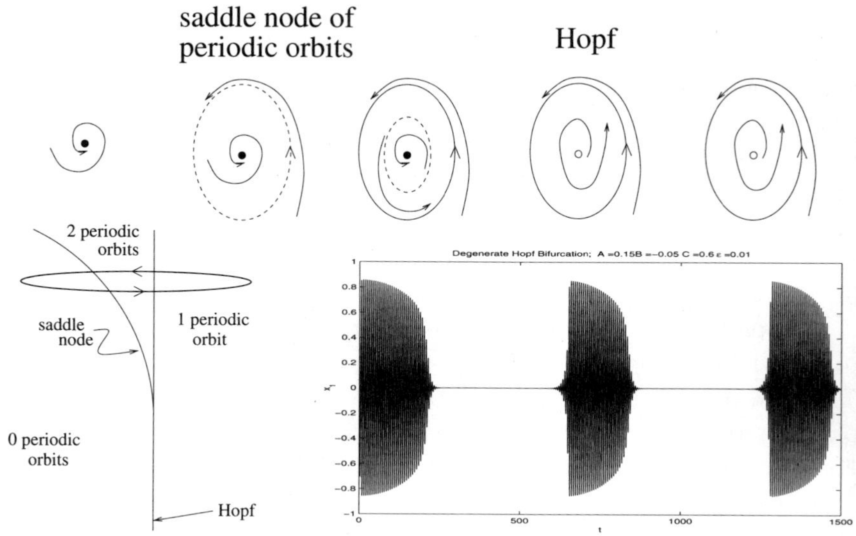

Fig. 8.1. A schematic representation of Type III elliptic bursting. The stable and unstable periodic orbits collide in a saddle-node of periodic orbits, causing the system to return to the quiescent state. The slow passage effect is manifested at the beginning of each active phase.

oscillations, we obtain the following equations for the slow variables

$$y_1' = \varepsilon g(\bar{x}, y_1, \bar{x}, y_2) \qquad\qquad y_2' = \varepsilon g(\bar{x}, y_2, \bar{x}, y_1).$$

The manifold $\Sigma_y = \{(y_1, y_2) : y_1 = y_2\}$ is invariant for this reduced system. Therefore, under these conditions, the slow variables can be expected to behave synchronously, even when the fast variables do not.

Alternatively, consider a coupled system depending on an ambient parameter which slowly changes (for instance an extracellular concentration of calcium which changes slowly compared to the internal dynamics of the two cells). Let us assume that the network consists of two identical, symmetrically coupled cells which depend in the same way on the ambient parameter.

In both of these cases it is reasonable to look at the following model

$$x_1' = f(x_1, x_2, p(\varepsilon t)) \qquad\qquad x_2' = f(x_2, x_1, p(\varepsilon t)). \tag{8}$$

In the first example, $p(\varepsilon t)$ corresponds to the synchronous slow variables. In the second it represents the slowly varying parameter. In many situations $p(\varepsilon t)$ is periodic in time. This occurs for many systems modeling bursting behavior. This is the type of model we will analyze.

Note that the diagonal $\Sigma_x = \{(x_1, x_2) : x_1 = x_2\}$ =Fix($\mathbf{Z}_2$) is an invariant submanifold for system (8) and contains the synchronous solutions of the system. We will concentrate on bifurcations from synchronous solutions, that is from different orbits contained in Σ_x.

We take the approach outlined in the previous section and developed in [6], and consider periodic paths through the unfolding of low codimension bifurcations. Since (8) is $\mathbf{Z}_2$-equivariant, this will be reflected in the unfoldings that we consider.

8.4. $\mathbf{Z}_2$-Equivariant Bifurcations

In this section we review the codmension one and codimension two $\mathbf{Z}_2$-equivariant local bifurcations from a $\mathbf{Z}_2$-invariant equilibrium x_0 of a system of differential equations $\dot{x} = h(x)$ where $x \in \mathbf{R}^n$.

There are four types of codimension one $\mathbf{Z}_2$-equivariant bifurcations: two steady-state and two Hopf bifurcations. These bifurcations are summarized in Table 8.1. Let γ be the nonidentity symmetry in $\mathbf{Z}_2$. Let $J = (dh)_{x_0}$ be the Jacobian matrix of the ODE system at x_0. It follows from the chain rule that $J\gamma = \gamma J$, and hence that

$$\mathbf{R}^n = \Sigma \oplus \Sigma^\perp$$

where Σ and $\Sigma^\perp$ are J-invariant, γ acts trivially on Σ and as $-I$ on $\Sigma^\perp$. More explicitly,

$$\Sigma = \{(x_1, x_1) : x_1 \in \mathbf{R}^k\} \quad \text{and} \quad \Sigma^\perp = \{(x_1, -x_1) : x_1 \in \mathbf{R}^k\}$$

Table 1: Codimension one $\mathbf{Z}_2$-equivariant bifurcations

Bifurcation	Type	Solution Type
steady-state	Σ	saddle-node of $\mathbf{Z}_2$-invariant states
steady-state	$\Sigma^\perp$	pitchfork to symmetry related pairs
Hopf	Σ	$\mathbf{Z}_2$-invariant periodic solutions
Hopf	$\Sigma^\perp$	half-period out of phase periodic solutions

Generically, the eigenspaces of J are contained either in Σ or $\Sigma^\perp$. The two steady-state bifurcations correspond to a simple zero eigenvalue with eigenvector in Σ or in $\Sigma^\perp$. Generically, the first case leads to a saddle node bifurcation of γ-invariant equilibria (that is, the steady states lie inside Fix(γ) $= \Sigma$). Generically, the second case leads to a pitchfork bifurcation (that is, to pairs of γ related equilibria bifurcating from a branch of γ-invariant equilibria).

The two Hopf bifurcations correspond to simple purely imaginary eigenvalues with two-dimensional critical subspace W in Σ or in $\Sigma^\perp$. Each of these bifurcations leads generically to a unique branch of periodic solutions from a branch of γ-invariant equilibria. In the first case the periodic solutions themselves are γ-invariant (that is, lie inside $\mathrm{Fix}(\gamma)$). In the second case, the periodic solutions $x(t)$ are half-period out of phase periodic solutions (that is, $\gamma x(t) = x(t + T/2)$ where T is the period of $x(t)$).

Codimension two bifurcations appear in two types: mode interactions and nonlinear degeneracies. In this paper we consider three types of mode interaction: steady-state/steady-state, steady-state/Hopf, and Hopf/Hopf. Each of these three types appear in three different ways: Σ-Σ, Σ-$\Sigma^\perp$, and $\Sigma^\perp$-$\Sigma^\perp$ mode interactions. So there are nine different mode interactions that can be considered. Note that generically the steady-state/steady-state mode interactions Σ-Σ and $\Sigma^\perp$-$\Sigma^\perp$ occur as Takens-Bogdanov codimension two bifurcations. We will not present detailed results from all nine of these different mode interactions. For the most part, the analyses of these codimension two bifurcations may be found in the literature or are simple adaptations of what is in the literature. See [8].

We end this section by commenting on what is needed for these various bifurcations to occur in a coupled cell system

$$\begin{aligned} \dot{x}_1 &= f(x_1, x_2) = \alpha x_1 + \beta x_2 + \cdots \\ \dot{x}_2 &= f(x_2, x_1) = \alpha x_2 + \beta x_1 + \cdots \end{aligned}$$

where $x_1, x_2 \in \mathbf{R}^k$, α and β are $k \times k$ matrices, and the assumed equilibrium is at $x_0 = (0, 0)$. Here α is the linearized internal dynamics and β is the linearized coupling. Moreover

$$J|\Sigma = \alpha + \beta \quad \text{and} \quad J|\Sigma^\perp = \alpha - \beta$$

Thus, a steady-state Σ bifurcation occurs when $\alpha + \beta$ has a zero eigenvalue, etc. In general, we will only consider bifurcations and mode interactions when the dimension k of each cell is minimum. For example, we take $k = 1$ for steady-state bifurcations and $k = 2$ for Hopf bifurcations. Note that we can assume $k = 2$ for Σ-Σ and $\Sigma^\perp$-$\Sigma^\perp$ Takens-Bogdanov singularities but we can take $k = 1$ for Σ-$\Sigma^\perp$ steady-state/steady-state mode interactions.

8.5. Pitchfork Bifurcation

Consider a system of the form (8) in which the two cells have one-dimensional internal dynamics. As discusses in section 8.3, if the system has a fixed point in Σ, two types of steady-state bifurcations will be typical, a bifurcation inside the synchrony subspace Σ which will generically be a saddle-node bifurcation, and a bifurcation in the direction normal to Σ which will typically be a pitchfork bifurcation.

The truncated normal form of the pitchfork bifurcation is given by

$$\xi' = \xi(p \pm \xi^2). \tag{13}$$

This bifurcation will occur in a direction tangent to the space $\Sigma^{\perp}$, and therefore we can think of ξ as a coordinate along the center manifold in which this bifurcation occurs. To examine the bifurcations it is therefore natural to write the normal form in the coordinates

$$\xi = \frac{x_1 - x_2}{2} \qquad \eta = \frac{x_1 + x_2}{2} \tag{14}$$

Note that η is the coordinate along the linear submanifold Σ corresponding to the synchronized state. The subspace $\Sigma^{\perp}$ must be stable for the bifurcation to be observable; therefore we assume that equation for η is

$$\eta' = -\lambda\eta \qquad\qquad \lambda > 0. \tag{15}$$

We can use (14) to rewrite the pitchfork bifurcation in the original network coordinates as[a]

$$\begin{aligned} x_1' &= (x_1 - x_2)\left(p - (\tfrac{x_1 - x_2}{2})^2\right) - \lambda(x_1 + x_2) \\ x_2' &= -(x_1 - x_2)\left(p - (\tfrac{x_1 - x_2}{2})^2\right) - \lambda(x_1 + x_2). \end{aligned} \tag{16}$$

As discussed in the introduction, we can observe bursting behavior if we let the bifurcation parameter vary slowly, and move through the bifurcation point $p = 0$. In particular, let

$$p = p(\varepsilon t) = C\sin(\varepsilon t) + A. \tag{17}$$

The state $x_1 = x_2$ becomes unstable as p becomes positive. Due to delayed passage [12], the system does not follow the branch of equilibria that would be obtained in the quasi-steady-state approximation. See Fig. 8.2.

Note that the manifold Σ is invariant for the system (16)-(17). Since this is a codimension one manifold in the phase space of the system, either x_1

[a]In writing equations (16), as well as equations (20), and (25), we omit certain constants that multiply the right hand side. This change corresponds to a reparametrization of time, and does not affect the solutions in any other way.

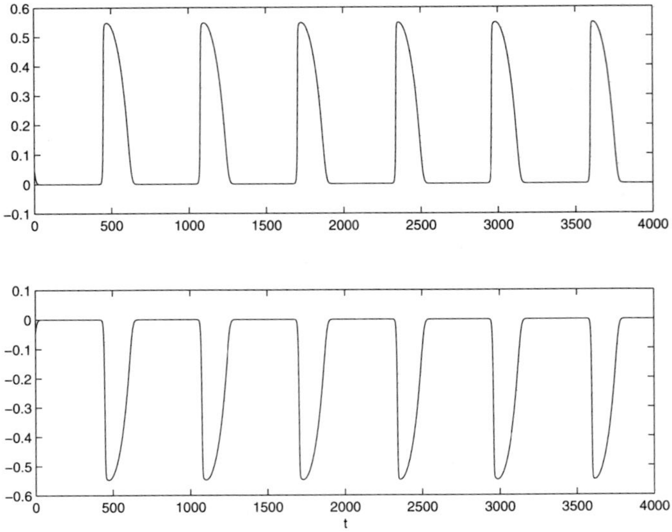

Fig. 8.2. The time series for x_1 (top) and x_2 (bottom) are half period out of phase in(16) with $p(\varepsilon t) = 0.4\sin(\varepsilon t) - 0.1$ and $\varepsilon = 0.001$.

will increase, and x_2 will decrease during the burst, if the initial conditions satisfy $x_1(0) - x_2(0) > 0$ (this is the situation in Fig. 8.2). If $x_2(0) - x_1(0) > 0$, the orbit is attracted to the symmetrical attractor, and x_1 and x_2 switch places.

If we look at the orbit in the (ξ, η, p) coordinates, then ξ is contracted exponentially to $\xi = 0$ when $p < 0$, that is before the onset of the pitchfork bifurcation. Since p evolves on a much longer timescale than ξ an exponentially small amount of noise can kick ξ across the manifold $\{\xi = 0\}$, which corresponds to the manifold Σ in the (x_1, x_2, p) coordinates.

Therefore in the cell coordinates, a small amount of noise will allow the trajectory to cross the synchronized state Σ. If the noise is small, the deterministic dynamics will eventually force the system into a burst. If the noise intensity is equal in both cells, the system will be equally likely to burst in the positive or negative ξ direction. As a result, the system will be equally likely to burst in either of the two modes. This is illustrated in Fig. 8.3. To create the figure we have added a small perturbation of the form $\delta \sin(t)$, with $\delta \ll 1$ to equation (13). Since the frequency of this perturbation is much higher than the frequency of p in (17), this term effectively acts like noise. For details on the slow passage through a pitchfork bifurcation in the presence of noise, we refer the reader to [1, 4].

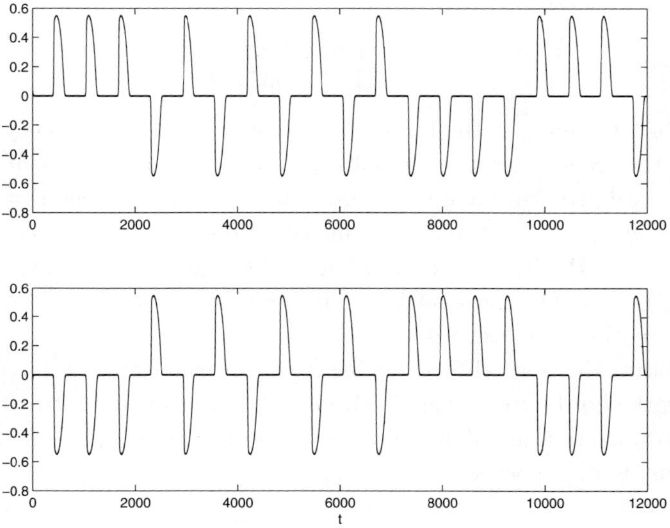

Fig. 8.3. The time series for x_1 (top) and x_2 (bottom) are half period out of phase, and randomly switch branches as noise ($0.01\sin(\pi t)$) is added to the pitchfork bifurcation (16); $p(\varepsilon t) = 0.4\sin(\varepsilon t) - 0.1$ and $\varepsilon = 0.001$.

8.6. Hopf / Hopf Mode Interactions

In this section we consider different phenomena that are possible when the network undergoes Hopf bifurcations. Harkin *et al.* [9] show that two bubbles in a fluid that descend under gravity can transition between in phase and out of phase oscillation. This observation motivates our discussion of bursting arising from Hopf / Hopf mode interactions. We suppose that two Hopf modes, one preserving $\mathbf{Z}_2$-symmetry and one breaking that symmetry, bifurcate simultaneously from a $\mathbf{Z}_2$-invariant equilibrium and show that bursting between in phase and out of phase oscillation can occur robustly in the unfoldings of this mode interaction.

We assume that the frequencies of the two modes are irrationally related. It follows that the Poincaré-Birkhoff normal form of the center manifold vector fields decouple into phase-amplitude equations [8] and that the amplitude equations have $\mathbf{Z}_2 \oplus \mathbf{Z}_2$-symmetry. We use the results in chapter X of [7] to describe the unfoldings of this mode interaction. The universal unfolding in the vicinity of a Hopf bifurcation of this mode interaction is given by

$$\begin{aligned} \xi' &= -i\xi - (|\xi|^2 + m|\eta|^2 - p)\xi \\ \eta' &= -\sqrt{2}\, i\eta - (n|\xi|^2 + |\eta|^2 - (p-\sigma))\eta \end{aligned} \tag{18}$$

where $\xi, \eta \in \mathbf{C}$, and p is the bifurcation parameter. The frequency of oscillation in the second equation is multiplied by $\sqrt{2}$ to avoid resonances. The equations are given in complex coordinates, and we can use $\xi = \xi_r + i\xi_i$ and $\eta = \eta_r + i\eta_i$ to transform the equations to the real coordinates $(\xi_r, \xi_i, \eta_r, \eta_i) \in \mathbf{R}^4$. The values of m and n determine several possible bifurcation scenarios. The parameter σ determines the location of a secondary Hopf bifurcation (see Fig. 8.4 and [7]).

To obtain the normal form of the $\mathbf{Z}_2$ equivariant Hopf bifurcations in the network coordinates we again think of ξ as a coordinate transversal to the synchronization manifold, and η as a coordinate along to the synchronization manifold. Therefore

$$\xi = \frac{z_1 - z_2}{2} \qquad \eta = \frac{z_1 + z_2}{2} \tag{19}$$

can be used to transform equation (18) into the network coordinates. In the new coordinates we have

$$\begin{aligned} z_1' = &-z_1\left[(2+m+n)\rho + (m-n)\tau - 4(2p-\sigma) + 4(\sqrt{2}+1)i\right] \\ &-z_2\left[(n-m)\rho + (2-m-n)\tau + 4\sigma + 4(\sqrt{2}-1)i\right], \\ z_2' = &-z_1\left[(n-m)\rho + (2-m-n)\tau + 4\sigma + 4(\sqrt{2}-1)i\right] \\ &-z_2\left[(2+m+n)\rho + (m-n)\tau - 4(2p-\sigma) + 4(\sqrt{2}+1)i\right]. \end{aligned} \tag{20}$$

where $\rho = |z_1|^2 + |z_2|^2$ and $\tau = z_1\bar{z}_2 + \bar{z}_1 z_2$.

In the following we let $m = 4$, $n = 1/2$, and $\sigma = 1/4$, which corresponds to case 2 on p. 434 of [7]. When $p < 0$ the origin is a globally attracting fixed point. The origin loses stability at $p = 0$ in a Hopf bifurcation which gives rise to a stable state in which the two systems are half period out of phase. This state remains stable in some interval $p > 0$, and loses stability in a subcritical Neimark-Sacker bifurcation at $p = p^2_{\mathrm{NS}}$.

Note that there is a Hopf bifurcation at the origin when $p = \sigma$ giving rise to an initially unstable periodic solution which lies inside

$$\Sigma = \{(z_1, z_2) \in \mathbf{C}^2 : z_1 = z_2\} = \{(\xi, \eta) \in \mathbf{C}^2 : \xi = 0\}\}$$

and therefore corresponds to the synchronous state. The unstable torus that is born at the Neimark-Sacker bifurcation at p^2_{NS} collides with this

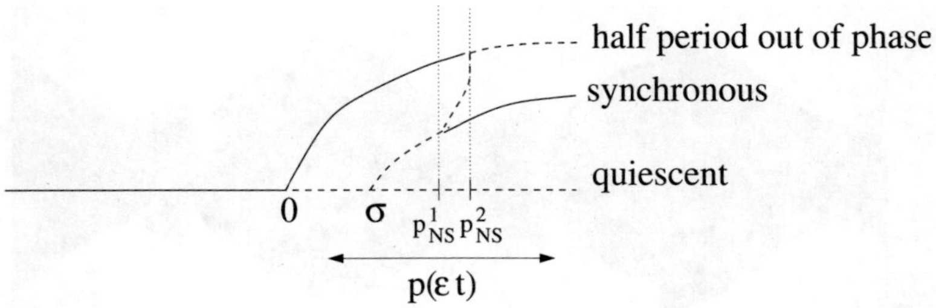

Fig. 8.4. Bifurcation diagram corresponding to equation (18). The solid and dashed lines represent stable and unstable states. The ξ state is synchronous and the η state is asynchronous.

synchronous state in a reverse Neimark-Sacker bifurcation at p^1_{NS} in which the synchronous state becomes stable.

We again assume that the bifurcation parameter p varies slowly in time. For the parameter values given above we let $p(\varepsilon t) = 0.3\sin(\varepsilon t) + 0.4$ and $\varepsilon = 0.005$ which corresponds to the path shown in Fig. 8.4.

As the parameter sweeps the diagram from left to right, the state in which the oscillators are half period out of phase loses stability at $p = p^2_{\text{NS}}$, and the system is attracted to the synchronous state. As the parameter evolves in the opposite direction, the synchronous state in turn loses stability at $p = p^1_{\text{NS}}$, and the system jumps back to the out of phase state. Therefore the system is observed to burst between an *in-phase* and an *out-of-phase* state (see Fig. 8.5).

Note that during the time $\eta \neq 0$, the variable ξ decays to 0 exponentially. Since the manifold Σ is invariant, orbits that come within numerical accuracy of the manifold will never leave it in a numerical simulation. To avoid such problems, as well as reduce the slow passage effects, we added a small sinusoidal term with frequency $\mathcal{O}(1)$ to the equations (20). The exact form of the term is not of importance.

8.7. Takens-Bogdanov Bifurcation with $\mathbf{Z}_2$ Symmetry

Consider the two-coupled cell system

$$\begin{aligned} x_1' &= f(x_1, x_2, p_1, p_2) \\ x_2' &= f(x_2, x_1, p_1, p_2) \end{aligned}$$

in which the two cells both have two-dimensional internal dynamics. We again consider systems which have equilibria on the diagonal Σ which are

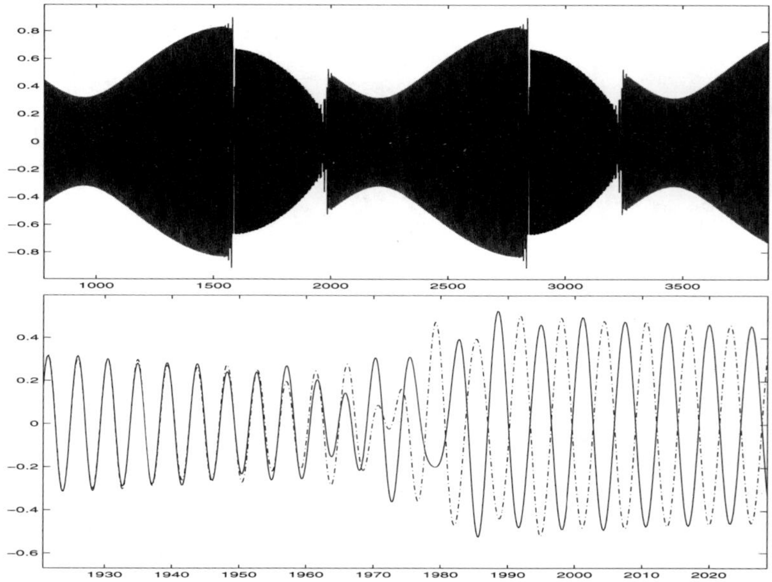

Fig. 8.5. Bursting corresponding to the path shown in Fig. 8.4. The timeseries of Re z_1 (solid line) and Re z_2 (dashed line) are shown in both figures. A portion of the top figure is enlarged in the bottom figure to illustrate the transition between the synchronous and the half period out of phase state.

close to a bifurcation. Without loss of generality, we assume the equilibrium is at the origin.

As in the case of the pitchfork bifurcation, we restrict our attention to bifurcations that break $\mathbf{Z}_2$-symmetry, that is, occur tangent to the space $\Sigma^{\perp}$. Again, we consider coordinates $\eta = x_1 + x_2$ and $\xi = x_1 - x_2$, where $\xi = (\xi_1, \xi_2)$. The normal form of the bifurcation will therefore be symmetric under the interchange of the two cells, which is equivalent to the transformation $\xi \mapsto -\xi$.

We consider the codimension two Takens-Bogdanov bifurcation that breaks the $\mathbf{Z}_2$-symmetry. The normal form of this bifurcation commutes with the symmetry $\xi \mapsto -\xi$, or equivalently, with rotation of phase space through π. The particular normal form that we discuss is

$$\begin{aligned} \xi_1' &= \xi_2 \\ \xi_2' &= p_1\xi_1 + p_2\xi_2 + a\xi_1^3 + \xi_1^2\xi_2, \end{aligned} \tag{23}$$

where p_1 and p_2 are the unfolding parameters. This particular normal form includes the coalescence of limit cycles (see [15] and section 7.3 of [8]). The two-parameter unfolding of this bifurcation is presented in Fig. 8.6.

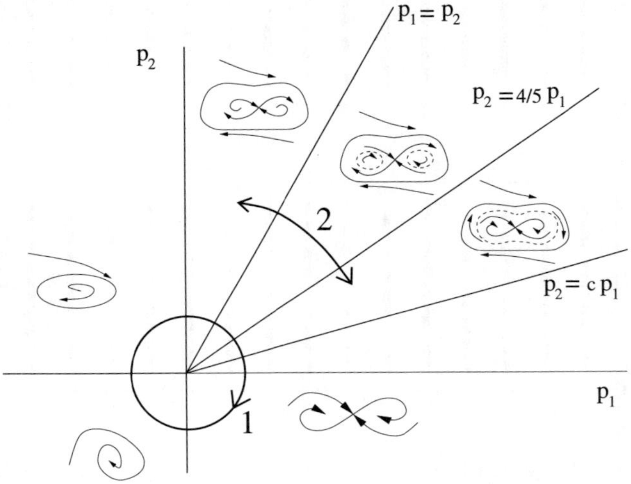

Fig. 8.6. The unfolding of the the $\mathbf{Z}_2$ symmetric Takens-Bogdanov bifurcation. Path 1 through the unfolding gives the bursting pattern shown in Fig. 8.7. After reversing the flow, path 2 results in the bursting pattern presented in Fig. 8.9. Stable limit cycles are shown by solid lines, while unstable ones are shown by dashed lines.

We assume that the center manifold in which the Takens-Bogdanov bifurcation occurs is stable. Let $\eta = x_1 + x_2 = (\eta_1, \eta_2)$ be the coordinate transverse to the center manifold. For simplicity, we assume that

$$\begin{aligned} \eta_1' &= -\lambda_1 \eta_1 \\ \eta_2' &= -\lambda_2 \eta_2 \end{aligned} \tag{24}$$

for $\lambda_1, \lambda_2 > 0$. By rewriting (23)-(24) in the x_1, x_2 coordinates we obtain a representative coupled cell system undergoing this type of bifurcation.

$$\begin{aligned} x_{11}' &= (-\lambda_1 x_{11} + x_{12} - \lambda_1 x_{21} - x_{22}) \\ x_{12}' &= (p_1 x_{11} + (p_2 - \lambda_2) x_{12} - p_1 x_{21} - (p_2 + \lambda_2) x_{22} \\ &\quad -(x_{11} - x_{21})^3 - (x_{11} - x_{21})^2 (x_{12} - x_{22})) \\ x_{21}' &= (-\lambda_1 x_{11} - x_{12} - \lambda_1 x_{21} + x_{22}) \\ x_{22}' &= (-p_1 x_{11} - (p_2 + \lambda_2) x_{12} + p_1 x_{21} + (p_2 - \lambda_2) x_{22} \\ &\quad +(x_{11} - x_{21})^3 + (x_{11} - x_{21})^2 (x_{12} - x_{22})) \end{aligned} \tag{25}$$

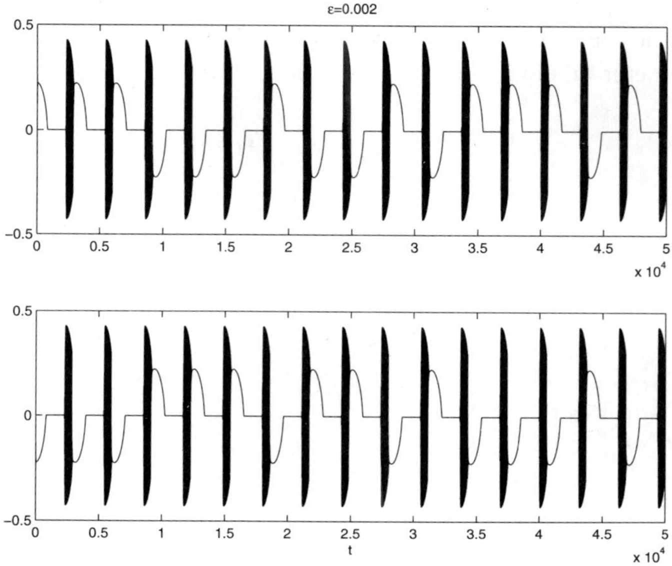

Fig. 8.7. Following path 1 in Fig. 8.6, the time series x_{11} (top) and x_{21} (bottom) are half period out of phase and attracted to the opposite limit cycles and equilibria.

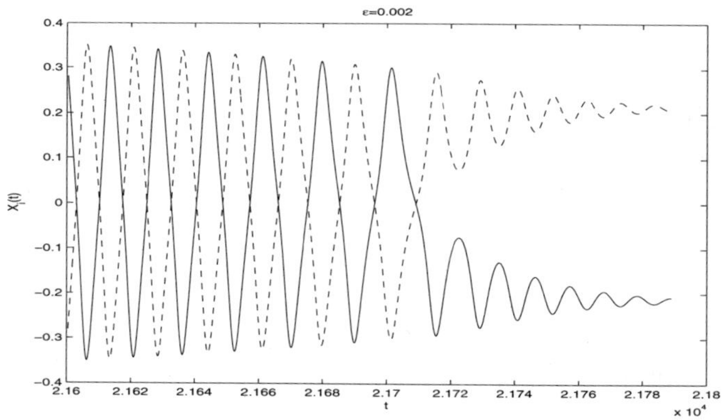

Fig. 8.8. An enlarged view of $x_{11}(t)$ and $x_{21}(t)$ together from Figure 8.7 shows the transition from antisychronous limit cycles to antisychronous equilibria.

Choosing different paths through the unfolding of this bifurcation leads to different types of bursting. Here we consider two choices leading to interesting behavior. Other paths through the unfolding can be analyzed similarly.

The first path, shown schematically as path 1 in Fig. 8.6, is given by $(p_1(\varepsilon t), p_2(\varepsilon t)) = 0.2(\cos(\varepsilon t), \sin(\varepsilon t))$. If we follow this path starting in the third quadrant, the oscillators are initially attracted to the equilibrium at the origin. This equilibrium undergoes a Hopf bifurcation at $p_2 = 0, p_1 < 0$. Since the resulting limit cycle bifurcates in the direction tangent to $\Sigma^{\perp}$, that is in the direction of $\xi = x_1 - x_2$, it leads to half period out of phase oscillations in the two cells x_1 and x_2.

This burst terminates near the line $p_2 = cp_1$ in which the stable outer limit cycle and the unstable inner limit cycle disappear in a saddle-node bifurcation. There are two stable equilibria, $(\xi^{\pm}, 0)$ with $\xi^+ = -\xi^- \neq 0$, that the system can tend to after this bifurcation. The point $(\xi^+, 0)$ corresponds to $x_{11} > x_{21}$ and $x_{12} = x_{22} = 0$, whereas the point $(\xi^-, 0)$ corresponds to $x_{11} < x_{21}$ and $x_{12} = x_{22} = 0$. Which point is chosen depends on whether the system is in the basin of attraction of the left hand or the right hand point after the attracting limit cycle disappears. Both choices are equally likely due to symmetry, and since the two basins are intertwined, one can expect different outcomes after each traversal of the path. Random switching between the two states can be seen in Figs. 8.7 and 8.8. Finally, the two points $(\xi^{\pm}, 0)$ coalesce in a subcritical pitchfork bifurcation as the slow variable re-enters the third quadrant at at $p_2 = 0, p_1 < 0$, and the entire process repeats.

In this example we observe random switching between the steady states $(\xi^{\pm}, 0)$ from one traversal of the path through the unfolding to the next. Consider the same system with time reversed (simply reverse all the arrows in Fig. 8.6). We need to compensate for the reversal of time by letting $\lambda_1 < 0$ and $\lambda_2 < 0$ in (24). In this system it is possible to observe random switching between limit cycles from burst to burst.

To illustrate this behavior we consider path 2 in Fig. 8.6, which is given by $(p_1, p_2) = 0.2(\cos(\frac{\pi}{4} + \delta \sin(\varepsilon t)), \sin(\frac{\pi}{4} + \delta \sin(\varepsilon t)))$ with $\delta = 0.1256$. The bursting resulting from this path is shown in Fig. 8.9. Note that the stable limit cycles are now denoted by dashed lines. Following the path starting in the region adjacent to the p_2 axis and proceeding clockwise, we start at one of the two stable fixed points. As in the previous examples, the two fixed points are given by $(\xi^{\pm}, 0)$. Both of these fixed points undergo a supercritical Hopf bifurcation at $p_1 = p_2$, which results in oscillations. Due to delayed passage, these oscillations are not very prominent in Fig. 8.9, but can be observed. Approximately at $p_2 = 4/5p_1$, the two limit cycles that arose in the Hopf bifurcation coalesce in a $\mathbf{Z}_2$ symmetric homoclinic bifurcation, and give rise to a limit cycle that encompasses the origin. Again, this limit cycle corresponds to half period out of phase oscillations. The detailed analysis of the slow passage through a homoclinic bifurcation is quite involved, and we refer the reader to [5], and references therein.

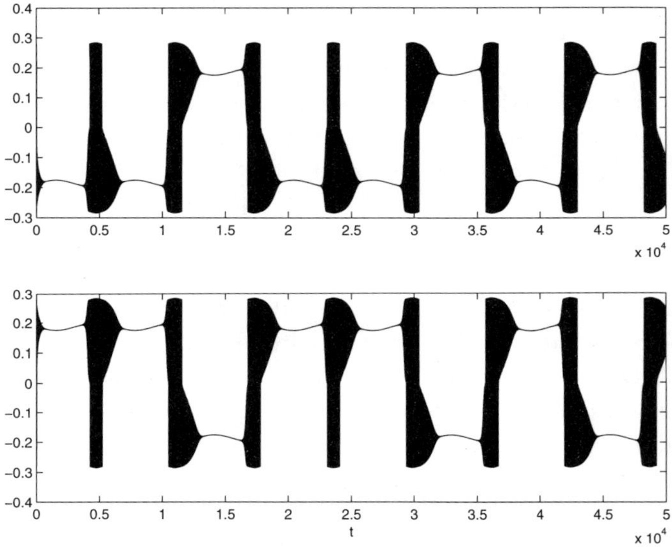

Fig. 8.9. Following path 2 (with reversal in time) in Fig. 8.6, $x_{11}(t)$ and $x_{21}(t)$, top and bottom respectively, are half period out of phase and attracted to the opposite limit cycles and equilibria.

After this bifurcation the path is traversed in the opposite direction. We first encounter the $\mathbf{Z}_2$ symmetric homoclinic bifurcation again. This bifurcation results in two limit cycles, one in the region $\xi_1 < 0$, and one in the region $\xi_1 > 0$. Which limit cycle is chosen depends on the state of the system prior to bifurcation. It is therefore expected that both limit cycles are equally likely and that it is possible to approach either. As shown in Fig. 8.9, this is indeed the case, and both types of oscillations are observed. The chosen limit cycle now disappears at a subcritical Hopf bifurcation, and the orbit settles at one of the fixed points $(\xi^-, 0)$ or $(\xi^+, 0)$ depending

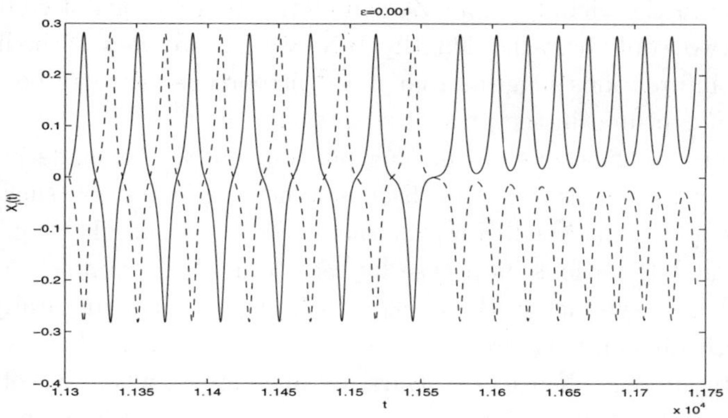

Fig. 8.10. A close view of $x_{11}(t)$ and $x_{21}(t)$ together from Fig. 8.9 shows the transition from an antisychronous limit cycle encompassing both the origin and the symmetric equilibria, to two disjoint, antisychronous limit cycles, each encompassing one of the symmetric equilibria.

on whether the system followed the left or the right limit cycle. The entire process repeats, and since, at each traversal of the path, both limit cycles arising in the $\mathbf{Z}_2$ symmetric homoclinic bifurcation are equally likely, we observe random switching between these two states from burst to burst.

8.8. Conclusion

In this chapter we have extended the ideas developed in [6] to the case of two coupled identical fast-slow systems. While these extensions are natural, the fact that we used an abstract, model independent approach may leave the reader wondering whether the phenomena we discussed can be observed in models that are used in practice.

It is natural to relate the likelihood of encountering a burster to the codimension of the bifurcation in whose unfolding it first appears. As was shown in [2, 6], the different single cell bursters most frequently encountered in applications, are, in fact, among the most likely bursters to be encountered from this viewpoint. In the present work, we have presented an overview of the phenomena that occur near low codimension bifurcations in a system of two coupled cells. In analogy to the single cell case, we can expect that these are the phenomena that are most likely to be encountered when such networks are modeled in practice.

As noted in section 8.4, a comprehensive catalog of bursting types that can occur in the vicinity of all $\mathbf{Z}_2$ symmetric bifurcations of codimension one and two would be rather lengthy. However, an overview of the literature on these bifurcations suggests that most phenomena that can be expected have been captured in the present chapter and in [6].

Similar classifications of bursting phenomena can be made in coupled systems with symmetry and our discussion here indicates how such a classification might be pursued. However, one needs to consider low codimension equivariant bifurcations on a case by case basis. For example, in rings of cells with $\mathbf{D}_n$ symmetry, Buono *et al.* [3] show that structurally stable, asymptotically stable heteroclinic cycles can appear in Hopf / steady-state mode interactions when $n \geq 5$. Bursting phenomena when one of the stable states in the fast equations is itself a heteroclinic cycle might be quite interesting.

Acknowledgments

We thank Tasso Kaper for pointing out that bursting between in phase and out of phase periodic solutions can occur in models with $\mathbf{Z}_2$ symmetry. This work was supported in part by NSF Grant DMS-0244529.

References

[1] N. Berglund and B. Gentz, Pathwise description of dynamic pitchfork bifurcations with additive noise, *Probab. Theory Related Fields* **122**(3), 341–388, (2002).

[2] R. Bertram, M. Butte, T. Kiemel, and A. Sherman, Topological and phenomenological classification of bursting oscillations, *Bull. of Math. Bio.* **57**, 413–439, (1995).

[3] P. L. Buono, M. Golubitsky, and A. Palacios, Heteroclinic cycles in rings of coupled cells, *Physica D* **143**, 74–108, (2000).

[4] H. Crauel, P. Imkeller, and M. Steinkamp, Bifurcations of one-dimensional stochastic differential equations, In: *Stochastic dynamics (Bremen, 1997)*, Springer, New York, 27–47, (1999).

[5] D. C. Diminnie and R. Haberman, Slow passage through homoclinic orbits for the unfolding of a saddle-center bifurcation and the change in the adiabatic invariant, *Physica D* **162**(1-2), 34–52, (2002).

[6] M. Golubitsky, K. Josić, and T. J. Kaper, An unfolding theory approach to bursting in fast-slow systems, In: *Global Analysis of Dynamical Systems*, Inst. Phys., Bristol, 277–308, (2001).

[7] M. Golubitsky and D. G. Schaeffer, *Singularities and groups in bifurca-*

tion theory, Vol. I, Applied Mathematical Sciences **51**, Springer-Verlag, New York, (1985).

[8] J. Guckenheimer and P. Holmes, *Nonlinear Oscillations, Dynamical Systems, and Bifurcations of Vector Fields*, Springer-Verlag, New York, (1983).

[9] A. Harkin, T. Kaper, and A. Nadim. Coupled pulsation and translation of two gas bubbles in a liquid, *J. Fluid Mech.* **445**, 377–411, (2001).

[10] M. G. Hayes, *Geometrical Analysis of Delayed Bifurcations*, PhD thesis, Boston University, (1999).

[11] E .M. Izhikevich, Neural excitability, spiking and bursting, *Internat. J. Bifur. Chaos Appl. Sci. Engrg.* **10**(6), 1171–1266, (2000).

[12] M. Krupa and P. Szmolyan, Extending slow manifolds near transcritical and pitchfork singularities, *Nonlinearity* **14**(6), 1473–1491, (2001).

[13] J. Rinzel, Bursting oscillations in an excitable membrane model, In: *Ordinary and Partial Differential Equations (Dundee, 1984)*, Springer, Berlin, 304–316, (1985).

[14] J. Su, The phenomenon of delayed bifurcation and its analyses, In: *Multiple-Time-Scale Dynamical Systems (Minneapolis, MN, 1997), IMA Vol. Math. Appl.* **122**, Springer, New York, 203–214, (2001).

[15] F. Takens, Forced oscillations and bifurcations, In: *Applications of Global Analysis, I (Sympos., Utrecht State Univ., Utrecht, 1973)*, Comm. Math. Inst. Rijksuniv. Utrecht, No. 3, 1–59. Math. Inst. Rijksuniv. Utrecht, Utrecht, (1974).

[16] D. Terman, Chaotic spikes arising from a model of bursting in excitable membranes, *SIAM J. Appl. Math.* **51**(5), 1418–1450, (1991).

CHAPTER 9

MODULATORY EFFECTS OF COUPLING ON BURSTING MAPS

Gerda de Vries

Department of Mathematical and Statistical Sciences
University of Alberta
Edmonton, AB, T6G 2G1, Canada
e-mail: devries@math.ualberta.ca

We treat one-dimensional and two-dimensional maps exhibiting bursting oscillations. These maps have been proposed as a computationally efficient alternative to conventional models based on the Hodgkin-Huxley formalism in studying the collective behaviour of networks of neurons. We review cobwebbing and bifurcation analyses which are used to reveal the mechanisms underlying the formation of the bursting oscillations. New and existing results on the synchronizing effect of mean-field and diffusive coupling are brought together, compared, and contrasted. We demonstrate that synchronization comes in the form of in-phase and anti-phase bursting oscillations, as well as in-phase and anti-phase spiking. We explain some coupling effects by extending the bifurcation analysis of a single cell to a two-cell system.

9.1. Introduction

There are many papers investigating the collective behaviour of networks of oscillators, with the aim of explaining synchronization in neurobiological systems. In most cases, each oscillator is represented by a high-dimensional system of nonlinear ordinary differential equations. Coupling many such systems together to study collective phenomena is computationally expensive, and mechanisms responsible for the phenomena are difficult to uncover.

In recent years, a number of authors have proposed the use of simple systems of discrete-time equations, or maps, to overcome these difficulties. The maps proposed have low dimension (one or two). Simple iteration, which is cheap computationally, is all that is required to generate wave-

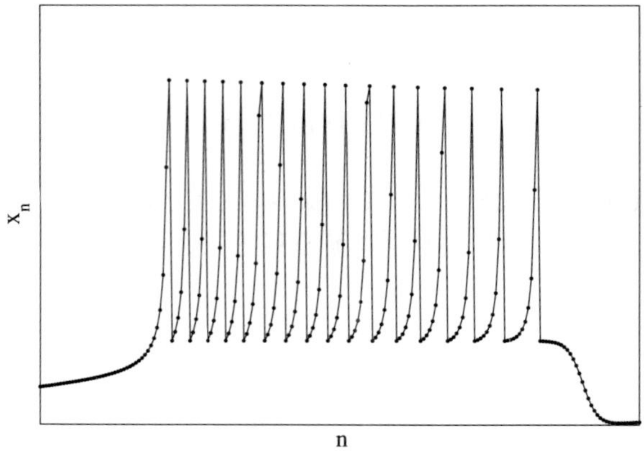

Fig. 9.1. An example of a bursting map, showing many iterates in a silent phase and several iterates within each spike in the active phase.

forms. Although the maps are derived without making any direct reference to neural mechanisms, their behaviour mimics that of real, physiological neurons. Further, networks of coupled maps can generate synchronized behaviour, as observed experimentally in networks of neurons.

In this chapter, we focus on so-called bursting maps. These maps generate a sequence of iterates which, when plotted, trace out a bursting oscillation, with many iterates occurring during the silent phase, and several iterates defining each spike in the active phase. An example of a bursting oscillation produced by such a map is shown in Fig. 9.1. There is a large body of work that deals with the reduction of systems of ordinary differential equations exhibiting bursting oscillations to maps via Poincaré sections (see for example the papers by Butera [1], Chay and Rinzel [3], Medvedev [12], and Terman [18]). Those maps are not explicit maps exhibiting bursting oscillations themselves, and are not of interest here. Here we bring together the most prominent bursting maps that have been proposed and summarize results on the effect of coupling. We will see that coupled maps of identical cells can exhibit a variety of synchronized behaviour, ranging from in-phase and anti-phase spiking to in-phase and anti-phase bursting, depending on the constituents of the coupled system and the form of the coupling. While some of the effects of coupling have been explained, others await further investigation.

In section 9.2, we introduce a number of one-dimensional and two-dimensional maps exhibiting bursting oscillations that have been proposed. The different synchronized responses of these maps to coupling are summarized in section 9.3. In section 9.4, we focus on one bursting map, and use a bifurcation analysis to uncover the mechanism underlying its response to coupling. Concluding remarks can be found in section 9.5.

9.2. Examples of Bursting Maps

There are several examples of discrete-time models exhibiting bursting oscillations, and we review these here. A disctinction is made between one-dimensional maps (section 9.2.1) and two-dimensional maps (section 9.2.2).

9.2.1. *One-dimensional maps*

The simplest maps exhibiting bursting oscillations are one-dimensional maps of the form

$$x_{n+1} = F(x_n) \tag{1}$$

which are near a homoclinic bifurcation of co-dimension one. These maps can be perturbed so that the resulting map has a homoclinic orbit to a fixed point x^*. For the given $F(x)$, the homoclinic orbit has given way to a periodic orbit. Izhikevich and Hoppensteadt [10] have classified one-dimensional maps of this form, and identified three distinct types, namely "node", "focus", and "fold". An example of each is shown in Fig. 9.2. Bursting ensues because the periodic orbit contains many subsequent iterates near an unstable fixed point (in the bursters of types "node" and "focus") or near the ghost of a fixed point (in the burster of type "fold"). These iterates create the so-called silent phase that is characteristic of bursting oscillations.

Cazelles *et al.* [2] introduced the following one-dimensional bursting map,

$$F(x) = \begin{cases} 0.0 + 1.05x & \text{when } 0.0 \le x \le 0.4, \\ 1.5 - 1.25x & \text{when } 0.4 < x \le 0.6, \\ -0.9 + 1.50x & \text{when } 0.6 < x \le 0.7, \\ 1.4 - 1.00x & \text{when } 0.7 < x \le 1.0, \end{cases} \tag{2}$$

to describe the chaotic activity of spiking-bursting neurons. This map is of "node" type. Cazelles *et al.* showed that two coupled maps can exhibit anti-phase bursting or in-phase bursting, depending on the sign of the coupling term, mimicking phenomena observed in experiments with central pattern generator chaotic neurons. We will examine the coupled map in section 9.3.1.

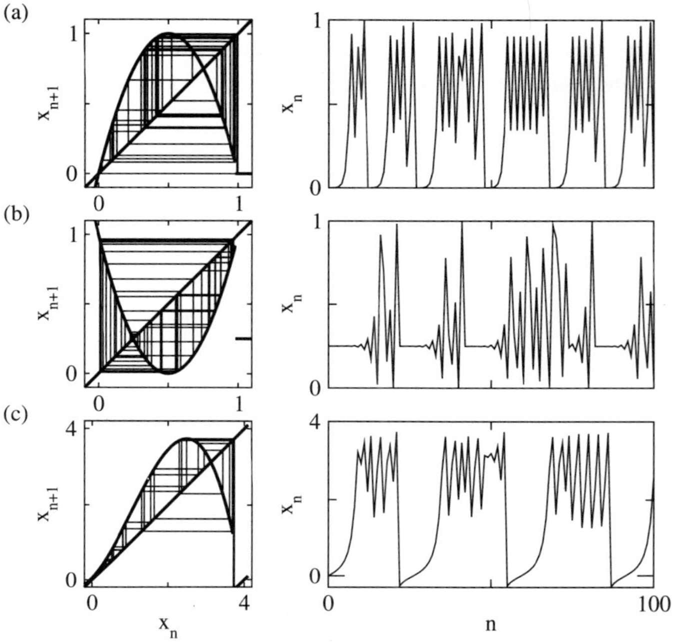

Fig. 9.2. Examples of one-dimensional maps of the form $x_{n+1} = F(x_n)$ exhibiting bursting oscillations. (a) Burster of "node" type; $F(x) = 4x(1-x)$ when $x \leq 0.98$ and $0.000098x$ when $x > 0.98$. (b) Burster of "focus" type; $F(x) = 1 - 4x(1-x)$ when $x \leq 0.98$ and $0.25 + 0.00003x$ when $x > 0.98$. (c) Burster of "fold" type; $F(x) = -0.25 + 2x - 0.3(x-1)^3$ when $x \leq 3.7$ and $x - 4$ when $x > 3.7$.

9.2.2. *Two-dimensional maps*

We now turn our attention to two-dimensional maps exhibiting bursting behaviour. In particular, we focus on those maps that are analogous to the classical continuous-time bursters that can be decomposed into a fast and a slow subsystem, and have the following form:

$$x_{n+1} = f(x_n, y_n), \tag{3}$$

$$y_{n+1} = y_n + \varepsilon g(x_n), \tag{4}$$

where x_n is the fast variable describing the spiking behaviour, y_n is the slow variable that modulates the spiking dynamics, and $0 < \varepsilon \ll 1$.

The analysis of such a system is analogous to Rinzel's classical analysis [13]. In particular, one first ignores the dynamics of the y-variable, and studies the behaviour of the fast subsystem, (3), for different values of the y-variable. As with continuous-time bursters, the fast subsystem exhibits

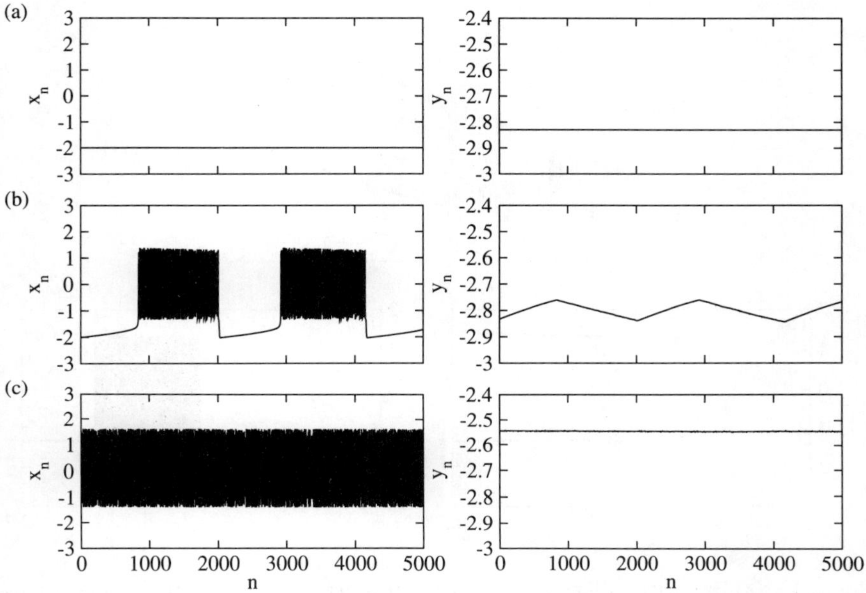

Fig. 9.3. Behaviour of system (3)–(6). (a) $\sigma = -2$; (b) $\sigma = -1$; (c) $\sigma = 0$. Other parameter values are $\alpha = 4.15$ and $\varepsilon = 0.0001$.

bistability for a range of values of the y-variable. In this case, the bistability is between a stable fixed point (responsible for the silent phase of the bursting oscillation) and a stable periodic or chaotic orbit (responsible for the active phase). The inclusion of the dynamics of the slow subsystem, (4), allows for bursting to take place, via hysteresis which periodically switches the orbit between the silent and active phases.

A specific example of such a two-dimensional map is taken from Rulkov [14], namely

$$f(x, y) = \frac{\alpha}{1 + x^2} + y, \tag{5}$$

$$g(x) = -(x - \sigma), \tag{6}$$

where α and σ are $\mathcal{O}(1)$ parameters. A few typical waveforms for (3)–(6) are shown in Fig. 9.3.

The bifurcation diagram of the fast subsystem is shown in Fig. 9.4(a). The curve of fixed points, given by

$$R(x; y) = \alpha/(1 + x^2) + y = x, \tag{7}$$

traces out an S shape. Thin solid portions indicate stable fixed points and

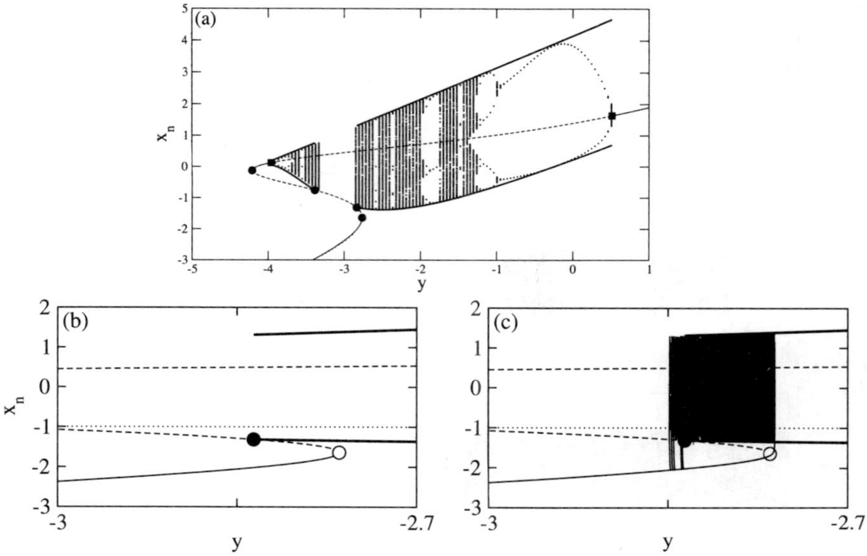

Fig. 9.4. (a) Bifurcation diagram for the fast subsystem of (3)–(4), with $f(x, y)$ given by (5) and $\alpha = 4.15$. Thin solid and dashed curves indicated stable and unstable fixed points, respectively. Thick solid curves represent $x = R(0)$ and $x = R(R(0))$, the theoretical maximum and minimum iterates, respectively. Small dots represent periodic and chaotic iterates of the one-dimensional map (shown for 100 values of y, with 300 iterates for each value of y). Open circles represent saddle-node bifurcations; filled squares represent period-doubling bifurcations; filled circles represent external crisis bifurcations. (b) Close-up of the region of bistability, with the nullcline $x = \sigma = -1$ superimposed (dotted line). (c) As (b), with the trajectory shown in Fig. 9.3(b) superimposed.

dashed portions indicate unstable fixed points. Saddle-node bifurcations, denoted by open circles, occur at the knees of this curve. The stability of the fixed points on the upper branch of the S-shaped curve changes at period-doubling bifurcations, denoted by filled squares. For 100 values of y lying between the period-doubling bifurcations, iterates of the slow subsystem are shown (300 iterates for each value of y). For values of y near the period-doubling bifurcations, stable two-cycles are observed. As the value of y is changed, two-cycles give way to four-cycles, eight-cycles, etc., similar to the cascade of period-doubling bifurcations observed in the well-known logistic map [11]. Periodic orbits give way to chaotic attractors, but periodic windows can be observed for small intervals of y. The thick solid curves indicate upper and lower bounds on the iterates, given by $x = R(0; y) = \alpha + y$ and $x = R(R(0; y); y) = \alpha/(1+(\alpha+y)^2)+y$, respectively. These curves terminate at external crisis (homoclinic) bifurcations, denoted by filled circles, when the curve $x = R(R(0;y);y)$ intersects the middle branch of the S-shaped curve.

Let y_{SN} and y_{EC} denote the values of y at which the right saddle-node and external crisis bifurcations occur, respectively. The bistability between stable fixed points on the bottom branch of the S-shaped curve and periodic and/or chaotic attractors surrounding the unstable fixed points on the upper branch for $y_{EC} < y < y_{SN}$ plays a key role in generating bursting oscillations when the dynamics of the slow subsystem are taken into account. This region of bistability is shown with better detail in Fig. 9.4(b). The slow subsystem, given by (4) and (6), implies that $y_{n+1} > y_n$ when $x_n < \sigma$, and $y_{n+1} < y_n$ when $x_n > \sigma$. Thus, during the silent phase, when iterates are at or near the stable fixed points on the bottom branch of the S-shaped curve, the y-variable is increasing. When $y_n > y_{SN}$, the switch to the active phase is made. During the active phase, iterates lie above the line $x_n = \sigma$ (on average), and the y-variable is decreasing. When $y_n < y_{EC}$, the switch back to the silent phase is made. In Fig. 9.4(c), the waveform that is shown in Fig. 9.3(b) and obtained from the full two-dimensional map is projected onto the bifurcation diagram of the fast subsystem. The agreement between the predicted dynamics and the actual dynamics of the full two-dimensional map is very good. As in the case of continuous-time bursters, the accuracy with which the dynamics of the full two-dimensional map are predicted by the fast/slow subsystem decomposition depends on the magnitude of the parameter ε. The smaller ε, the better the prediction.

The burster exemplified by equations (3)–(6) can be characterized as being of the "fold/homoclinic" type, referring to the two bifurcations that underlie the transitions between the active and silent phases, with "fold" referring to the saddle-node bifurcation that underlies the transition from the silent to the active phase, and "homoclinic" referring to the external crisis or homoclinic bifurcation that underlies the transition from the active to the silent phase. Izhikevich and Hoppensteadt [10] have classified all 20 combinations of bifurcations in two-dimensional maps of the form (3)–(4) that can lead to bursting oscillations of co-dimension one. The classification is in the same vein as the earlier classification by Izhikevich [9] of bursting in systems of ordinary differential equations.

The discrete-time burster discussed here exhibits chaotic spiking during the active phase, and often leads to irregular bursting oscillations. Modifications of $f(x,y)$ can be made to create regular spiking during the active phase. Rulkov [15] has introduced a second discrete-time burster in which

$f(x, y)$ is piecewise continuous to accomplish this, namely

$$f(x,y) = \begin{cases} \alpha/(1-x) + y & \text{when } x \le 0, \\ \alpha + y & \text{when } 0 < x < \alpha + y, \\ -1 & \text{when } x \ge \alpha + y. \end{cases} \tag{8}$$

$$g(x) = -(x - \sigma) - 1. \tag{9}$$

This bursting map also is of "fold/homoclinic" type. We will compare the response of both bursting maps to coupling in section 9.3.2.

9.3. Effects of Coupling

In this section, we investigate systems of two coupled cells, and summarize the modulatary effects of coupling on bursting oscillations in both one-dimensional maps (section 9.3.1) and two-dimensional maps (section 9.3.2). One can think of many types of coupling. Here, we focus on two types of coupling, namely mean-field and diffusive coupling, often used in creating neurobiological networks.

9.3.1. *Effects of coupling on one-dimensional maps*

In this section, we give examples of the effect that coupling may have on one-dimensional maps of the form (1) which exhibit bursting oscillations. We couple two maps as follows:

$$x_{n+1} = F(x_n) + g_c G(x_n, y_n), \tag{10}$$

$$y_{n+1} = F(y_n) + g_c G(y_n, x_n), \tag{11}$$

where g_c represents coupling strength. Note that the two elements being coupled are identical, and the coupling terms are symmetrical. The coupling function $G(x, y)$ can take a variety of forms, a few of which will be discussed below.

Many different coupling responses can be observed, depending on the form of the coupling function and the maps being coupled. We examine two different bursting maps, both of "node" type, namely the one introduced by Cazelles *et al.* [2], (2), and the one shown in Fig. 9.2(a). We demonstrate four synchronized responses, namely anti-phase and in-phase bursting, as well as anti-phase and in-phase spiking.

We begin with an examination of coupling two units of the map introduced by Cazelles *et al.* They suggested that the coupling function is of the following form,

$$G(x, y) = x^2 + y, \tag{12}$$

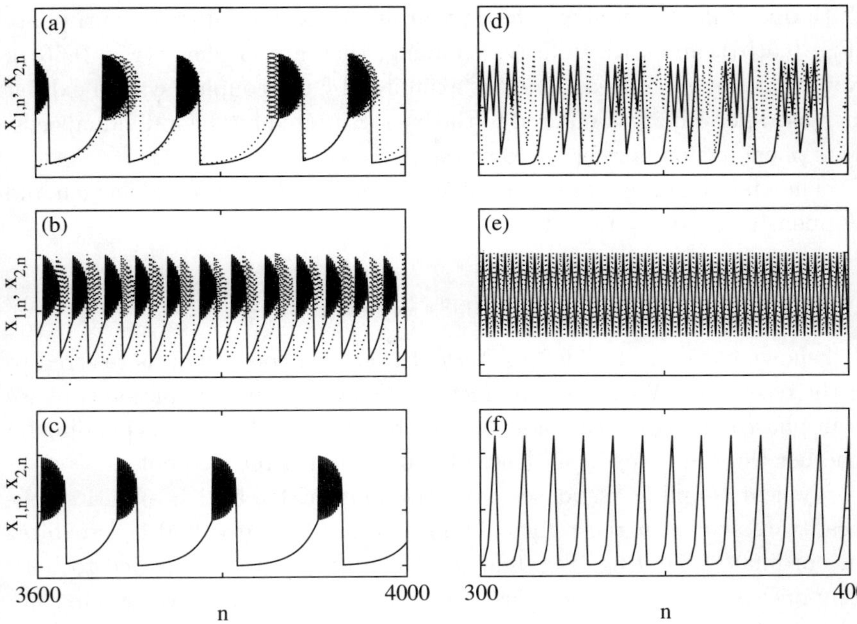

Fig. 9.5. Behaviour of coupled one-dimensional bursting maps, (10)–(11). In each case, the solid curve represents x_1 and the dotted curve represents x_2. Left column: the map of Cazelles *et al.* [2], with $F(x)$ given by (2). (a) No coupling; (b) mean-field coupling ($G(x, y)$ given by (13), with $g_c = 0.03$); (c) diffusive coupling ($G(x, y)$ given by (14), with $g_c = 0.15$). Right column: the map of "node" type from Fig. 9.2(a). (d) No coupling; (e) mean-field coupling ($G(x, y)$ given by (13), with $g_c = 0.4$); (f) partial mean-field coupling ($G(x, y)$ given by (16), with $g_c = 0.4$).

and referred to maps coupled this way as synaptically coupled maps, corresponding phenomenologically to the reciprocal excitatory synaptic connection between neurons. Using $g_c = 0.016$, the system of two coupled maps, (10)–(11), exhibits anti-phase bursting oscillations. We will use a variant of this coupling term, namely

$$G(x, y) = \frac{x + y}{2}, \tag{13}$$

which we will refer to as *mean-field coupling*, as well as

$$G(x, y) = y - x, \tag{14}$$

which we will refer to as *diffusive coupling*.

Typical coupling responses with the map of Cazelles *et al.* are shown in the left column of Fig. 9.5. Individual cells exhibit uncoordinated bursting (Fig. 9.5(a)). Coupling results in synchronized bursting oscillations.

With mean-field coupling, the synchronized oscillations are anti-phase (Fig. 9.5(b)), and with diffusive coupling, they are in-phase (Fig. 9.5(c)). Note that the bursting oscillations exhibited by the coupled system exhibit increased periodicity compared to the ones exhibited by the individual cells. This phenomenon is referred to as regularization.

The one-dimensional map of "node" type introduced by Izhikevich and Hoppensteadt [10] is given by

$$F(x) = \begin{cases} 4x(1-x) & \text{when } x \le 0.98, \\ 0.000098x & \text{when } x > 0.98, \end{cases} \tag{15}$$

and shown earlier in Fig. 9.2(a). Here, the second component is referred to as the reset step. With this map, mean-field coupling may induce anti-phase or in-phase spiking instead of anti-phase bursting oscillations, depending on whether the reset step is subjected to the coupling term or not.

Typical coupling responses with the map of Izhikevich and Hoppensteadt are shown in the right column of Fig. 9.5. Individual cells exhibit uncoordinated bursting (Fig. 9.5(d)). Mean-field coupling applied to both components of $F(x)$ induces fast, small-amplitude anti-phase spiking behaviour (Fig. 9.5(e)), and partial mean-field coupling, using

$$G(x,y) = \begin{cases} \frac{x+y}{2} & \text{when } x \le 0.98, \\ 0 & \text{when } x > 0.98, \end{cases} \tag{16}$$

induces slow, large-amplitude in-phase spiking behaviour (Fig. 9.5(f)).

9.3.2. *Effects of coupling on two-dimensional maps*

We now return to two-dimensional maps, and examine the effect of simple coupling terms on the behaviour of the bursting oscillations. In particular, we couple two maps of the form (3)–(4) as follows:

$$x_{i,n+1} = f(x_{i,n}, y_{i,n}) + g_c h(x_{i,n}, x_{j,n}, y_{i,n}, y_{j,n}), \tag{17}$$

$$y_{i,n+1} = y_{i,n} + \varepsilon g(x_{i,n}), \tag{18}$$

for $i, j = 1, 2$ and $i \neq j$. As before, the two coupled maps are identical, and the coupling terms are symmetrical.

We first examine the effect of mean-field coupling on Rulkov's first map [14]. For this map, $f(x, y)$ and $g(x)$ are given by (5)–(6), and

$$h(x_1, x_2, y_1, y_2) = \frac{x_1 + x_2}{2}. \tag{19}$$

Results are shown in Fig. 9.6. Without coupling, the maps exhibit un-

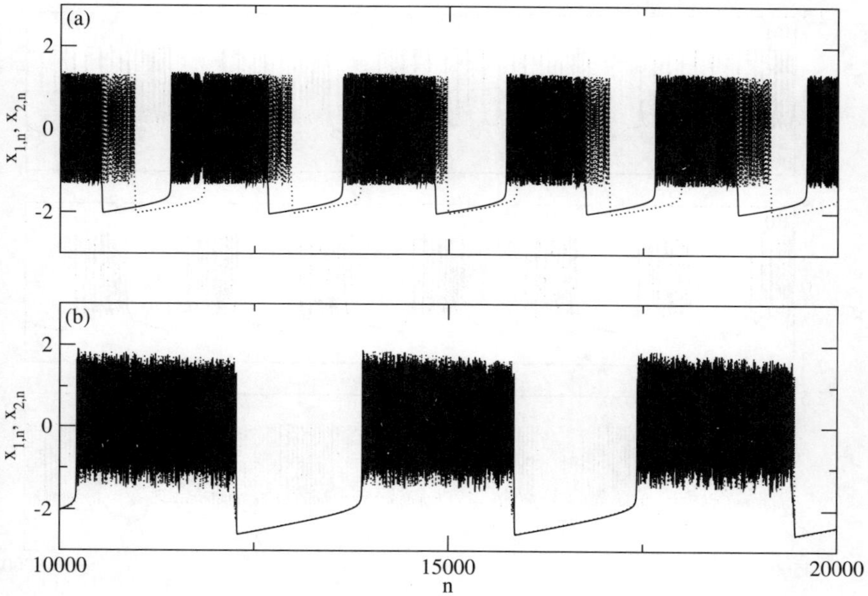

Fig. 9.6. Behaviour of coupled two-dimensional bursting maps, (17)-(18), with $f(x, y)$ and $g(x)$ given by (5)-(6), $\alpha = 4.15$, $\sigma = -1$, $\varepsilon = 0.001$, and $h(x_1, x_2, y_1, y_2)$ given by (19). (a) $g_c = 0$; (b) $g_c = 0.2$.

coordinated bursting oscillations (Fig. 9.6(a)). With coupling, bursts are synchronized (Fig. 9.6(b)). In general, the spikes within the bursts are not synchronized, unless the same initial conditions are used for both maps. Note that mean-field coupling extends the burst period and increases the amplitude of the burst oscillations. These observations can be explained using a fast/slow decomposition and a bifurcation analysis of the coupled fast subsystem, which we do in section 9.4.

Applying diffusive coupling to Rulkov's first map destroys the bursting oscillations. Rulkov's second map [15] responds well to both mean-field and diffusive coupling, in the sense that bursting oscillations are preserved. We focus on the response to diffusive coupling. For this map, $f(x, y)$ and $g(x)$ are given by (8)–(9), and

$$h(x_1, x_2, y_1, y_2) = \begin{cases} x_{2,n} - x_{1,n} & \text{when } \ x < \alpha + y_1, \\ 0 & \text{when } \ x \geq \alpha + y_1. \end{cases} \tag{20}$$

The diffusive coupling used here is slightly different from that used by Rulkov [15] (in particular, only the equations for x_i are coupled instead of the equations for both x_i and y_i; in addition, the coupling terms are added

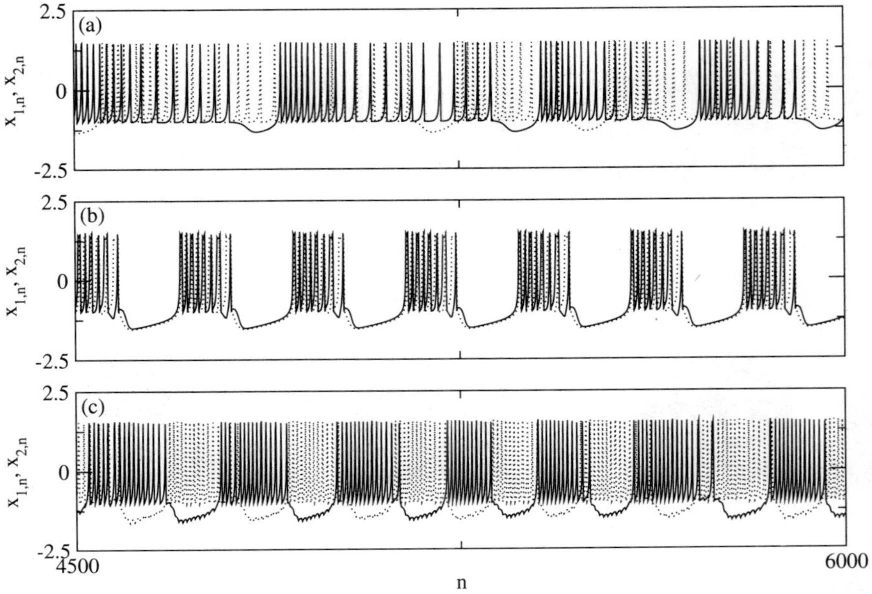

Fig. 9.7. Behaviour of coupled two-dimensional bursting maps, (17)-(18), with $f(x,y)$ and $g(x)$ given by (8)-(9), $\alpha = 4.9$, $\sigma = 0.24$, $\varepsilon = 0.001$, and $h(x_1, x_2, y_1, y_2)$ given by (20). (a) $g_c = 0$; (b) $g_c = 0.05$; (c) $g_c = -0.03$.

externally rather than incorporated into the definition of $f(x,y)$). Results are shown in Fig. 9.7. Without coupling, the maps exhibit uncoordinated bursting oscillations (Fig. 9.7(a)). With $g_c > 0$, bursts are synchronized and in-phase (Fig. 9.7(b). With $g_c < 0$, bursts again are synchronized but anti-phase (Fig. 9.7(c). Note that coupling leads to regularization of the bursting oscillations, as we observed earlier in the context of coupled one-dimensional maps.

9.4. Rulkov's First Bursting Map: Explaining the Effect of Coupling

In the previous section, we observed a number of responses to coupling, depending on the maps being coupled and the form of the coupling. Most of the phenomena observed await further investigation. The one case which has been studied in detail is the effect of mean-field coupling on Rulkov's first map [4, 14], and we review the results here.

We return to the system of two coupled maps, (17)–(18), with $f(x,y)$ and $g(x)$ given by (5)–(6), and $h(x_1, x_2, y_1, y_2)$ given by (19), and extend

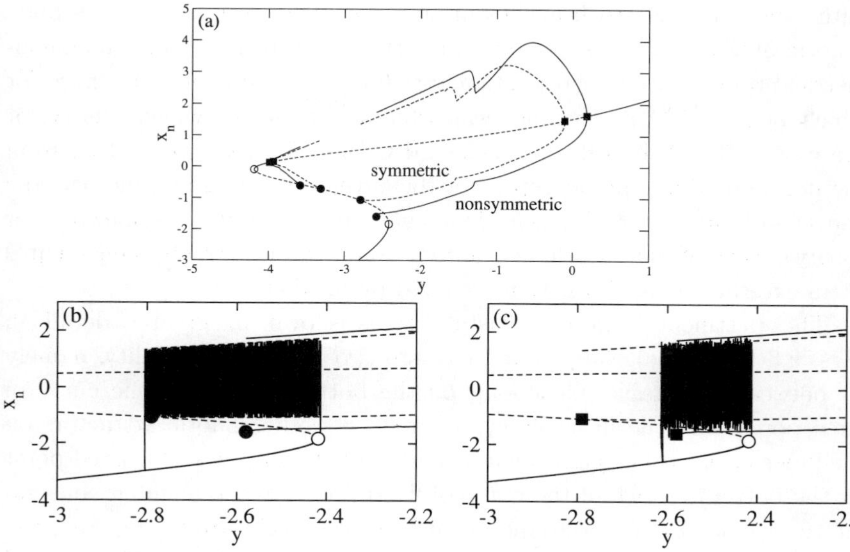

Fig. 9.8. (a) Bifurcation diagram for the two-cell fast subsystem, (21)–(22), with $\alpha = 4.15$ and $g_c = 0.2$. The C-shaped and backward C-shaped curves emanating from the period-doubling bifurcation points represent the envelopes containing the stable (solid) and unstable (dashed) periodic/chaotic orbits of the map. (b) Close-up of the region of bistability, with a trajectory of the full two-cell system superimposed. The two cells were given identical initial conditions. (c) As (b), but now the two cells were given non-identical initial conditions.

the bifurcation analysis of the single-cell fast subsystem to the coupled fast subsystem. In the coupled fast subsystem, there are two slow variables, $y_{1,n}$ and $y_{2,n}$. However, simulations reveal that $y_{1,n} \approx y_{2,n}$, justifying the study of the following coupled fast subsystem:

$$x_{n+1,1} = \frac{\alpha}{1 + x_{n,1}^2} + y + \frac{g_c}{2}(x_{n,1} + x_{n,2}), \tag{21}$$

$$x_{n+1,2} = \frac{\alpha}{1 + x_{n,2}^2} + y + \frac{g_c}{2}(x_{n,1} + x_{n,2}). \tag{22}$$

The bifurcation diagram for (21)–(22), using y as the bifurcation parameter, is shown in Fig. 9.8(a). As before, the curve of fixed points traces out an S-shaped curve. Thin solid portions indicate stable fixed points, and dashed portions indicated unstable fixed points. On the upper branch of fixed points, both period-doubling bifurcations that were seen in the bifurcation diagram for the single-cell fast subsystem have been replaced by a pair of period-doubling bifurcations, denoted by filled squares. The outer ones give rise to branches of stable nonsymmetrical n-cycles and chaotic attractors; the inner ones give rise to branches of unstable symmetrical n-cycles and chaotic attractors (symmetrical orbits are those for which $x_{1,n} = x_{2,n}$; nonsymmetrical orbits are those for which this is not the case). The C-shaped and backward C-shaped curves emanating from the period-doubling points represent the envelopes containing the periodic and chaotic attractors (the envelopes have been smoothed somewhat for clarity). Each of the branches of periodic and chaotic attractors terminates at an external crisis bifurcation, denoted by filled circles.

The pertinent region of bistability is shown in greater detail in Figs. 9.8(b) and (c). Note that there are two types of bistability, namely (i) between the stable fixed point on the bottom branch of the curve of fixed points and the unstable symmetrical periodic/chaotic attractors on the inner backward C-shaped curve, and (ii) between the stable fixed point on the bottom branch of the curve of fixed points and the stable nonsymmetrical periodic/chaotic attractors on the outer backward C-shaped curve. Either type of bistability can give rise to bursting oscillations. If the initial conditions of the two cells are identical, ($x_{1,0} = x_{2,0}$ and $y_{1,0} = y_{2,0}$), then bursting is characterized by bistability of type (i) (Fig. 9.8(b)); if the initial conditions of the two cells are not identical, then bursting is characterized by bistability of type (ii) (Fig. 9.8(c)).

The observations made earlier about the effect of coupling on the burst period and amplitude now can be explained. Both are determined by the size of the region of bistability, $M_b = y_{SN} - y_{EC}$, where y_{SN} is the value of y at the right saddle-node bifurcation, and y_{EC} is the value of y at the rightmost external crisis bifurcation (assuming that nonsymmetrical bursting oscillations are of interest). The value of M_b for the coupled system is significantly larger than that for the single cell. Thus, both the silent and active phases, as well as the burst period, are prolonged with coupling, as observed earlier. Since y decreases more during the active phase in the coupled system compared to the single-cell system, the value of x is smaller upon return to the silent phase, explaining the increased burst amplitude observed earlier.

A two-parameter bifurcation diagram that summarizes the effect of coupling strength, g_c, on the locations of the bifurcation points is shown in Fig. 9.9. Note that as g_c increases, both pertinent external crisis and saddle-node bifurcation points move to the right. However, the saddle-node bifurcation point moves to the right faster than the external crisis bifurcation point. Hence M_b increases with coupling strength.

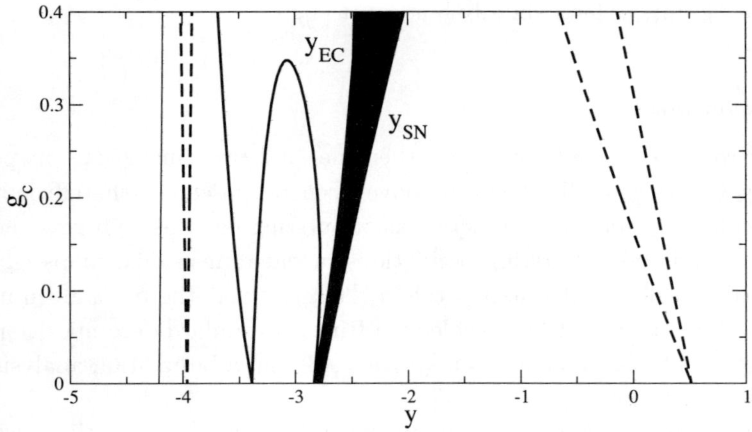

Fig. 9.9. Two-parameter bifurcation diagram, summarizing the effect of the coupling strength, g_c, on the locations of the bifurcation points from the diagram in Fig. 9.8(a). The thin solid curves, with the right one labelled y_{SN}, represent the saddle-node bifurcations. The thick dashed curves represent the period-doubling bifurcations. The thick solid curves, with the rightmost one labelled y_{EC}, represent the external crisis bifurcations. The shaded region indicates the region of bistability for values of y between y_{EC} and y_{SN}.

Bifurcation analyses of an analogous continuous bursting system [5, 6, 17] revealed the possibility of emergent bursting oscillations, meaning bursting oscillations that emerge through coupling cells which are incapable of bursting individually. A similar phenomenon can be demonstrated with the map being studied here. In particular, nonbursting cells can be created by a small change in the model parameters, for example by setting $\alpha = 8\sqrt{3}/3$, so that the pertinent external crisis and saddle-node bifurcation points coincide and $y_{EC} = y_{SN}$. This change destroys the region of bistability. Individual cells no longer burst; they are either at rest or spiking continuously, depending on the value of the parameter σ in the slow subsystem, given by (4) and (6). As before, coupling results in both the external crisis and saddle-node bifurcation points moving to the right, but because the saddle-node bifurcation point moves to the right faster than the external crisis bifurcation point, the region of bistability is reintroduced. Thus, the coupled system can exhibit bursting oscillations, whereas individual cell cannot.

In the analogous continuous bursting system, heterogeneity in the model parameters enhanced the phenomenon of emergent bursting [6]. Interestingly, heterogeneity in the map being studied here does not promote emergent bursting but, in fact, slightly hinders it [4].

9.5. Discussion

In this chapter, we have brought together one- and two-dimensional maps exhibiting bursting oscillations that have been proposed for the efficient study of collective behaviour in networks of bursting neurons. Whereas the mechanism underlying bursting oscillations in one-dimensional maps can be revealed in a plot of the map in the (x_n, x_{n+1}) plane, the mechanism in two-dimensional maps is best revealed via Rinzel's standard decomposition of the system into fast and slow subsystems [13] and a bifurcation analysis of the fast subsystem.

The coupling of two bursting maps can take several forms. Here, we have focussed on mean-field and diffusive coupling, forms of coupling which often are used in creating neurobiological networks. In all cases discussed, coupling serves to synchronize the behaviour of the two cells, either in an anti-phase or an in-phase fashion.

In particular, the one-dimensional map of Cazelles, which is of "node"-type, responds to mean-field coupling with anti-phase bursting oscillations, and to diffusive coupling with in-phase bursting oscillations. Curiously, the one-dimensional map of "node"-type introduced by Izhikevich and Hoppensteadt responds differently to mean-field coupling, namely with large anti-phase spikes. When the mean-field coupling is partial (not applied to the reset step), then the two-cell system responds with large in-phase spikes. These results raise two immediate questions, namely (1) what are the mechanisms underlying the responses, and (2) what are the characteristic features of the map, other than its classification type, that favour a particular outcome? In general, can a particular outcome be predicted, given the characteristics of the map and the form of the coupling?

The effect of coupling on two-dimensional maps has been studied in more detail, although the results are not yet complete, and questions similar to the ones posed above in the context of one-dimensional maps can be raised here. In particular, both of Rulkov's bursting maps are of "fold/homoclinic" type. However, whereas Rulkov's first map responds well only to mean-field coupling, Rulkov's second bursting map responds well to both mean-field and diffusive coupling. Why is this the case? Rulkov's first bursting map responds to mean-field coupling with in-phase bursting oscillations. The reasons for this can be understood via a bifurcation analysis of the coupled fast subsystem. Rulkov's second bursting map responds to diffusive coupling with either in-phase or anti-phase bursting oscillations, depending on the sign of the coupling strength. The reasons for this are not yet understood.

Often, a bursting map exhibits irregular bursting oscillations, which become regular upon coupling (see for example Figs. 9.5 and 9.6). The increased periodicity or the formation of periodic temporal patterns in chaotic systems is referred to as regularization. In the case of Rulkov's first bursting map, regularization results from an increased burst period in the coupled system, so that small variations in the timing of the return from the active phase back to the silent phase are not nearly as significant as they are in single cells. Regularization serves to make the system less susceptible to the disruptive effects of noise, and is of interest in information processing.

The effects of noise on bursting maps has been studied by Hilborn [7] and Hilborn and Erwin [8]. They have shown that Rulkov's first bursting map exhibits both stochastic resonance and stochastic coherence, which are widely studied noise-induced phenomena. Stochastic resonance refers to the enhancement of the response of the system to a small external periodic signal with an appropriate, intermediate amount of noise. Stochastic coherence refers to the enhanced periodicity of the behaviour of the system when noise is added. Hilborn and Erwin [8] discovered that Rulkov's first bursting map exhibits stochastic resonance when noise is added to either the fast or the slow subsystem, but that the effect is significantly pronounced when the noise is added to the fast subsystem. How other bursting maps, including coupled systems, respond to noise remains to be seen.

In this chapter, we have focussed on the modulatory effects of coupling in systems of two cells. As with continuous bursting models, it is implied that the results carry over to larger neurobiological networks, where the advantage of computational efficiency can come to its full right. For example, Rulkov's second bursting map was used by Rulkov *et al.* [16] to simulate oscillations in large-scale cortical networks, with up to 100,000 neurons. The neurons were coupled via synaptic currents, a type of coupling not discussed here, where the form of the term that represents the synaptic current has been adapted from the usual form used in models based on the Hodgkin-Huxley formalism. Responses of the network of map-based models were similar to those found in networks of biophysically-based models and in experiments, but obtained in a fraction of the time required with the more elaborate Hodgkin-Huxley models.

Although the bursting maps discussed in this chapter can reproduce many phenomena that have been observed in neurobiological systems, they were derived without any direct reference to the biophysical properties of the neuron. As such, there are some difficulties with tuning model parameters (and equations) in order to endow the map with certain desired behavioural properties. This is a disadvantage that must be weighed carefully against the advantage of computational efficiency.

The results highlighted in this chapter are unified through the theme of synchronization. However, it is clear that we currently lack general results with respect to being able to predict a certain synchronization outcome given the characteristics of the bursting map and the form of the coupling terms. The results collected here, and the questions they raise, may well serve to stimulate further research into this area of nonlinear dynamics.

Acknowledgments

This work was supported in part by the Natural Sciences and Engineering Research Council of Canada.

References

[1] R. J. Butera, Multirhythmic bursting, *Chaos.* **8**, 274–284, (1998).

[2] B. Cazelles, M. Courbage, and M. Rabinovich, Anti-phase regularization of coupled chaotic maps modelling bursting neurons, *Europhys. Lett.* **56**, 504–509, (2001).

[3] T. R. Chay and J. Rinzel, Bursting, beating, and chaos in an excitable membrane model, *Biophys. J.* **47**, 357–366, (1985).

[4] G. de Vries, Bursting as an emergent phenomenon in coupled chaotic maps, *Phys. Rev. E.* **64**, 051914(9), (2001).

[5] G. de Vries and A. Sherman, Channel sharing in pancreatic β-cells revisited: Enhancement of emergent bursting by noise, *J. Theor. Biol.* **207**, 513–530, (2000).

[6] G. de Vries and A. Sherman, From spikers to bursters via coupling: Help from heterogeneity, *Bull. Math. Biol.* **63**, 371–391, (2001).

[7] R. C. Hilborn, A simple model for stochastic coherence and stochastic resonance, *Am. J. Phys.* **72**, 528–533, (2004).

[8] R. C. Hilborn and R. J. Erwin, Coherence resonance in models of an excitable neuron with noise in both the fast and slow dynamics, *Phys. Lett. A.* **322**, 19–24, (2004).

[9] E. M. Izhikevich, Neural excitability, spiking and bursting, *Int. J. Bifurcation and Chaos.* **10**, 1171–1266, (2000).

[10] E. M. Izhikevich and F. Hoppensteadt, Classification of bursting mappings, *Int. J. Bifurcation and Chaos.* **14**, 3847–3854, (2004).

[11] R. M. May, Simple mathematical models with very complicated dynamics, *Nature (London).* **261**, 459–467, (1976).

[12] G. S. Medvedev, Reduction of a model of an excitable cell to a one-dimensional map, *Physica D.* **202**, 37–59, (2005).

[13] J. Rinzel. Bursting oscillations in an excitable membrane model. In eds. B. D. Sleeman and R. J. Jarvis, *Ordinary and Partial Differential Equations, Lecture Notes in Mathematics, Vol. 1151*, pp. 304–316. Springer, New York, (1985).

[14] N. F. Rulkov, Regularization of synchronized chaotic bursts, *Phys. Rev. Lett.* **86**, 183–186, (2001).

[15] N. F. Rulkov, Modeling of spiking-bursting neural behavior using two-dimensional map, *Phys. Rev. E.* **65**, 041922(9), (2002).

[16] N. F. Rulkov, I. Timofeev, and M. Bazhenov, Oscillations in large-scale cortical networks: map-based model, *J. Comput. Neurosci.* **17**, 203–223, (2004).

[17] A. Sherman, Anti-phase, asymmetric and aperiodic oscillations in excitable cells - I. coupled bursters, *Bull. Math. Biol.* **56**, 811–835, (1994).

[18] D. Terman, Chaotic spikes arising from a model of bursting in excitable membranes, *SIAM J. Appl. Math.* **51**, 1418–1450, (1991).

CHAPTER 10

BEYOND SYNCHRONIZATION: MODULATORY AND EMERGENT EFFECTS OF COUPLING IN SQUARE-WAVE BURSTING

Gerda de Vries
Department of Mathematical and Statistical Sciences
University of Alberta
Edmonton, AB, T6G 2G1, Canada
e-mail: devries@math.ualberta.ca

Arthur Sherman
Laboratory of Biological Modeling, NIDDK
National Institutes of Health
Bethesda, MD 20892, USA.
e-mail: asherman@nih.gov

We show that diffusive coupling of square-wave bursters, beyond the expected effect of synchronization, can greatly influence the characteristics of the oscillations. For cells that are already bursters, coupling tends to increase burst period. Cells that are not bursters, but near a bursting regime, can be induced to burst by coupling; we call this emergent bursting. Both effects require that coupling be strong enough to synchronize the slow bursts but not the fast spikes. We therefore review in detail the transitions of the fast subsystem from out-of-phase spiking to in-phase spiking as coupling strength is increased and the consequences for the full fast-slow bursting system. The beginnings of an extension of the theory to synaptic coupling are indicated.

10.1. Introduction

In many respects, type I bursting (also known as square wave or fold-homoclinic bursting) can be understood as a minor variant of a relaxation oscillator. By averaging over the spikes of the active phase, the oscillatory plateau is replaced by an equivalent quasi-steady level (voltage, for a neural-type system). However, this erases the information contained in the homoclinic termination, effectively replacing it by a saddle-node bifurcation. In the terminology of Izhikevich [17], one could say that the point-cycle burster is converted to a degenerate point-point burster with no spikes.

One situation in which this is particularly pertinent is when two or more bursters are coupled. One expects electrical (diffusive) coupling to synchronize a population of bursters, and one is not disappointed. However, for a common sub-class of square-wave bursters, to be defined below (see Fig. 10.6), one finds additional effects. For cells that are already bursters, the burst period is generically larger for the coupled population than for the individual cells. A more extreme form of this phenomenon occurs when two cells that are not bursters, but spikers, are coupled. Under certain conditions the coupled pair can burst. If one defines "oscillation" as the slow oscillation or bursting, then in such cases coupling does more than just synchronize or prolong the oscillations; it is essential for the oscillations to exist. We call this "emergent bursting." In this chapter we will describe how these phenomena can be explained by appropriate bifurcation analyses of the coupled system. Both prolonged bursting and emergent bursting turn out to result from out-of-phase spiking with reduced amplitude. Both phenomena disappear for coupling that is strong enough to synchronize the spikes as well as the bursts. Thus, we will pay particular attention to the transition from out-of-phase to in-phase spiking as coupling is increased. We will discuss only two-cell networks, but the results have been seen empirically to carry over for networks of many cells.

The model and the questions addressed were originally motivated by our study of insulin-secreting pancreatic β-cells [6]. There has been a long debate over whether bursting is found in isolated cells or only in electrically coupled populations of cells. The natural setting for β-cells is indeed such coupled populations, namely the islets of Langerhans that make up the endocrine component of the pancreas. Views on this point are still in flux, but current work suggests that part of the confusion stems from the existence of two distinct oscillatory mechanisms in islets, a faster, electrical oscillation with a period of 10 – 60 sec, and a slower metabolic oscillation with a period of several minutes [5]. While the metabolic oscillation is often seen in isolated cells, the electrical oscillation patterns in isolated cells are disorganized, likely due to effects of channel noise [33] and heterogeneity [34, 37]. Some cells do exhibit a form of bursting, but it is much faster than that seen in islets, with a period of at most a few seconds [19, 36]. The remainder of the cells do not burst at all, but rather exhibit fast (1 Hz), large amplitude spiking. The idealized models considered in this chapter can be considered to represent those isolated β-cells, exhibiting fast spiking or fast bursting. We analyze one way in which those cells could approach the behaviour of islets solely by virtue of the dynamical influence of electrical coupling. Occupying a strategic middle ground between the specificity of β-cells and the generality of square-wave bursters, we hope the results will prove useful in advancing our understanding of both extremes.

10.2. The Model

For the purposes of this review, we will examine the following representative model of a square-wave burster:

$$\tau \frac{dv}{dt} = -I_{Ca}(v) - I_K(v,n) - I_s(v,s), \tag{1}$$

$$\tau \frac{dn}{dt} = \lambda[n_\infty(v) - n], \tag{2}$$

$$\tau_s \frac{ds}{dt} = s_\infty(v) - s, \tag{3}$$

where

$$I_{Ca}(v) = g_{Ca} m_\infty(v)(v - v_{Ca}), \tag{4}$$

$$I_K(v) = g_K n(v - v_K), \tag{5}$$

$$I_s(v) = g_s s(v - v_K), \tag{6}$$

$$x_\infty(v) = \frac{1}{1 + \exp[(v_x - v)/\theta_x]}, \quad x = m, n, s. \tag{7}$$

Values for the model parameters are shown in Table 10.1.

Table 10.1. Parameter values for the β-cell model, (1)–(7), unless specified otherwise in the figure captions.

$\bar{g}_{Ca} = 3.6$	$v_{Ca} = 25$ mV	$v_m = -20$ mV	$\theta_m = 12$ mV	$\tau = 20$ msec
$\bar{g}_K = 10$	$v_K = -75$ mV	$v_n = -17$ mV	$\theta_n = 5.6$ mV	$\lambda = 0.9$
$\bar{g}_s = 4$		$v_s = -38$ mV	$\theta_s = 10$ mV	$\tau_s = 35,000$ msec

This model is a simplified and scaled version of a biophysically based model for bursting in pancreatic β-cells [33]. Equation (1) is the current balance equation according to the Hodgkin-Huxley formalism [16], with v representing the membrane potential, and t the time. The right-hand side of the equation consists of terms for the currents thought to play an important role in the bursting oscillations. Here, $I_{Ca}(v)$ represents the current flowing through fast voltage-gated calcium channels, and $I_K(v,n)$ represents the current flowing through slower voltage-gated potassium channels. The last term, $I_s(v,s)$, represents a current that is slowly modulated. In this case, the current is a slowly activating potassium current, but it is easy to change it so that it represents, for example, a slowly inactivating calcium current.

The dynamics of the currents are governed by equations (2) and (3), with n and s representing the fractions of open channels. The parameters λ, τ, and τ_s control the time scale of the dynamics.

Using the parameter values listed in Table 10.1, the single-cell model, (1)–(7), exhibits bursting oscillations, as shown in Fig. 10.1(a). Since $\tau_s \gg \tau$, the dynamics of s are much slower than the dynamics of v and n. Thus, the bursting oscillation can be understood via the standard geometrical perturbation analysis pioneered by Rinzel [26]. In particular, (1)–(3) is decomposed into a fast subsystem, consisting of (1) and (2), and a slow subsystem, consisting of (3). A bifurcation analysis of the fast subsystem, using s as the bifurcation parameter, reveals that the single-cell model can exhibit square-wave bursting oscillations [3, 27], also known as fold/homoclinic bursting oscillations [17], as shown in Fig. 10.2(a). The key to bursting is the region of bistability that exists for the range of s values between the left saddle-node bifurcation and the homoclinic bifurcation. There is bistability between a stable steady state on the bottom branch of the curve of steady states (corresponding to the silent phase of bursting) and a stable limit cycle (corresponding to the active phase). When the dynamics of the slow subsystem are tuned appropriately, a hysteresis loop ensures periodic switching between the silent and active phases. With regards to the bifurcation diagram shown in Fig. 10.2(a), the slow subsystem needs to be tuned such that s decreases when the full system is operating near the stable steady state of the fast subsystem and s increases when it is operating near the limit cycle regime.

To study the effect of coupling on bursting, we use the following two-cell model,

$$\tau \frac{dv_j}{dt} = -I_{Ca}(v_j) - I_K(v_j, n_j) - I_s(v_j, s_j) - g_c(v_j - v_k), \tag{8}$$

$$\tau \frac{dn_j}{dt} = \lambda[n_\infty(v_j) - n_j], \tag{9}$$

$$\tau_s \frac{ds_j}{dt} = s_\infty(v_j) + \beta_j - s_j, \tag{10}$$

for $j,k = 1,2$, where g_c represents the coupling strength. The parameters β_j in the equations governing the dynamics of $s_{1,2}$ are included to allow

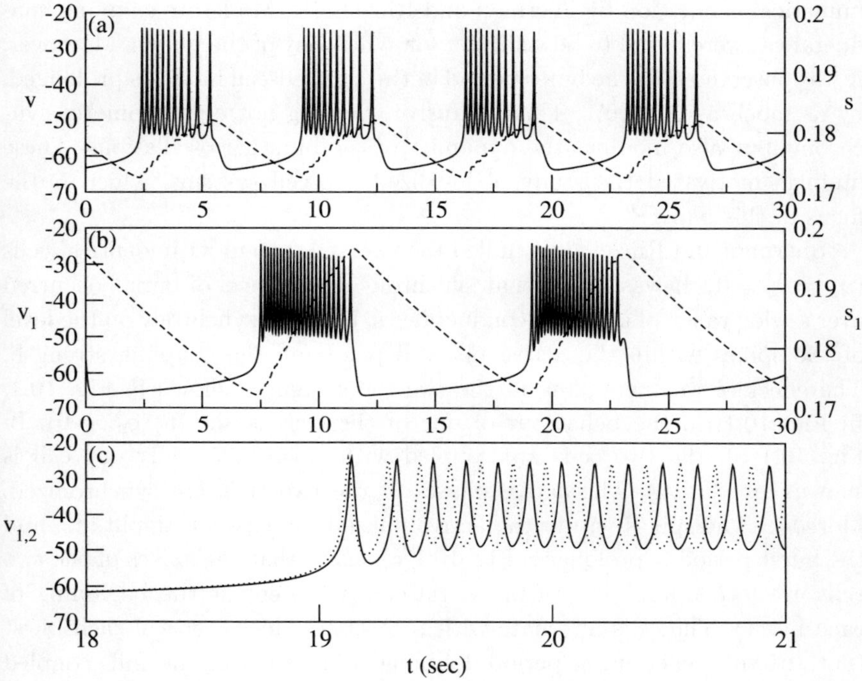

Fig. 10.1. Effect of weak coupling on the two-cell system, (8)–(10), using two identical cells ($\beta_1 = \beta_2 = 0$). **(a)** Behaviour of an uncoupled cell ($g_c = 0$). **(b)** Behaviour of one cell when the system is coupled ($g_c = 0.05$). The solid curves represent the membrane potential (v or $v_{1,2}$), and the dashed curves represent the slow variable (s or $s_{1,2}$). In **(b)**, the bursts of the two cells are in-phase, but the spikes during the active phases are anti-phase. Only one cell is shown for clarity. **(c)** Expanded view of the initial portion of the second active phase in **(b)**, with the solid line representing cell 1 and the dotted line representing cell 2, showing that the spikes of the two cells are antiphase.

for the possibility of heterogeneity in the system when $\beta_1 \neq \beta_2$. Varying the parameter β_j shifts the position of the slow nullcline for s_j relative to the Z-shaped curve of steady states in the bifurcation diagram for the fast subsystem. Note that the linear transformation $\tilde{s}_j = s_j - \beta_j$ transfers the heterogeneity to the fast subsystem, namely to the v_j equation, where it appears as an additional linear potassium current. Thus, the heterogeneity is more general than it appears at first glance.

10.3. Effect of Coupling: Identical Cells

The role of gap-junctional coupling in synchronizing electrical activity within small clusters ($5 \times 5 \times 5$ cells) of identical cells was studied via numerical simulation by Sherman and Rinzel [31]. Moderate coupling conductances were found to be sufficient for synchrony of the bursts. Moreover, it was observed that the burst period in the coupled-cell model is prolonged, by as much as 50–100%. Thus, diffusive coupling not only promotes synchrony, but also modifies the dynamics of the bursting oscillations. These findings motivated the study of idealized two-cell systems, which is the focus in this paper.

Sherman and Rinzel [32] studied the two-cell system with identical cells ($\beta_1 = \beta_2 = 0$). It was shown that synchrony on the level of bursts occurred over a wide range of coupling conductances, but that synchrony on the level of the spikes within the active phase depends on the coupling strength. The effect of weak coupling in the two-cell system is shown in Fig. 10.1. In Fig. 10.1(a), the behaviour of one of the cells is shown ($g_c = 0$). In Fig. 10.1(b), the two cells are coupled with $g_c = 0.05$ (only one cell is shown, for clarity). The active phases of the two cells are synchronized. Moreover, the spikes within the active phase have smaller amplitude, and the burst period is prolonged. Fig. 10.1(c) shows that the spikes of the two cells are locked 180° out of phase (after a transient at the beginning of each burst). The cells alternate with respect to which leads in each burst (not shown), reflecting a period-doubling bifurcation of the full, coupled bursting system; this will be discussed a little further in section 10.3.2.

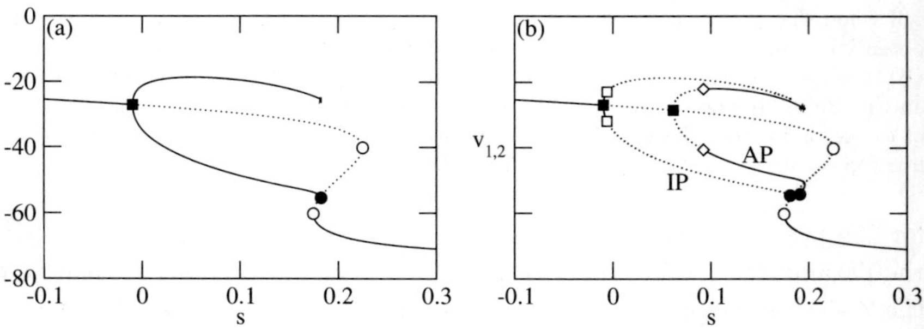

Fig. 10.2. One-parameter bifurcation diagrams for the fast subsystems. **(a)** Bifurcation diagram for the fast subsystem of the single-cell model, (1)–(2). **(b)** Pertinent branches of the bifurcation diagram for the fast subsystem of the two-cell model, (8)–(9), using $s = s_1 = s_2$ as the bifurcation parameter, with $\beta_1 = \beta_2 = 0$, and $g_c = 0.05$. All other parameter values are as listed in Table 10.1. IP refers to the branch of in-phase oscillations, and AP refers to the branch of anti-phase oscillations. Symbols represent bifurcations, as listed in Table 10.2.

Sherman [30] extended the fast-slow decomposition for the single-cell case to the two-cell case. The fast subsystem, (8)–(9), is four-dimensional, and there are two candidates for the bifurcation parameter, namely s_1 and s_2. However, $s_1 \approx s_2$, and so the bifurcation structure of the fast subsystem can be revealed with the single bifurcation parameter $s = s_1 = s_2$, as shown in Fig. 10.2(b). Instead of one Hopf bifurcation on the upper branch of the Z-shaped curve of steady states, there now are two Hopf bifurcations. The left-most gives rise to a branch of in-phase (IP) oscillations, while the other Hopf bifurcation gives rise to a branch of anti-phase (AP) oscillations. (See Han *et al.* [14] for a phase-plane analysis of how AP oscillations arise.) For values of s near the left-most saddle-node bifurcation, the in-phase oscillations are unstable, while the anti-phase oscillations are stable. Moreover, there is bistability between the stable anti-phase oscillations and the stable steady states on the lower branch of the Z-shaped curve, so that square-wave bursting is possible. The active phase of the bursts is carried by the branch of anti-phase oscillations, resulting in spikes with smaller amplitude, and a larger increase of s during the active phase, thus explaining the increased period in Fig. 10.1(b). (See also section 10.3.2.)

Table 10.2. Explanation of symbols and abbreviations used to represent bifurcations in the figures.

Symbol	**Bifurcation**	
	open	filled
circle	saddle-node (SN)	homoclinic (HC)
square	pitchfork (PF) (or pitchfork of periodics)	Hopf (HB)
diamond	torus (TR)	saddle-node on an invariant circle (SNIC)
triangle up	period-doubling (PD)	saddle-node of periodics (SNP)
triangle down	Takens-Bogdanov (TB)	cusp
star	saddle-node-loop (SNL)	

10.3.1. *Effects of coupling on spike patterns*

When coupling strength increases, the branch of anti-phase oscillations destabilizes and disappears, while the branch of in-phase oscillations restabilizes. Thus, as coupling strength increases, phase relationships other than anti-phase occur. Different phase relationships are illustrated in Fig. 10.3. Here, the dynamics of s are suppressed by fixing the value of s, and the spiking behaviour of the coupled fast subsystem, (8)–(9), is investigated for four different values of the coupling strength, g_c. With weak coupling, anti-phase oscillations are observed (Fig. 10.3(a)). Increasing the coupling strength leads to quasi-periodic oscillations during which both the spike amplitude and the phase difference vary (Fig. 10.3(b)). Increasing the coupling strength further yields asymmetrically phase-locked oscillations (Fig. 10.3(c)). In this case, the spike amplitude is constant, but different for each cell. The phase difference is constant, but the cells are neither perfectly in phase nor perfectly out of phase. Increasing the coupling strength even further causes the two-cell system to behave as a single cell, that is, the two cells are spiking in phase, with the spike amplitude equal to that of the single cells (Fig. 10.3(d)).

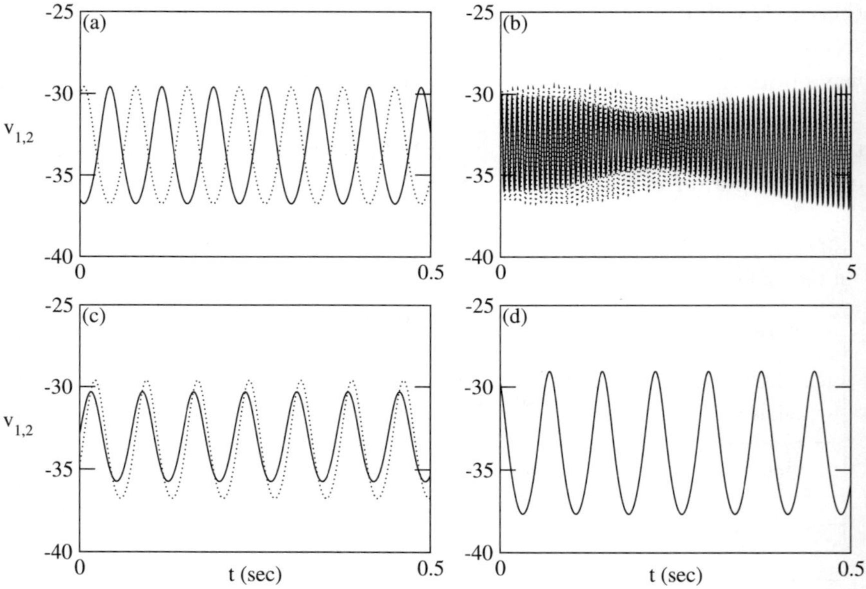

Fig. 10.3. Solution types for the coupled fast subsystem, (8)–(9), using identical cells ($\beta_1 = \beta_2 = 0$), with $\lambda = 1.1$, and $s_1 = s_2 = 0.1751$. **(a)** anti-phase (AP) spiking with $g_c = 0.003$; **(b)** quasi-periodic (QP) spiking with $g_c = 0.012$; **(c)** asymmetric (AS) spiking with $g_c = 0.05$; **(d)** in-phase (IP) spiking with $g_c = 0.1$.

The spiking behaviour can be summarized in a one-parameter diagram, where we track the amplitude of the oscillations, using coupling strength g_c as the bifurcation parameter, as shown in Fig. 10.4(a). The branch of anti-phase (AP) oscillations is stable for small values of g_c and unstable for larger values of g_c. The stability changes at a torus bifurcation. The amplitude of the oscillations decreases, until the anti-phase oscillations disappear at a Hopf bifurcation. The branch of in-phase (IP) oscillations is unstable initially, and gains stability via a pitchfork bifurcation. Branches of asymmetric (AS1 and AS2) oscillations emerge from the pitchfork bifurcation; these branches are symmetrically related, with cell 1 having larger amplitude on one branch and cell 2 having larger amplitude on the other. These branches are stable for large coupling strengths and unstable for small coupling strengths. Stability changes at a torus bifurcation. Quasi-periodic oscillations are not labelled on the bifurcation diagram because the software we use (XPPAUT) cannot track them. They exist for intermediate coupling strengths, when none of the other oscillatory branches are stable, in the gap between the torus bifurcations on the branches of anti-phase and asymmetric oscillations.

The qualitative nature of the bifurcation diagram shown in Fig. 10.4(a) persists for different values of s, but is not generic. In particular, the pitchfork bifurcation on the branch of in-phase oscillations exists because of the symmetry of the two-cell system when the two cells are identical. In section 10.4, we investigate the case where the cells no longer are identical. Before we do so, we investigate the effects of coupling on burst period.

10.3.2. *Effects of coupling on burst period*

Figs. 10.1 and 10.2 show that out-of-phase spiking results in increased burst period that goes along with reduced spike amplitude. Geometrically, the period increases because the homoclinic termination of the relevant spiking branch is shifted to the right and hence the slow variable s has to increase further. A more biophysical interpretation is that the mean v is increased. This happens even though the minima are pulled up and the maxima are pulled down because the spikes spend more time near their minima than near their peaks. Consequently, s has to increase further to offset the increased inward current. However, there is a counter-effect as well because s will tend to increase more rapidly. The net effect in this model is increased period, but this is mostly due to the increased duration of the silent phase, as the larger value of s at the beginning of the silent phase takes longer to relax back to the threshold for active phase re-initiation (cf. Fig. 10.1(b)). Thus, typically in models like this the increase in period is accompanied by a decrease in the fraction of the burst period spent in the active phase.

Figs. 10.3 and 10.4(a) show that as g_c increases, and the spike pattern runs through AP, QP, and AS, the spike amplitude first decreases and then

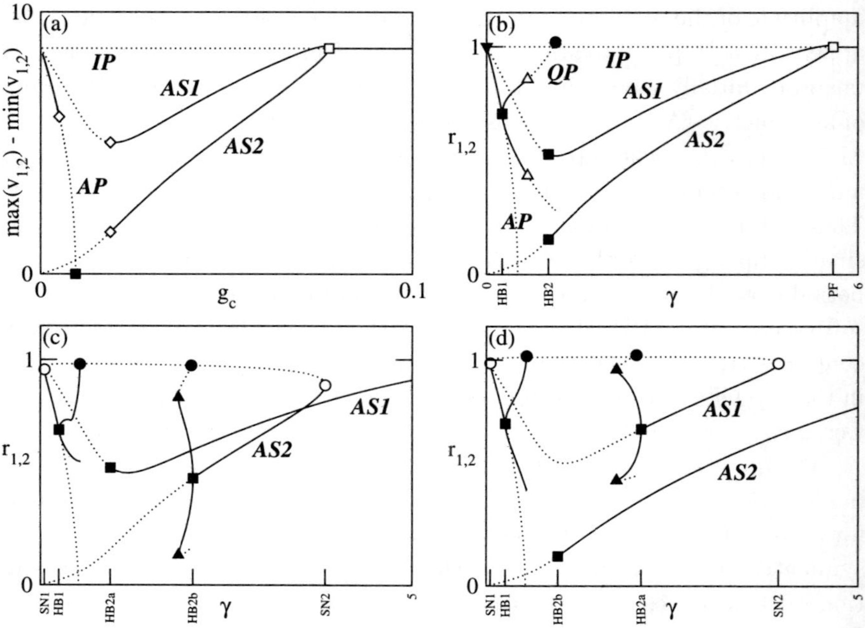

Fig. 10.4. One-parameter bifurcation diagrams, using coupling strength as the bifurcation parameter. **(a)** Diagram for the fast subsystem of the two-cell model, (8)–(9), using identical cells ($\beta_1 = \beta_2 = 0$), showing the steady-state amplitude of limit cycle oscillations as a function of coupling strength, g_c ($\lambda = 1.1$, and $s_1 = s_2 = 0.1751$). **(b)** Diagram for the reduced equations, (11)–(13), showing the steady-state behaviour of $r_{1,2}$ as a function of the coupling strength, γ. In this case, the two cells are identical, that is, $\Delta = 1$. **(c)** and **(d)** As in (b), but the cells are no longer identical ($\Delta = 0.98$ for (c) and $\Delta = 1.02$ for (d)).

recovers back to the IP level. Thus, one expects that burst period should also increase and then decrease with g_c. This is confirmed in Fig. 10.5(a). For the parameters used, bursting carried by asymmetric spiking is not seen, but it does occur if λ is increased slightly to 1.0 (see Fig. 7 in Sherman, 1994 [30]). We will see below that asymmetric spiking becomes much more prevalent when cells are heterogeneous and plays an important role in emergent bursting.

Although on average the period is larger when the spikes are out-of-phase, the bursts actually become aperiodic, as shown by the error bars in Fig. 10.5(a). This is especially prominent in the quasi-periodic regime. A more detailed view is afforded by Fig. 10.5(b), which displays Poincaré sections defined by the peak values of s at the end of the active phase. The period seems to follow well the variation in amplitude of s, suggesting that this is more significant than the increased rate of rise of s during the active phase.

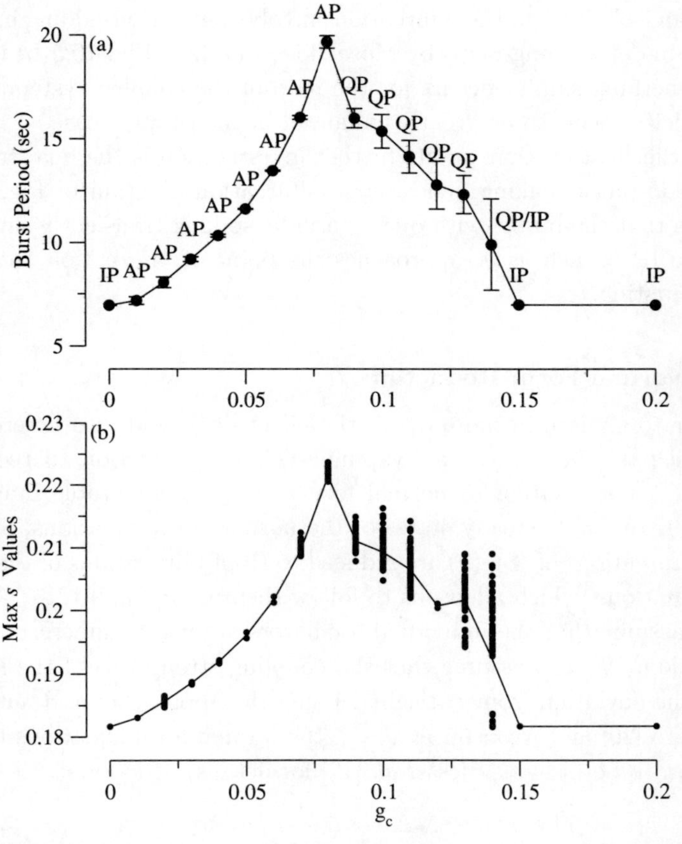

Fig. 10.5. **(a)** Burst period for two identical bursters, (8)–(10), with $\beta_1 = \beta_2 = 0$, coupled with the indicated g_c; other parameters as in Fig. 10.1. Points are labeled with the spike pattern at that value of g_c; IP = in-phase; AP = anti-phase; QP = quasi-periodic. The point labeled "QP/IP" exhibits irregular alternation between quasi-periodic and in-phase spiking. **(b)** Values of s at the end of the active phase (defined as v_1 decreases through -58 mV). This Poincaré section defines a map which can be periodic (e.g., for IP), doubly-periodic (e.g., the AP solution at $g_c = 0.05$) or aperiodic. The aperiodicity accounts for the large error bars in (a).

Note also that for very weak coupling, the map has period 2, with alternating longer and shorter bursts. This is another manifestation of the alternation in which cell leads, mentioned in the discussion of Fig. 10.1.

Closer investigation indicates that this is the beginning of a sequence of period doubling bifurcations of the map leading to chaos. As the mean period increases with g_c, the number of spikes increases, and each new spike is similarly associated with period-doubling and other bifurcations. For the case of an isolated cell, the bifurcations involved in period-adding have been studied in detail using maps by Mosekilde *et al.* [22]. Fig. 10.5(b) indicates that something similar occurs for the map of the coupled system. Indeed, aperiodicity seems to be greatly enhanced in the coupled case.

Another feature that merits further investigation is the final transition back to in-phase spiking. The coarse bifurcation diagram of Fig. 10.5(b) suggests that the bursts with quasi-periodic spiking transiently sample the unstable IP branch as g_c approaches the point of bifurcation back to in-phase bursting.

10.4. Normal Form Reduction

In order to explore in more detail the effect of g_c and also heterogeneity on spike patterns, we use a Lyapunov-Schmidt reduction to reduce the coupled fast subsystem to normal form. This reduces stable limit cycles of (8)–(9) to stable steady states of the normal form equations. Similarly, torus bifurcations of (8)–(9) are reduced to Hopf bifurcations of the normal form equations, which allows us to follow them with XPPAUT.

We assume that the individual oscillators are near a supercritical Hopf bifurcation. We also assume that the coupling strength is of the same order as the deviation from criticality. Using the approaches and notation in Kuramoto [20] and Aronson *et al.* [2], the normal form equations then can be shown to be (see de Vries *et al.* [12] for details) as follows:

$$\dot{r}_1 = r_1(1-r_1^2) + \gamma\sqrt{\Delta}(\cos\phi - \alpha\sin\phi)r_2 - \gamma r_1, \tag{11}$$

$$\dot{r}_2 = \Delta r_2(1-r_2^2) + \frac{\gamma}{\sqrt{\Delta}}(\cos\phi + \alpha\sin\phi)r_1 - \gamma r_2, \tag{12}$$

$$\begin{aligned}\dot{\phi} &= \beta(\Delta - 1) + \eta(r_1^2 - \Delta r_2^2) - \gamma\sqrt{\Delta}(\sin\phi + \alpha\cos\phi)\frac{r_2}{r_1} \\ &\quad - \frac{\gamma}{\sqrt{\Delta}}(\sin\phi - \alpha\cos\phi)\frac{r_1}{r_2}.\end{aligned} \tag{13}$$

The polar variables r_1 and r_2 represent the amplitude of the two oscillators, and $\phi = \theta_2 - \theta_1$ represents their phase difference, where θ_1 and θ_2 are the phase variables of the two oscillators, respectively.

The parameters α, β, and η are determined by the particular choice of model parameters in the original equations. With the parameter values as given in Table 10.1, but $\lambda = 1.1$, we find $\alpha = -0.522$, $\beta = -23.55$, and $\eta = 15.555$. The remaining two parameters, Δ and γ, are free. Δ measures the relative difference between the two oscillators (within the constraints of the assumptions mentioned above, the deviation from criticality may differ for the two oscillators) and γ represents the coupling strength.

We proceed to use the normal form equations to characterize the behaviour of the original coupled fast subsystem, (8)–(9).

10.4.1. *Identical cells:* $\Delta = 1$

The normal form equations, (11)–(13), admit two symmetrical steady states, corresponding to the IP and AP oscillations shown in Fig. 10.4(a), namely the in-phase (IP) steady state, characterized by $r_1 = r_2 = 1$ and $\phi = 0$, and the anti-phase (AP) steady state, characterized by $r_1 = r_2 = \sqrt{1 - 2\gamma}$ and $\phi = \pi$.

The stability of these steady states depends on the value of the coupling parameter γ, as shown in Fig. 10.4(b). The AP steady state exists only over a limited range of γ. It is stable for very weak coupling, and unstable for stronger coupling. The stability changes at a Hopf bifurcation, at $\gamma = \gamma_{HB1}$. In contrast, the IP steady state exists for all values of γ. It is unstable for weak coupling, and stable for strong coupling. The stability changes at a pitchfork bifurcation, at $\gamma = \gamma_{PF}$.

Two asymmetrically phase-locked steady states, corresponding to the AS1 and AS2 oscillations shown in Fig. 10.4(a), emerge from the pitchfork bifurcation on the branch of IP steady states. The AS1 and AS2 steady states are unstable for weak coupling, and stable for intermediate coupling. The stability of these steady states changes at a Hopf bifurcation, at $\gamma = \gamma_{HB2}$ of the reduced equations, which corresponds to the torus bifurcations of the limit cycles in Fig. 10.4(a).

Limit cycle solutions, characterized by oscillations in r_1, r_2, and ϕ, emerge from the Hopf bifurcations on both the branch of AP steady states and the branches of AS1 and AS2 steady states. These solutions correspond to the QP oscillations not shown (but implied) in Fig. 10.4(a). The main branch of limit cycles, emerging from the Hopf bifurcation at $\gamma = \gamma_{HB1}$, is shown in Fig. 10.4(b). The branch is stable initially, and loses stability at a period-doubling bifurcation.

The pitchfork bifurcation at $\gamma = \gamma_{PF}$ occurs because of the symmetry in the normal form equations. We will break the symmetry by setting $\Delta \neq 1$ in the next section. First, we investigate how the essential features of the bifurcation diagram in Fig. 10.4(b) depend on the values of α, β, and η.

10.4.1.1. *Stability of the in-phase and anti-phase steady states*

A change in the model equations or parameters results in different values of the normal form coefficients α, β, and η. Here, we investigate the effect of a change in these parameters on the relative locations of the pitchfork and Hopf bifurcations on the branches of IP and AP steady states. We will see that the appearance of stable AP steady states for weak coupling is not guaranteed, but depends on the choice of model and parameters. Similar results were obtained by Morita [21] for a ring of n coupled oscillators.

Since $\Delta = 1$, the only term containing β in (13) vanishes, that is, the value of β is inconsequential. Thus, we only need to consider α and η.

Examination of the Jacobian of the normal form equations at the two symmetrical steady states reveals that the pitchfork bifurcation occurs on the branch of IP steady states when $1 + \alpha\eta < 0$, at

$$\gamma_{IP} = -\frac{1+\alpha\eta}{1+\alpha^2}.$$

When $1 + \alpha\eta > 0$, the pitchfork bifurcation appears on the branch of AP steady states, at

$$\gamma_{AP} = \frac{1+\alpha\eta}{1+\alpha^2+2(1+\alpha\eta)}.$$

Independent of the pitchfork bifurcation, there is a Hopf bifurcation on the branch of AP steady states, at

$$\gamma_{HB} = \frac{1}{4},$$

unless the pitchfork is on the branch of AP steady states and $\gamma_{AP} > 1/4$.

The curves $\gamma_{IP} = 1/4$, $\gamma_{IP} = \gamma_{AP} = 0$, and $\gamma_{AP} = 1/4$ are shown in Fig. 10.6; they divide (α, η)-space into four different regions within which the relative locations of the pitchfork and Hopf bifurcations are the same. Stable AP steady states exist for very weak coupling in regions A and B only.

For the original model, the coefficients of the normal form equations are such that we land in region A, even with a significant change in the value of the model parameters. That is, the behaviour of the model is very robust. Many other models exhibiting bursting oscillations also lie in region A, and the results discussed here should carry over. However, the normal form parameters for the Hindmarsh-Rose model [15] lie in region B

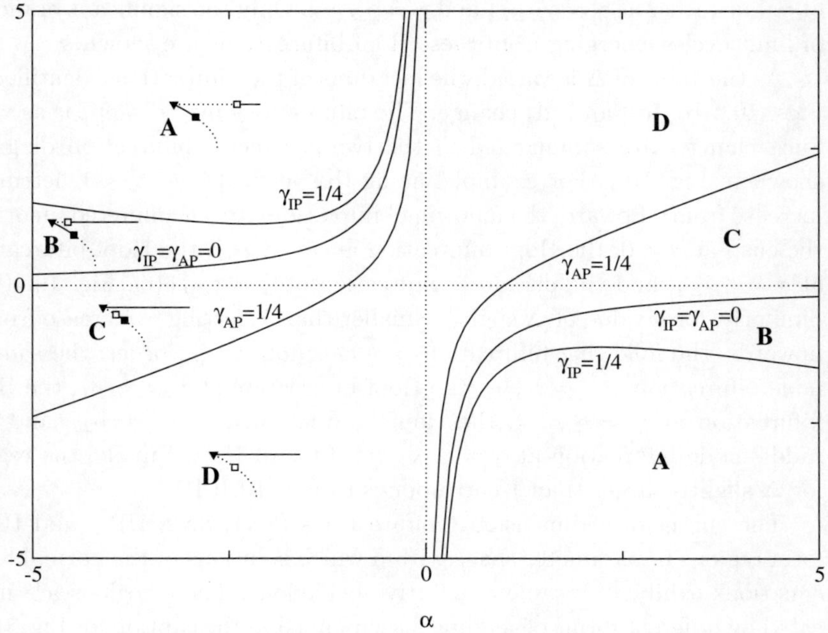

Fig. 10.6. Stability of the in-phase and anti-phase steady states of the reduced equations, (11)–(13), for the case of identical cells ($\Delta = 1$). Insets show the branches of IP and AP steady states as they would appear in a one-parameter bifurcation diagram as shown in Fig. 10.4(b). Region A: the pitchfork appears on the branch of IP steady states, with $\gamma_{IP} > 1/4$. Region B: the pitchfork appears on the branch of IP steady states, with $0 < \gamma_{IP} < 1/4$. Region C: the pitchfork appears on the branch of AP steady states, with $0 < \gamma_{AP} < 1/4$. Region D: the pitchfork appears on the branch of AP steady states, with $1/4 < \gamma_{AP} < 1/2$.

or C. The results of this chapter may apply in region B, where out-of-phase spiking can also occur, but we expect not in region C, where the in-phase oscillations are always stable.

10.4.2. *Non-identical cells:* $\Delta \neq 1$

When $\Delta \neq 1$, the symmetry in the normal form equations, (11)–(13) is broken. Consequently, the pitchfork bifurcation at $\gamma = \gamma_{PF}$ and the cusp at $\gamma = 0$ in Fig. 10.4(b) break, giving way to two saddle-node bifurcations, as shown in Figs. 10.4(c) and (d). The IP and AP steady states no longer exist; they have been perturbed to near-in-phase steady states for strong coupling and near-anti-phase steady states for weak coupling. The two Hopf bifurcations at $\gamma = \gamma_{HB2}$ in Fig. 10.4(b) no longer exist at the same value of γ, but rather at $\gamma = \gamma_{HB2a}$ and $\gamma = \gamma_{HB2b}$. Only the significant branches of limit cycles emerging from these Hopf bifurcations are shown.

As the value of Δ is varied, the locations of the bifurcations identified in Figs. 10.4(b), (c), and (d) change. The bifurcations may disappear as well. Such changes are summarized in the two-parameter bifurcation diagram shown in Fig. 10.7. For example, along the vertical line $\Delta = 1$, letting γ increase from 0 upward, the following bifurcations are encountered, in order: the cusp at $\gamma = 0$, the Hopf bifurcation at $\gamma = \gamma_{HB1}$, the Hopf bifurcation at $\gamma = \gamma_{HB2}$, and the pitchfork bifurcation at $\gamma = \gamma_{PF}$ (cf. Fig. 10.4(b)). Similarly, for a value of Δ slightly smaller than 1, letting γ increase from 0 upwards, the following bifurcations are encountered, in order: the saddle-node bifurcation at $\gamma = \gamma_{SN1}$, the Hopf bifurcation at $\gamma = \gamma_{HB1}$, the Hopf bifurcation at $\gamma = \gamma_{HB2a}$, the Hopf bifurcation at $\gamma = \gamma_{HB2b}$, and the saddle-node bifurcation at $\gamma = \gamma_{SN2}$ (cf. Fig. 10.4(c)). Finally, the region for Δ slightly larger than 1 corresponds to Fig. 10.4(d).

The curves of codimension-1 bifurcations (SN1, SN2, HB1, and HB2) form regions in parameter space within which solutions of the normal form equations exhibit the same qualitative behaviour. These regions are indicated by different forms of shading, as explained in the caption for Fig. 10.7. The white regions represent oscillator death, not mentioned previously. Oscillator death refers to the situation in which the two cells are sufficiently different that coupling causes the rest state ($r_1 = r_2 = 0$) to become stable (via a reverse Hopf bifurcation).

Fig. 10.7 indicates that the prevailing types of solution behaviour are asymmetrically phase-locked and nearly in-phase, provided coupling is not extremely weak (in which case quasi-periodic behaviour is seen), and the two coupled cells are not too different from each other (in which case oscillator death is seen).

10.5. Enhancement of the Period Extension with Heterogeneity

We now return to the full two-cell bursting system (8)–(10), and introduce heterogeneity by taking $\beta_1 \neq \beta_2$. Further, we consider relatively strong coupling ($g_c = 1$) to ensure synchronized bursts with asymmetric spikes (nearly in-phase). A sample solution is shown in Figs. 10.8(a) and (b). Relative to the case of identical cells, the spike amplitude is reduced, and the burst period is lengthened.

As before, these observations can be explained with a bifurcation study

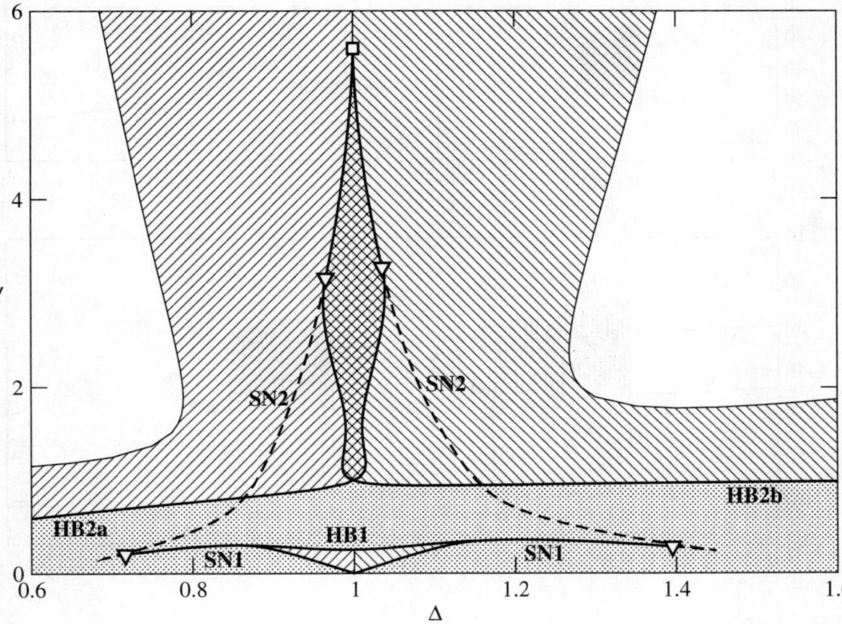

Fig. 10.7. Two-parameter bifurcation diagram for the reduced equations, (11)–(13), identifying regions of uniform qualitative solution behaviour. Regions with positively sloped diagonal lines: asymmetrically phase-locked solution (AS1); Regions with negatively-sloped diagonal lines: asymmetrically phase-locked solution (AS2); Hatched region: bistability of AS1 and AS2; Dotted region: non-phase-locked solution (QP); White regions: oscillator death (OD). The labelled curves defining the boundaries between the different regions are continuations of the saddle-node bifurcations (SN1 and SN2) and Hopf bifurcations (HB1, HB2a, and HB2b) identified in Fig. 10.4.

of the coupled fast subsystem. From Fig. 10.8(b), it is clear that the approximation $s_1 \approx s_2$, valid when the two cells are identical, no longer holds. However, $s_2 - s_1 \approx$ constant. We let

$$\delta = (s_2 - s_1)/2, \tag{17}$$

$$s = (s_2 + s_1)/2, \tag{18}$$

so that we can write $s_1 = s - \delta$ and $s_2 = s + \delta$, and compute the bifurcation diagram for the coupled fast subsystem with respect to s, holding δ fixed. The fixed value of δ is taken to be the average value of $(s_2 - s_1)/2$, based on a long-time solution of the full two-cell system. The resulting bifurcation diagrams, with the trajectories from Figs. 10.8(a) and (b), are shown in Fig. 10.8(c). (An asymptotic method can be used to approximate δ using only knowledge of the behaviour of an isolated cell [11]).

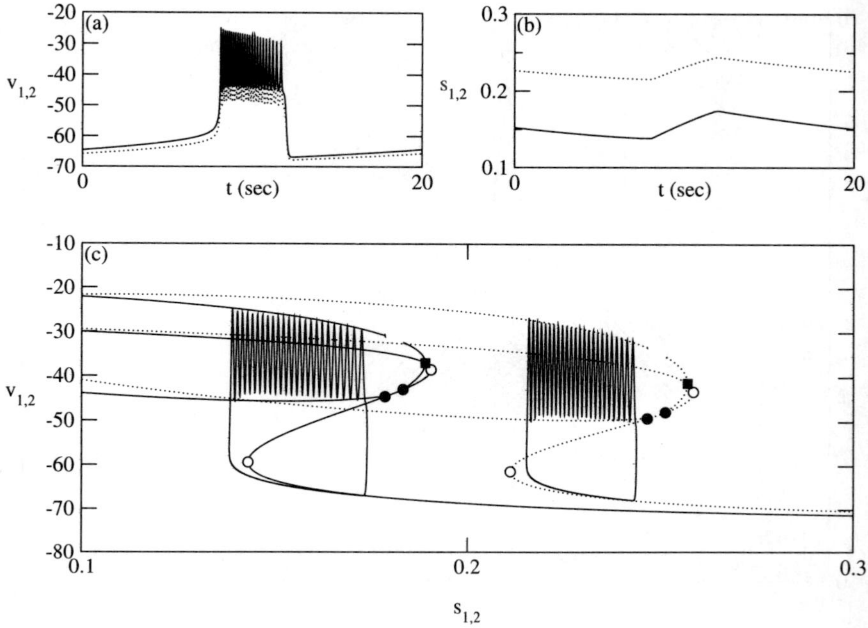

Fig. 10.8. **(a)** and **(b)** Numerical solution of the two-cell system, (8)–(10), using $g_c = 1$, for two non-identical cells ($\beta_1 = 0$, and $\beta_2 = 0.1$). **(c)** Projection of the solution trajectories, v_1 vs s_1 and v_2 vs s_1, onto the bifurcation diagrams for the coupled fast subsystem, (8)–(9), using $\delta = 0.034$.

The trajectories obtained from the full two-cell system follow the fast subsystem bifurcation structure nicely, *a posteriori* justifying the symmetric treatment of s_1 and s_2. We can now study the effect of varying δ. The larger the difference between β_1 and β_2, the more heterogeneous the cells, and the larger the value of $|\delta|$. Using δ as the secondary bifurcation parameter, we can address how varying δ affects the relative position of the pertinent bifurcations in the one-parameter bifurcation diagram.

The resulting bifurcation diagram is shown in Fig. 10.9(a). For a given value of $\delta \approx 0$, reading from left to right, the bifurcations encountered are the Hopf bifurcation (HB), a saddle-node bifurcation (SN), the homoclinic bifurcation (HC), and another saddle-node bifurcation (SN). For a given horizontal cut through this diagram, the distance between the intersections with the first SN and the HC curves indicates the size of the region of bistability in the fast subsystem – the larger this is, the longer both the active and silent phases, and the longer the period of the bursting oscillation. The bifurcation diagram thus shows that increasing $|\delta|$ enlarges the region of bistability, that is, increasing heterogeneity in the system prolongs the bursting period, as observed in Fig. 10.8. Increasing $|\delta|$ further leads to a loss of the homoclinic and Hopf bifurcations (at the codimension-2 Takens-Bogdanov bifurcation labelled with an open triangle), and a concurrent loss of spikes during the active phase (not shown). (This corresponds to the oscillator death region in Fig. 10.7 where the two cells are very different). Thus, while a moderate amount of heterogeneity is beneficial in that it generates more robust spiking with longer burst period, a large amount of heterogeneity is harmful in that it eliminates spiking activity.

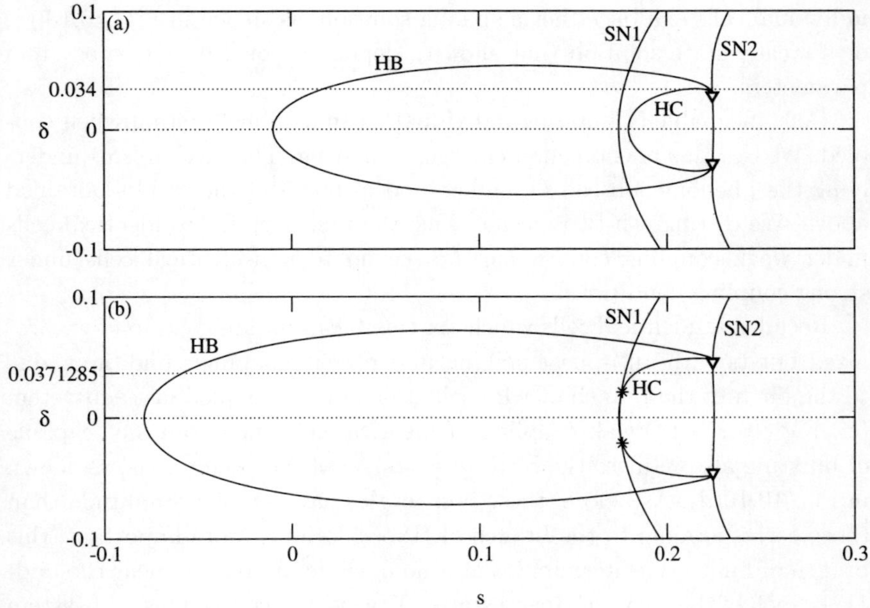

Fig. 10.9. Two-parameter bifurcation diagrams for the fast subsystem, (8)–(9), using s as the primary bifurcation parameter, and δ as the secondary bifurcation parameter. Coupling strength is held fixed at $g_c = 1$. **(a)** $\lambda = 0.9$, dotted line at δ=0.034 corresponds to Fig. 10.8; **(b)** $\lambda = 0.8$, dotted line at δ=0.0371285 corresponds to Fig. 10.10(g), (h).

10.6. Emergent Bursting

So far, bursting has depended fundamentally on two properties, namely 1) the presence of bistability in the fast subsystem between a stable steady state (quiescence) and a stable limit cycle (spiking), and 2) the presence of a slow process on the time scale of the bursting period. In cells possessing these two properties, the slow variable parameters can be tuned so that the cell periodically switches between quiescence and spiking, that is, such cells are capable of bursting.

When treating two-cell systems above, we implicitly assumed that the individual cells are capable of bursting. We now turn our attention to the case in which individual cells no longer are capable of bursting. In particular, we remove the first property, bistability, by moving the homoclinic bifurcation so that it co-exists with the left saddle-node bifurcation in a codimension-1 saddle-node-on-an-invariant-circle bifurcation (SNIC), as shown in Fig. 10.10(b). (This is done by reducing λ to 0.8.) In this case, individual cells exhibit either a spiking solution, as shown in Fig. 10.10(a), or a steady-state solution (not shown), depending on the slow subsystem parameters.

Cells incapable of bursting individually can exhibit bursting when coupled. We call this phenomenon emergent bursting. The mechanisms underlying the phenomenon can be understood in terms of the results obtained above. We distinguish two mechanisms: the first pertains to identical cells under weak coupling conditions; the second to non-identical cells under strong coupling conditions.

Recall that identical cells which are capable of bursting exhibit synchronized bursts with anti-phase spiking under weak coupling conditions, due to the birth of the branch of AP oscillations in the coupled fast subsystem (cf. Fig. 10.2(b)). Weak coupling of identical cells which are not capable of bursting also induces the birth of a branch of AP oscillations, as shown in Fig. 10.10(d). As before, these limit cycles have smaller amplitude than those corresponding to the branch of IP oscillations. More important, this branch of limit cycles terminates at a homoclinic bifurcation near the middle branch of the curve of steady states. That is, the coupled fast subsystem exhibits bistability between stable steady states (on the bottom branch of the curve of steady states) and AP oscillations, and bursting is possible, as shown in Fig. 10.10(c).

Emergent bursting exists for only a small range of coupling strengths, and is lost well before the branch of AP oscillations becomes irrelevant due to destabilization. This early loss of emergent bursting is due to the stabilization of the branch of IP oscillations near the SNIC as coupling strength is increased, as shown in Figs. 10.10(e) and (f). Trajectories of the full system are captured by the stable portion of the branch of IP oscillations, and trapped there.

The addition of small amounts of noise can enhance this form of burst-

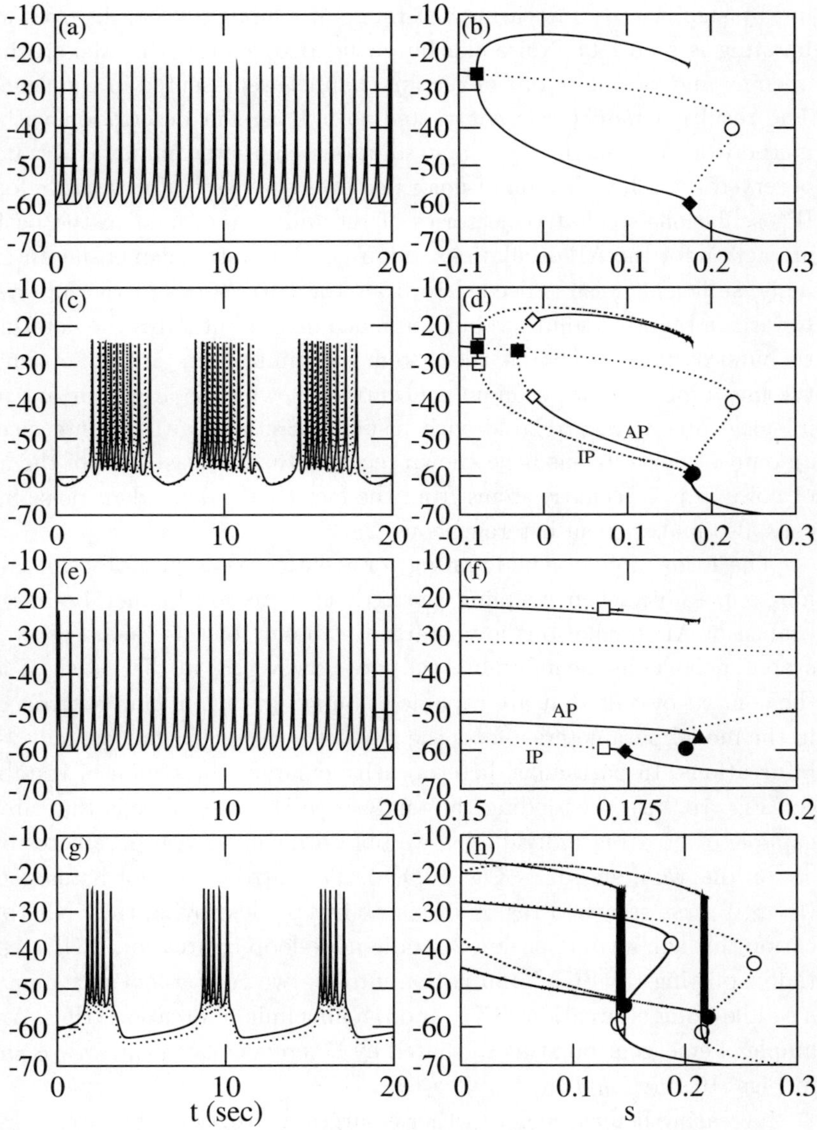

Fig. 10.10. Emergent bursting from non-bursting cells ($\lambda = 0.8$). Left: numerical simulations of the two-cell system, (8)–(10). Right: one-parameter bifurcation diagrams for the corresponding fast subsystem, (8)–(9). **(a)** and **(b)**: Individual cells are non-bursters ($g_c = 0$). **(c)** and **(d)**: Identical non-bursting cells burst with weak coupling ($g_c = 0.035$, $\beta_1 = \beta_2 = 0$). **(e)** and **(f)**: Emergent bursting with identical cells exists over a small range of coupling strengths only ($g_c = 0.07$). **(g)** and **(h)**: Emergent bursting with strong coupling ($g_c = 1$) and heterogeneity ($\beta_1 = 0, \beta_2 = 0.1$). In (h), $\delta = 0.0371285$.

ing by significantly increasing the range of coupling strengths over which bursting is seen [10]. Noise can be included by considering the stochastic opening and closing of one of the ion channels represented in equation (1). The resulting model was contracted to a Langevin description with the method of Fox and Lu [13], and solutions computed numerically. It was observed that the addition of noise perturbs the basin of attraction for the IP oscillations so that trajectories of the full system land in the basin of attraction for the AP oscillations, upon which bursting can ensue. Interestingly, sufficient noise is needed to draw the trajectories of the full system towards a bursting solution, but too much noise obliterates the deterministic burst dynamics. That is, the system is optimized (in terms of optimizing the mean intracellular calcium concentration, which is an important physiological quantity correlated with insulin secretion) with an intermediate amount of noise. It has been shown recently that at least part of the effect of noise in this scenario stems from the fact that independent noise in the cells also makes them heterogeneous [23].

The form of emergent bursting for identical cells just described is no longer possible when coupling strength is increased further because the branch of AP oscillations is unstable or absent. In this case, the two-cell system behaves as the individual cells do. However, as we discussed earlier in the context of cells that are capable of bursting, introducing heterogeneity in the model parameters affects the relative locations of the fast subsystem bifurcations. In particular, heterogeneity enlarges the region of bistability (cf. Fig. 10.9(a)). Extending the analysis to the case of cells that are not capable of bursting individually, we obtain a similar two-parameter bifurcation diagram, shown in Fig. 10.9(b). The introduction of heterogeneity ($|\delta| > 0$) first creates a region of bistability by destroying the SNIC bifurcation through a codimension-2 saddle-node-loop bifurcation (SNL), essentially splitting the SNIC bifurcation into its two constituent parts, namely a saddle-node bifurcation (SN1) and a homoclinic bifurcation (HC). An example of emergent bursting mediated by heterogeneity in this way is shown in Figs. 10.10(g) and (h).

Increasing heterogeneity further enlarges the region of bistability as before. The larger the heterogeneity in the system, however, the larger the incongruity between the bursting solutions of the two cells (in particular, the amplitude of the spikes of the two cells may differ significantly). Consequently, heterogeneity is beneficial in generating a bursting solution, but only up to a point.

10.7. Synaptic Coupling

In order to demonstrate the broader applicability of the phenomena discussed above, we have reconfigured the coupled-cell model, (8)–(10), as a pair of neurons coupled by fast, mutual excitation. We replace the diffusive coupling current with the fast synaptic current in the v equation for cell j:

$$\tau \frac{dv_j}{dt} = -I_{Ca}(v_j) - I_K(v_j, n_j) - I_s(v_j, s_j) - g_{Syn} e_j (v_j - v_{Syn}), \tag{19}$$

$$\tau_{Syn} \frac{de_j}{dt} = e_\infty(v_k) - e_j, \tag{20}$$

and similarly for cell k. Note that the activation of e_j depends on cell k, and *vice versa.* Values of the additional parameters are as shown in Table 10.3.

Table 10.3. Values of the parameters appearing in the synaptic coupling equations, (19)–(20).

$\tau_{Syn} = 10$ msec	$v_{Syn} = 0$ mV	$g_{Syn} = 0.25$
$v_e = -30$ mV	$\theta_e = 9$ mV	

In Fig. 10.11(a), the two cells are started off out-of-phase but uncoupled with the same parameters (and the same bifurcation diagram) as in Figs. 10.10(a) and (b). There is no bistability in the fast subsystem of these cells, and both cells exhibit spiking. At $t = 10$ sec, the mutual excitation is turned on, and bursting with anti-phase spikes immediately begins, similar to the case shown in Fig. 10.1 for identical cells coupled diffusively. Indeed, the bifurcation diagram for the corresponding fast subsystem, shown in Fig. 10.11(b), is topologically equivalent to that in Fig. 10.2(b). Thus, the synaptic coupling induces emergent bursting carried by anti-phase spikes. Note, however, that in Fig. 10.11(b), the homoclinic termination of the IP branch has moved away from the left saddle-node, and rightward on the middle branch of the curve of steady states. With the weak coupling used in Fig. 10.11, this has no consequence as the branch of IP oscillations is unstable. However, as g_{Syn} is increased, the branch of AP oscillations shrinks and disappears while the branch of IP oscillations restabilizes. The same sequence of bifurcations occurs as in the diffusive coupling case (cf. Fig. 10.3), and each type of out-of-phase spiking can carry emergent bursting. The new feature is that for stronger coupling, emergent bursting can be carried by *in-phase* spiking. The mutual excitation is able to lift the mean membrane potential and induce bistability, which did not occur in the diffusive case. Emergent oscillations are thus more robust for excitatory synaptic coupling in the sense that they can persist even for arbitrarily large coupling. However, the branch of IP oscillations also shrinks in amplitude and eventually disappears, leaving emergent relaxation oscillations rather than bursting.

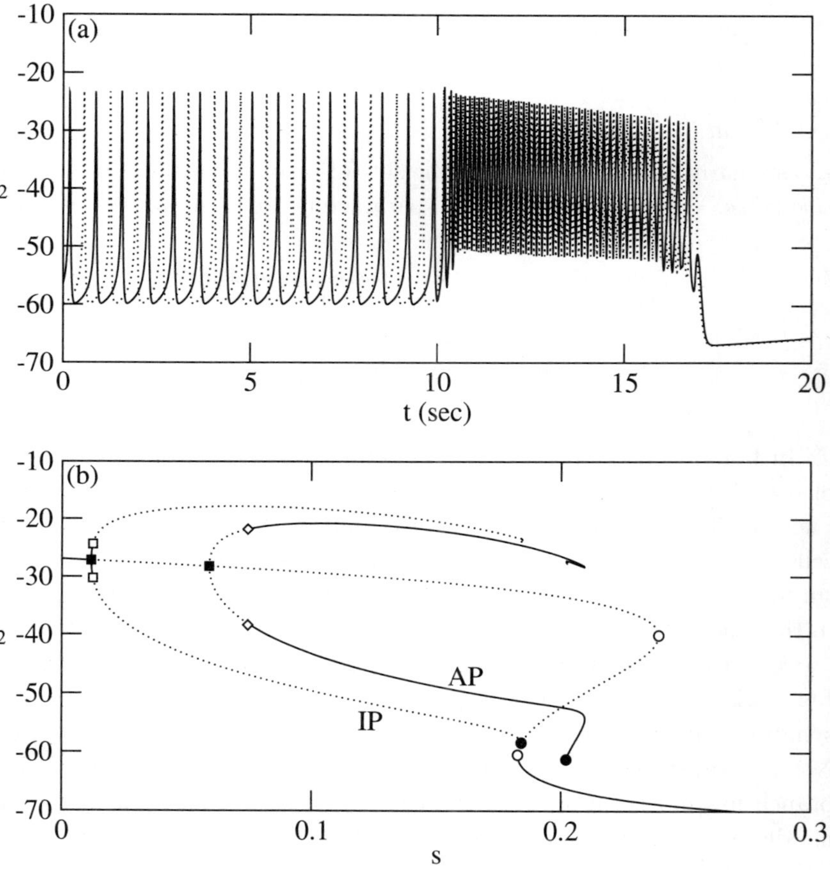

Fig. 10.11. Emergent bursting with synaptic coupling, using (8)–(9) and (19)–(20). The two cells are non-bursting ($\lambda = 0.8$) and identical ($\beta_1 = \beta_2 = 0$). **(a)** In the absence of coupling, bursting is precluded (left half). Mutual synaptic excitation is turned on at $t = 10$ sec with strength $g_{Syn} = 0.25$, which induces emergent bursting. **(b)** Bifurcation diagram for the corresponding fast subsystem, with coupling turned on. Compare with Fig. 10.2(b). Note that the homoclinic termination of the branch of IP oscillations has migrated rightward on the middle branch of the curve of steady states.

10.8. Discussion

We have reviewed established results showing that diffusive coupling of square-wave bursters can lead to longer period and, in extreme cases, increase burst period from essentially 0 to a significant finite value (emergent bursting). We have also summarized new results indicating that synaptic coupling leads to increased burst period (not shown) and emergent bursting. Our results are more general than the examples discussed, but one would not expect them to apply to arbitrary square-wave bursters, because they depend on out-of-phase spiking, which is only guaranteed to occur if the normal form of the fast subsystem lies in an appropriate region of parameter space (Fig. 10.6).

Emergent bursting for either type of coupling must be interpreted in a limited sense, as all of our examples involve systems that possess the required slow negative feedback process and lack only bistability between a steady state and an oscillation. However, they are near the right parameter regime for bistability such that they need only a modest perturbation from the coupling currents. We are unaware of examples of emergent bursting of any type found in neurons or other excitable cells where the bursting is truly manufactured out of whole cloth.

We regret that we cannot yet report any experimental evidence confirming the predictions of the analysis in coupled neurons or other bursting cells. However, confirmation of a sort has been obtained for another physical system, in which two electronic neurons, designed to implement a version of the Hindmarsh-Rose model [24], were coupled. Figures 4 and 5 of that paper show that as coupling conductance increased, the burst pattern underwent a transition from synchronized bursts with unsynchronized spikes to synchronized bursts with synchronized spikes. Burst period was longer when the spikes were out of phase, in accordance with the results summarized here. The same group also coupled a chaotically firing electronic Hindmarsh-Rose neuron to an irregularly spiking PD neuron from the lobster stomatogastric ganglion via an electronic gap junction [35]. The coupled pair switched to robust square-wave bursting, but it is difficult to evaluate how this relates to our model.

10.8.1. *Limitations and extensions*

One way to view the lessons of this chapter is that one must couple the system first, and then carry out averaging. If done in the reverse order, the wrong answer may be obtained. Specifically, since information about the homoclinic termination of the spiking branch is lost, the effects of coupling to increase burst period and mediate emergent bursting, which depend on a shift in the homoclinic, will be overlooked. This raises a practical question for future investigation. Numerical simulations of large populations of bursters are time-consuming because of the need to follow events on both the fast time scale of spiking and the slow time scale of bursting, requiring small time steps. Several attempts have been made to reduce the computational complexity of simulating individual bursters by reducing the dynamics to a map [9, 29]. It is not obvious how to model the effects of coupling on spike amplitude and burst period in such reduced systems. However, the extended integrate-and-fire system described in [18] retains a piece-wise continuous description of membrane potential and may thus preserve the features described in this chapter.

We have reported analysis using a "classical" bursting model with a single slow variable. More recent models for β-cells have introduced a second, much slower, slow variable [4, 6, 37]. In such models, the time scale of bursting is a mixture of the time scales of the two slow variables and has therefore been called "phantom bursting". Phantom bursters exhibit period extension just as the classical models do when coupled, but the increase can be exaggerated because the establishment of an out-of-phase spiking branch by coupling can engage a very slow variable that was pre-empted by the faster slow variable when the system was uncoupled. It is also possible for coupling to dramatically reduce burst period, which we have not seen in classical models. This phenomenon involves disengaging the very slow variable, typically in the transition region between moderate and very strong coupling where quasi-periodic spiking prevails [37].

All of the analysis presented here has been limited to the case of two cells. However, we have seen the same apparent phenomena in large networks with or without noise [31] and in the presence of heterogeneity [11]. Conversely, we have not seen any obvious phenomena in the n-cell case not already present with two cells, but without a theory one cannot be sure. It might be easier to extend the analysis to the continuum limit rather than consider large n directly. The inclusion of synaptic coupling opens up the possibility of long-range, not merely nearest neighbor coupling, and might lead to genuinely new phenomena.

We have considered coupling only via the membrane potential as this seemed most relevant to the original problem of interest, the islet of Langherhans. However, coupling through the slow variable s is also plausible if interpreted as, for example, intracellular calcium or a diffusible metabolite such as ATP. Limited work has been done in this area, but Postnov *et al.* [25] have applied phase reduction [20] to weak coupling of the full bursting system through both v and s and found multiple stable patterns of asynchronous behaviour.

In the interests of brevity and thematic unity we have not said much about channel-gating noise. See the reference list for some studies of the ways that noise can both help and hinder bursting [1, 11, 33].

10.8.2. *Comparison to other emergent oscillations*

Other scenarios have been considered for emergent bursting. One is based on a heterogeneous population in which the cells are conditional bursters, meaning they have an appropriate slow negative feedback variable and are bistable, but may be below the lower threshold or above the upper threshold for oscillation. A mix of such cells can oscillate if sufficiently strongly coupled even if no individual cell lies in the intermediate parameter regime for oscillation because, at very strong coupling, the network will behave like a single cell with average properties [34]. This scenario does not exploit the detailed properties of the burster, specifically the location or even existence of a homoclinic orbit of the fast subsystem, and has been analyzed using networks of relaxation oscillators [8]. One might object that it seems contrived for cells to be either too active or not active enough but unable to sit in the middle. We have shown recently that such a bimodal distribution can be generated naturally using a unimodal distribution of a membrane conductance when the oscillatory regime is narrow [37].

A more subtle case has arisen in a network of respiratory neurons modeled as synaptically coupled square-wave bursters [7]. The coupling was not extremely strong, allowing the network to oscillate (i.e., burst) at levels of tonic drive both below and above the oscillatory range for a single cell, and also to exhibit other more exotic dynamics. Analysis by Rubin and Terman [28] showed that this phenomenon again depended only on the relaxation oscillator character of the bursters, not on induction of bistability. However, homogeneous respiratory networks and pairs of cells were found similarly to oscillate at levels of tonic drive above the upper limit for single cells. See chapter 12, this volume, for detailed analysis of synaptic coupling in the respiratory model.

References

[1] J. Aguirre, E. Mosekilde, and A. F. Sanjuan, Analysis of the noise-induced bursting-spiking transition in a pancreatic β-cell model, *Physical Review E.* **69**, 041910(16), (2004).

[2] D. Aronson, G. Ermentrout, and N. Kopell, Amplitude response of coupled oscillators, *Physica D.* **41**, 403–449, (1990).

[3] R. Bertram, M. Butte, T. Kiemel, and A. Sherman, Topological and phenomenological classification of bursting oscillations, *Bull. Math. Biol.* **57**, 413–439, (1995).

[4] R. Bertram, J. Previte, A. Sherman, T. A. Kinard, and L. S. Satin, The phantom burster model for pancreatic β-cells, *Biophys. J.* **79**, 2880–2892, (2000).

[5] R. Bertram, L. Satin, M. Zhang, P. Smolen, and A. Sherman, Calcium and glycolysis mediate multiple bursting modes in pancreatic islets, *Biophys. J.* **87**, 3074–3087, (2004).

[6] R. Bertram and A. Sherman. Negative feedback by calcium: The road from Chay-Keizer. In eds. S. Coombes and P. Bressloff, *Bursting: The Genesis of Rhythm in the Nervous System.* World Scientific, Singapore, (2005). This volume, chapter 2.

[7] R. J. Butera, J. Rinzel, and J. C. Smith, Models of respiratory rhythm generation in the pre-Bötzinger complex. II. Populations of coupled pacemaker neurons, *J. Neurophysiol.* pp. 398–415, (1999).

[8] J. H. E. Cartwright, Emergent global oscillations in heterogeneous excitable media: The example of pancreatic β cells, *Physical Review E.* **62**(1), 1149–1154, (2000).

[9] G. de Vries, Bursting as an emergent phenomenon in coupled chaotic maps, *Physical Review E.* **64**, 051914(9), (2001).

[10] G. de Vries and A. Sherman, Channel sharing in pancreatic β-cells revisited: Enhancement of emergent bursting by noise, *J. Theor. Biol.* **207**, 513–530, (2000).

[11] G. de Vries and A. Sherman, From spikers to bursters via coupling: Help from heterogeneity, *Bull. Math. Biol.* **63**, 371–391, (2001).

[12] G. de Vries, A. Sherman, and H.-R. Zhu, Diffusively coupled bursters: effects of cell heterogeneity, *Bull. Math. Biol.* **60**, 1167–1200, (1998).

[13] R. Fox and Y.-N. Lu, Emergent collective behavior in large numbers of globally coupled independently stochastic ion channels, *Physical Review E.* **49**, 3421–3431, (1994).

[14] S. K. Han, C. Kurrer, and Y. Kuramoto, Dephasing and bursting in

coupled neural oscillators, *Physical Review Letters.* **75**(17), 3190–3193, (1995).

[15] J. Hindmarsh and R. Rose, A model of neuronal bursting using three coupled first order differential equations, *Proc. R. Soc. Lond. B.* **221**, 87–102, (1984).

[16] A. Hodgkin and A. Huxley, A quantitative description of membrane current and its application to conduction and excitation in nerve, *J. Physiol. (London).* **117**, 500–544, (1952).

[17] E. Izhikevich, Neural excitability, spiking and bursting, *Int. J. Bifurcation and Chaos.* **10**, 1171–1266, (2000).

[18] E. Izhikevich, Which model to use for cortical spiking neurons?, *IEEE Trans. on Neural Networks.* **15**, 1063–1070, (2004).

[19] T. Kinard, G. de Vries, A. Sherman, and L. Satin, Modulation of the bursting properties of single mouse pancreatic β-cells by artificial conductances, *Biophys. J.* **76**, 1423–1435, (1999).

[20] Y. Kuramoto, *Chemical Oscillations, Waves, and Turbulence.* (Springer, Berlin, 1984).

[21] Y. Morita, A periodic wave and its stability to a circular chain of weakly coupled oscillators, *SIAM J. Math. Anal.* **18**(6), 1681–1698, (1987).

[22] E. Mosekilde, B. Lading, S. Yanchuk, and Y. Maistrenko, Bifurcation structure of a model of bursting pancreatic cells, *BioSystems.* **63**, 3–13, (2001).

[23] M. G. Pedersen, A comment on enhanced bursting in pancreatic beta-cells, *J. Theor. Biol.* **235**, 1–3, (2005).

[24] R. D. Pinto, P. Varona, A. R. Volkovskii, A. Szücs, H. D. I. Abarbanel, and M. I. Rabinovich, Synchronous behavior of two coupled electronic neurons, *Physical Review E.* **62**(2), 2644–2656, (2000).

[25] D. E. Postnov, O. V. Sosnovtseva, S. Y. Malova, and E. Mosekilde, Complex phase dynamics in coupled bursters, *Physical Review E.* **67**, 016215(10), (2003).

[26] J. Rinzel. Bursting oscillations in an excitable membrane model. In eds. B. D. Sleeman and R. J. Jarvis, *Ordinary and Partial Differential Equations, Lecture Notes in Mathematics 1151*, pp. 304–316. Springer, New York, (1985).

[27] J. Rinzel. A formal classification of bursting mechanisms in excitable systems. In eds. E. Teramoto and M. Yamaguti, *Mathematical Topics in Population Biology, Morphogenesis, and Neurosciences, Lecture Notes in Biomathematics 71*, pp. 267–281. Springer-Verlag, New York,

(1987).

[28] J. Rubin and D. Terman, Synchronized bursts and loss of synchrony among heterogeneous conditional oscillators, *SIAM J. Applied Dynamical Systems.* **1**, 146–174, (2002).

[29] N. F. Rulkov, Regularization of synchronized chaotic bursts, *Physical Review Letters.* **86**, 183–186, (2001).

[30] A. Sherman, Anti-phase, asymmetric and aperiodic oscillations in excitable cells - I. coupled bursters, *Bull. Math. Biol.* **56**, 811–835, (1994).

[31] A. Sherman and J. Rinzel, Model for synchronization of pancreatic β-cells by gap junctions, *Biophys. J.* **59**, 547–559, (1991).

[32] A. Sherman and J. Rinzel, Rhythmogenic effects of weak electrotonic coupling in neuronal models, *Proc. Natl. Acad. Sci. USA.* **89**, 2471–2474, (1992).

[33] A. Sherman, J. Rinzel, and J. Keizer, Emergence of organized bursting in clusters of pancreatic β-cells by channel sharing, *Biophys. J.* **54**, 411–425, (1988).

[34] P. Smolen, J. Rinzel, and A. Sherman, Why pancreatic islets burst but single β cells do not: the heterogeneity hypothesis, *Biophys. J.* **64**, 1668–1680, (1993).

[35] A. Szücs, P. Varona, A. R. Volkovskii, H. D. I. Abarbanel, M. I. Rabinovich, and A. I. Selverston, Interacting biological and electronic neurons generate realistic oscillatory rhythms, *NeuroReport.* **11**(3), 563–569, (2000).

[36] M. Zhang, P. Goforth, A. Sherman, R. Bertram, and L. Satin, The Ca^{2+} dynamics of isolated mouse β-cells and islets: Implications for mathematical models, *Biophys. J.* **84**, 2852–2870, (2003).

[37] C. Zimliki, D. Mears, and A. Sherman, Three roads to islet bursting: Emergent oscillations in coupled phantom bursters, *Biophys. J.* **87**, 193–206, (2004).

CHAPTER 11

BURSTING IN EXCITATORY NEURAL NETWORKS

Joël Tabak

Department of Biological Sciences, Florida State University
Tallahasse, FL 32306, USA
email: joel@neuro.fsu.edu

John Rinzel

Center for Neural Science and Courant Institute of Mathematical Sciences
New York University, NY 10003, USA
e-mail: rinzel@cns.nyu.edu

Rhythmic activities underly many crucial functions such as locomotion, respiration, secretion, etc. Models of network rhythmicity have generally included cellular oscillators or inhibitory connections between antagonistic centers. Here, we present a model of the spontaneous episodic activity in developing spinal cord networks that include neither of these two components. This model only represents the averaged activity and excitability in the network, assumed purely excitatory. In our model, positive feedback through excitatory connections generates episodes of activity, which are terminated by a slow, activity-dependent depression of network activity (slow negative feedback). This idealized model allowed a qualitative understanding of the network dynamics which lead to prediction and comprehension of experimental observations. Although the complexity of the system has been restricted to the interactions between fast positive and slow negative feedback, the emergent feature of the network rhythm was captured, and it applies to many developing/excitatory networks. Finally, we show that this model of network rhythmicity behaves similarly to models of repetitive bursting in single cells.

11.1. Introduction

In this chapter, we present a network model that generates periodic activity using dynamical principles already described for some cellular bursters (cf. chapter 2). Indeed, many networks generate rhythmic activity, such as locomotor networks or the respiratory network described chapter 12. Although mechanisms for network rhythmicity often involve pacemaker cells or inhibitory connections as essential components [27, 33], it has recently been recognized that purely excitatory networks with no pacemaker cells could generate bursts of activity. Here we describe a model of the spontaneous activity in a developing network

11.2. Spontaneous Activity in the Developing Spinal Cord

Early in development, neuronal networks of the central nervous system generate spontaneous activity. This activity is not evoked by sensory inputs or inputs from other parts of the nervous system, but is generated within each of these circuits in isolation, hence the term "spontaneous." Spontaneous activity has been well characterized in the developing spinal cord, hippocampus, and retina and has also been described in other circuits. Although they have widely different architectures, the features of the spontaneous activity are similar in all these networks [29]. The most characteristic feature of this activity is its episodic nature: most if not all neurons of the network become active together for several seconds to a minute, then the network becomes silent for intervals that can last up to several minutes, as illustrated in Fig. 11.1.

Because spontaneous activity is so widespread in the developing nervous system and with striking similarities between different circuits, understanding its mechanisms of generation may provide some general principles of neuronal network function. Furthermore, there is evidence that spontaneous activity can drive the refinement of neuronal circuits [22, 51], as this activity usually involves large populations of neurons in a highly correlated fashion (see below) and therefore may lead to strengthening/weakening of synaptic connections through Hebbian mechanisms [32, 51]. Finally, the temporal pattern of activity may also regulate the electrical properties of the individual neurons [17, 25]. It is therefore important to understand the mechanisms of generation of spontaneous activity in the developing nervous system. In the following, we focus on the temporal organization of activity through activity-dependent synaptic depression in the developing spinal cord, but suggest that the same features are common to other neural networks.

Spontaneous activity was first observed as spontaneous movements in embryos of diverse animals. Embryonic motility was extensively studied in the chicken embryo [18], as it was easy to observe spontaneous movements through the egg shell, and later to record electrical activity through a small window in the shell. It was shown that these episodic movements were caused by spontaneous electrical activity in the neuronal networks of the spinal cord. More recently, an isolated in vitro preparation of the embryonic chick spinal cord was developed [30], allowing one to record the activity and to manipulate the network (by lesions or pharmacology) at different stages of development.

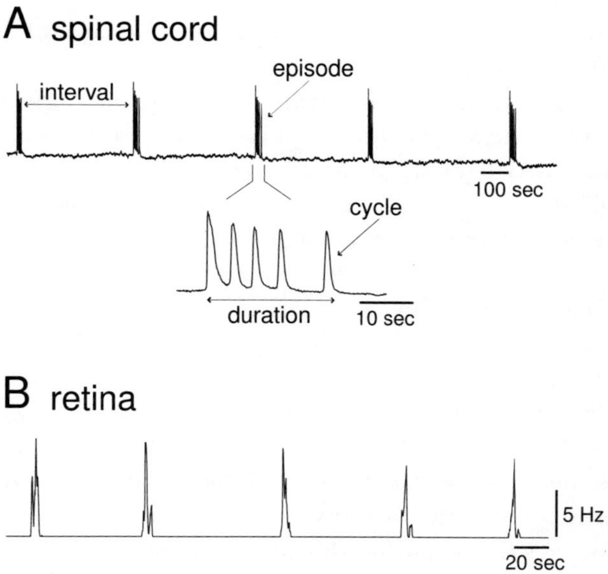

Fig. 11.1. Episodic activity in developing networks. A) Spontaneous activity recorded from the isolated spinal cord of a 7.5 day old chick embryo. The activity is recorded from a ventral root and represents the synaptic drive received by a population of motoneurons. It is characterized by rhythmic episodes lasting up to a minute which are separated by silent intervals lasting up to 20 minutes. Modified from [43]. B) Spontaneous activity recorded from the isolated retina of a 9 day old mouse (postnatal). This signal is the rate of neuronal discharge averaged over 29 cells. Note the difference in the time scale with the recording in A. Data courtesy of J. Demas, S.J. Eglen and R.O.L. Wong.

We can record this activity from a population of motoneurons (the output neurons projecting to the muscles) by suctioning a ventral root (axons from the motoneurons) into an electrode. The activity recorded this way is illustrated in Fig. 11.1(A). It represents the depolarization (increase of membrane potential) of the motoneurons, propagating passively along the axons. This signal is a good indicator of the activity in the whole network, since motoneuron depolarization is caused by synaptic inputs from other neurons in the network. The activity is episodic, with episodes lasting up to a minute separated by intervals of up to 20 minutes. Within an episode, the activity is rhythmic with a cycle frequency of 0.2-1.0 Hz, markedly decreasing toward the end of the episode. Each cycle can be seen as a network "spike", representing the depolarization of the whole neuronal population. Although the neurons are activated in synchrony, their action potentials are not synchronized.

How is this activity generated? Several key experimental findings provide a working hypothesis.

The first thing to note is that many developing networks can be considered as purely excitatory circuits. This is because the inhibitory neurotransmitters GABA and glycine have excitatory effects early in development [2, 7]. Indeed, blocking the action of excitatory neurotransmitters acetylcholine and glutamate does not prevent the spinal cord from generating episodic activity [8]. It is therefore easy to understand the presence of spontaneous activity in immature circuits. Any event such as a few neurons randomly firing can be amplified by positive feedback through the recurrent excitatory projections, leading to massive activity in the whole network. This explains the activity, but not its episodic pattern. How are the episodes terminated, in the absence of inhibitory connections?

One possibility is that the network "fatigues" during activity, until it is no longer able to sustain activity. In other words, there is an activity-dependent process that depresses the excitability of the network. To demonstrate the presence of such activity-dependent depression process, we have stimulated populations of interneurons through sensory or propriospinal afferents and observed the evoked synaptic response on the motoneurons [13]. The synaptic potentials recorded on the motoneurons are decreased after an episode of activity, and progressively increase during the interval between episodes. This suggests that network excitability is depressed by the episodes of activity and that it recovers in the interval between episodes. This depression may be synaptic, that is, activity decreases synaptic efficacy. An activity-dependent synaptic depression process, by reducing the strength of the connections between neurons, would effectively decrease the positive feedback. Another possibility is that this depression acts on the neurons to decrease their intrinsic excitability, making them less likely to fire action potentials. Such activity-dependent cellular adaptation process would shift the input/output function of the neurons and make them less responsive to inputs.

Finally, it must be stressed that no particular network structure or cellular properties are thought to underlie the pattern of activity. As mentioned above, spontaneous episodic activity is observed in developing networks with a great variety of structure, and a similar type of activity is observed in dissociated cultures of spinal neurons for which inhibitory transmission has been blocked [40]. In the chick embryo, lesion studies have shown that ventral networks of the spinal cord can generate the activity despite transversal or horizontal sectioning [20] and pharmacological studies have shown that episodic activity is still generated when individual neurotransmitters are blocked [8]. In addition, there is no evidence that cellular pacemaker properties underlie the rhythmic activity. It is through (excitatory) network interactions that the rhythm arises, i.e. the rhythmic activity is an emergent property of the network and the dynamics of the recurrent connections.

The main hypothesis is therefore that the spontaneous, episodic activity is generated by a purely excitatory network. This activity depresses network excitability and when excitability is too low the activity stops. In the silent period, network excitability recovers and eventually a new episode begins. In order to test this hypothesis, we have built a very idealized model (schematized in Fig. 11.2(A)) based on these observations. This differential equation model can be analyzed qualitatively using geometric and fast/slow dissection methods, so we can understand its dynamical behavior. It allowed us to explain some experimental results and make some predictions, some of which are presented below.

11.3. Model of the Spontaneous Activity in the Embryonic Chick Spinal Cord

According to the experimental findings presented above, we model a purely excitatory network whose detailed structure (connectivity pattern, heterogeneity of cell types) is not known but does not seem to be important. We also assume that the details of the neurons' membrane properties are not important either and that all the neurons are active or inactive together. We therefore use a "mean field" representation of the activity and depression variables, as used by Wilson and Cowan [49]. According to this formulation, the activity $a(t)$ of the network is an average of the neuronal firing rate over the population of neurons (see Fig. 11.2(A), (B)). Individual spikes are not modeled (and assumed not to occur synchronously). The firing rate is a temporally coarse-grained representation, that is, averaged over a short period of time. Thus, a can be related to the (pre)synaptic drive, i.e. the amount of synaptic input exciting neurons in the network [34]. The model consists of three equations: [43]

$$\tau_a \, \dot{a} = a_\infty(w \cdot s \cdot d \cdot a) - a \tag{1}$$

$$\tau_d \, \dot{d} = d_\infty(a) - d \tag{2}$$

$$\tau_s \, \dot{s} = s_\infty(a) - s. \tag{3}$$

The first equation describes how activity evolves in a recurrent excitatory network. Basically, a tends to a_∞ with a time constant τ_a. The function a_∞ represents the input-output function of the network. This function depends on the input-output functions of the individual neurons, their distribution across the population, and the dynamics of the synaptic signals. For simplicity we have chosen a sigmoidal function $a_\infty(i) = 1/(1 + e^{4(\theta_0 - i)/k_a})$, as illustrated in Fig. 11.2(C). For low inputs to the network, there is very little output ($a_\infty \simeq 0$) until a threshold (θ_0) is reached, the output then quickly reaches its maximal value ($a_\infty \simeq 1$); θ_0 can be seen as an average firing threshold in the neuronal population. Note that the activity a is itself the input to the network – modulated by the effective connectivity $w \cdot s \cdot d$ – because of the recurrent excitatory connections. The parameter w is the network connectivity, a composite measure of the number of connections per neuron and synaptic strength which determines the maximal gain of the positive feedback loop created by excitatory connections. As described below, the activity defined by this equation is bistable over a wide range of parameters. The time constant τ_a is set to 1, that is, time is expressed relative to τ_a. It represents the time scale of network recruitment, which is on the order of 100 ms [26].

The second equation describes the evolution of the synaptic variable d, which represents a fast depression of the effective connectivity; τ_d was chosen to be on the order of 100 ms (like τ_a, but slightly larger), as in cortical networks [6]. When $d = 0$ all synapses are totally depressed while synapses have full strength when $d = 1$; d_∞ is a decreasing function of a, also chosen to be sigmoidal for convenience. The interplay between a and d can create oscillations of the activity; these oscillations correspond to the cycling that is observed during an episode (see Fig. 11.1). Finally,

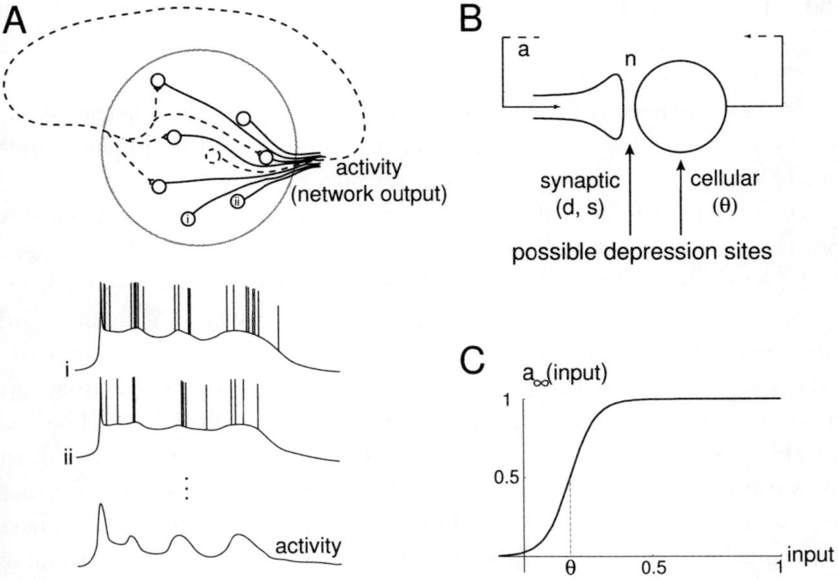

Fig. 11.2. Model of the network generating episodic activity. A) Justification for a mean field formulation. Neurons are connected to each other through random excitatory connections. Neurons i, ii, ... are active together but their spikes are not synchronized. Spike rate can thus be averaged, giving a smooth curve, the "activity", which represents the population signal shown in Fig. 11.1(A). B) Schematic representation of the model network. Network output (a) is fed back to the neuron population through recurrent excitatory synapses. The amount of feedback is proportional to the connectivity (w) and can be reduced by fast (d) and/or slow (s) synaptic depression. Network output can also be modulated by slow variations of the average cellular threshold (θ). C, sigmoidal input-output function of the network. Note that, since $a_\infty(0) \neq 0$ we are implicitly assuming that some few cells in the network are spontaneously discharging at low rate, providing a background "input" to the network. Modified from [43].

Eq. (3) describes the variations of the slow ($\tau_s \gg \tau_a$) synaptic variable s. This variable also decreases when a is large and increases for low activity, but on a much slower time scale. A possible biophysical mechanism for this slow (timescale minutes) synaptic depression involves the loss of chloride ions by the neurons during an episode, decreasing the excitatory action of GABAergic and glycinergic connections [9, 26]. Alternatively, the slow depression could be due to a cellular process (instead of a synaptic process) that increases the cellular firing threshold for high levels of activity. In that case, Eq. (1) would be replaced by

$$\tau_a \, \dot{a} = a_\infty(w \cdot d \cdot a - \theta) - a \tag{4}$$

and Eq. (3) would be replaced by

$$\tau_\theta \, \dot{\theta} = \theta_\infty(a) - \theta, \tag{5}$$

θ_∞ being an increasing function of a. The slower depression, whether synaptic (s) or cellular (θ), is responsible for the episodic nature of the activity (see below).

By reducing the network to a system of three differential equations, we lose the complexity of a population of neurons and only study the mean-field (deterministic) interactions between the fast positive feedback and the slower negative feedback in generating this activity. The advantage is that we are able to qualitatively analyze the dynamics of the system with fast/slow dissection techniques (see, e.g., [35]). We present this dissection in the next section, but in brief the methodology is as follows. The slow variable s is first considered as a parameter, and the dynamic states of the one-variable (a) (or the two-variable a, d) fast subsystem are fully described; the steady state (and oscillatory, in the case of a two-variable fast subsystem) solutions are obtained as a function of s. Then when s is free to follow its autonomous dynamics the full system has solutions that evolve on the slow time scale of s, sampling the solution states of the fast subsystem and at critical (bifurcation) points executing rapid transitions between states. This analysis involves numerical bifurcation and branch-tracking methods and forward-in-time integrations, which were carried out using the XPPAUT package [12]. A 4th-order Runge-Kutta scheme with time step of 0.1 was used to numerically integrate the differential equations. Parameter values used in the simulations are given in Table 11.4.

11.4. Properties and Applications of the Model

11.4.1. *Bistability of the excitatory network with fixed synaptic efficacy*

We first analyze the properties of the network without depression. That is, we study Eq. (1) with the depression variables frozen ($s = d = 1$). Such a system will reach a steady state ($\dot{a} = 0$) for which the activity is defined by $a = a_\infty(w \cdot a)$ (from Eq. (1)). The steady states can be determined graphically as the intersections of the straight line and the curve shown in Fig. 11.3(A) for any value of w. When connectivity is low ($w = 0.3$ in Fig. 11.3(A)), there is only one intersection for a low value of a. Thus the connectivity is too small to sustain a high level of activity. Even if the network is transiently stimulated, activity will quickly go back to its low

Table 11.4. Definition and value of the parameters used for each model, unless otherwised mentioned in text or figure.

parameter	s-model	θ-model
w, network connectivity	1	1
τ_a, network recruitment time constant	1	1
θ_0, average firing threshold (half activation)	0.18	0
k_a, reciprocal of slope of a_∞ at half activation	0.2	0.2
τ_d, time constant of fast synaptic depression	2	2
θ_d, half activation of d	0.5	0.5
k_d, reciprocal of slope of d_∞ at half activation	-0.8	-0.8
τ_s, time constant of slow synaptic depression	500	
θ_s, half activation of s	0.14	
k_s, reciprocal of slope of s_∞ at half activation	-0.08	
τ_θ, time constant of slow cellular adaptation		1000
θ_θ, half activation of θ		0.15
k_θ, reciprocal of slope of θ_∞ at half activation		0.2

level state. On the other hand, for large values of w ($w = 0.9$ in Fig. 3A), there is one intersection but at a high activity level. Connectivity in the network is so high that activity is self-sustained. This is expected from an excitatory network: for very low connectivity the network is inactive, while for high connectivity, the activity is maintained through positive feedback. But for intermediate connectivity, the low and high activity states can both exist [49], as described below.

For intermediate values of connectivity ($w = 0.5$ in Fig. 11.3(A)), we find three intersections. There are steady states at low, high and intermediate levels. Note that the middle steady state is unstable. This can be easily seen since the slope of a_∞ is greater than 1 at this point. Therefore if a is slightly increased (respectively decreased) its derivative will become positive (respectively negative) which will tend to further increase (respectively decrease) a. The slightest movement away from this steady state will therefore be amplified. This is illustrated in Fig. 11.3(B). If the network activity is perturbed from the low state to just below the middle state level (dashed line), activity will decrease back to its low level (i). On the other hand, if the network is kicked to just above the middle state, activity will jump to the high steady level (ii). The middle steady state is thus a *network* threshold, separating the low (inactive) and high (active) states.

We can summarize these results by plotting the activity levels (steady states) calculated when w is varied continuously. We obtain the important diagram shown in Fig. 11.3(C). The resulting "S-shaped" curve has three branches: the lower branch (solid) corresponds to the low activity states, the

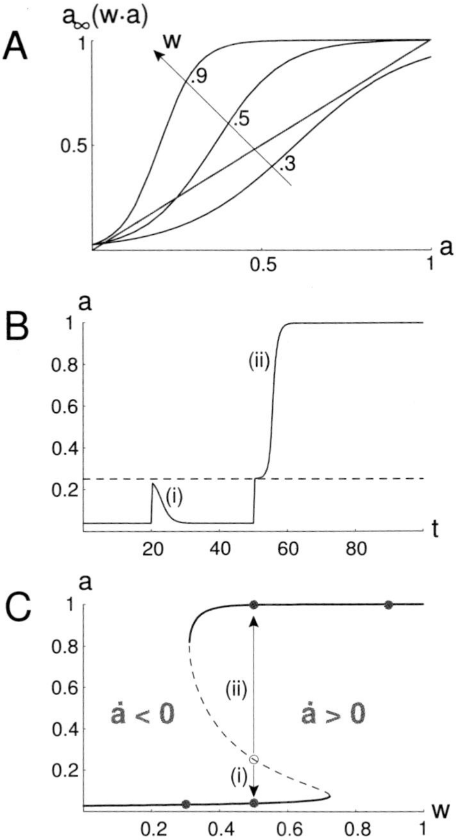

Fig. 11.3. Bistability from recurrent excitation, depression frozen. A) Graphical solutions of the equation $a = a_\infty(w \cdot a)$. Depending on the value of connectivity (w), there can be 1 or 3 solutions. B) Time course of network activity for $w = 0.5$. The network receives external inputs at $t = 20$ and $t = 50$ (dimensionless time, relative to τ_a). The first input (i) brings the activity just below the middle state (network threshold, dashed line) so activity decreases back to the low state. The second input brings activity just above the network threshold, it then jumps up to the high steady state. C) Diagram showing the possible steady state values of activity for all values of w between 0 and 1. The dashed curve (middle branch) indicates unstable states. The steady states determined in A) are represented on the curve by filled (stable) or open (unstable) circles. Modified from [43].

middle branch (dashed) corresponds to the unstable states and the upper branch (solid) corresponds to the high activity states. The S-curve defines two domains in the (w, a) plane. For any value of w, if the activity is such that the point (w, a) is rightward of the curve, then activity will increase until the system reaches the upper branch (high state). Conversely, if (w, a) is leftward of the S-curve, activity will decrease until it reaches the low state.

We can see that for a range of values of w (approximately between 0.31 and 0.73) there are two possible stable states. The network is bistable. As we have seen for $w = 0.5$, a perturbation strong enough to cross the middle branch allows to switch between the two stable states. This bistability is the basis for the oscillatory and episodic behavior described below. Imagine the network is in the high activity state and we slowly decrease the connectivity. The state of the system, defined by a point in the (w, a) plane will be on the upper branch and slowly move to the left, with a minimal decrease of activity. However, when w passes below a critical value around 0.31 where the upper and middle states coincides (the "left knee" of the S-curve) the only remaining state is the low activity state and the network crashes to that state. Now, we slowly increase w, so the state of the system tracks the lower branch, drifting to the right. The activity slowly increases but only slightly until the "right knee" is reached where middle and lower states coalesces. Once w is above that point, only the high state remains and the network will jump to its high activity state, terminating the cycle.

11.4.2. *Episodic and rhythmic behavior due to activity-dependent depression of network excitability*

The network can switch spontaneously between the high and low states according to the above mechanism if we include an activity-dependent mechanism that can slowly modulate the connectivity. With this insight we now let the slow variable s vary according to Eq. (3) (for now, the fast depression variable is still frozen: $d = 1$). Because s_∞ is a decreasing function of a, the new variable s and therefore the effective connectivity $w \cdot s$ will tend to decrease when the network is in the high state and increase when the network is in the low state. This may lead to slow oscillations between the high and low states as explained in the previous paragraph and illustrated in Fig. 11.4(A).

We can explain the episodic behavior of the system geometrically as shown in Fig. 11.4(B). This treatment is similar to the phase plane analysis of single neuron excitability pioneered by Fitzhugh [14, 35]. The variations of the variables a and s (activity and fraction of synapses not affected by slow depression) define a trajectory in the (s, a) phase plane. The S-curve in Fig. 11.4(B) defines the states of the system for which $\dot{a} = 0$ (cf.

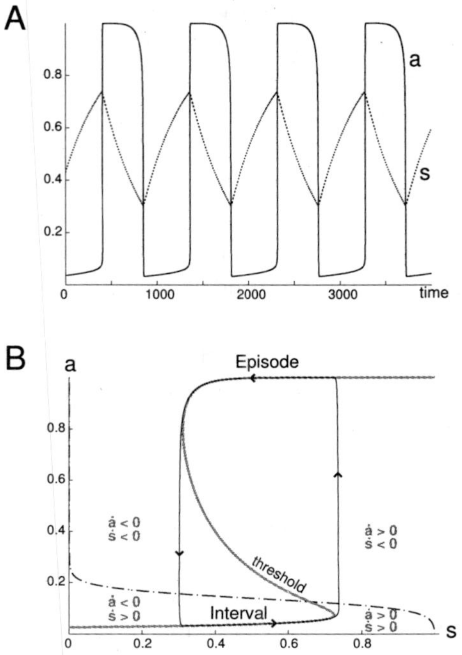

Fig. 11.4. Episodic behavior of the network (Eqs. (1) and (3) with d frozen, $d = 1$). A) Slow oscillatory variations of activity (a, solid curve) and slow depression variable (s, dotted curve) with time. Time is dimensionless, relative to τ_a. B) Phase plane representation of the episodic behavior. The trajectory continuously cycles through the high (Episode) and low (Interval) activity states. The transitions between the two activity levels are very fast because they are governed by the small time constant while the evolution at either level is slow because governed by the large time constant. S-shaped curve: a-nullcline; Dashed curve: s-nullcline.

Fig. 11.3(C)), the a-nullcline. The dashed curve defines the s-nullcline (it is simply the curve $s = s_\infty(a)$). For any pair of values (s, a) that is below the s-nullcline s will be increasing, while s will be decreasing if a is above it. The steady states of the system (comprised of Eqs. (1) and (3)) are the intersections of the two nullclines. In the case of Fig. 11.4(B), there is only one steady state and it is unstable. A necessary condition for the steady state to be unstable is that the intersection occurs on the middle branch of the a-nullcline. If there was an intersection on the upper or lower branch, that intersection would define a stable steady state at high or low activity, which would prevent the episodic behavior. This immediately imposes a constraint on the parameters of the model if episodes are to occur.

Imagine the system begins in a state (s, a) below the a-nullcline and to the right of the "S" switchback. The trajectory will quickly ascend as if s was constant (because $\tau_a \ll \tau_s$), until it reaches the upper branch of the a-nullcline. Then activity will remain high and nearly constant, while s decreases slowly, since the system is now above the s-nullcline. The trajectory will thus track the upper branch, drifting slowly leftward. As it reaches the a-nullcline's left knee $\dot{s}$ is still < 0 driving the trajectory just beyond the knee and forcing the system to leave the a-nullcline. Now, being on the leftward of the a-nullcline, activity decreases so that the trajectory quickly falls down to the lower branch of the a-nullcline. During this transition, the trajectory crosses the s-nullcline, so s starts increasing. The trajectory will thus track the lower branch going right, until it passes the right knee, causing a new transition upward to the upper state.

So far, the combination of the bistability of the activity (Eq. (1)) and the slow, activity-dependent variations of the effective connectivity (due to Eq. (3)) creates slow, spontaneous oscillations between low and high states that mimic the episodic activity observed experimentally. Now, if we allow the fast depression variable, d, to vary according to Eq. (2), the system may oscillate quickly during each episode. The system then generates rhythmic episodes as shown in Fig. 11.5. For a complete analysis of the full system using fast/slow dissection technique, see [43]. Briefly, if we follow the same procedure as above to demonstrate network bistability, freezing s but considering the fast (a, d) subsystem, the steady states for different s values are again on an S-shaped curve (Fig. 11.5(A)). Now, however, there is a range of values for which the upper states are unstable, with stable oscillations around these unstable steady states (these oscillations are represented by the gray curve showing the high and low points during the oscillations and they have the faster time scale of τ_a and τ_d). Thus, when s is allowed to vary, the system can switch periodically between a low state and a high, oscillatory state, as shown on Fig. 11.5. Note that the episodes terminate when the oscillatory state meets an unstable middle state, i.e., before reaching the left knee. Thus episode duration is much shorter in the presence of oscillations during the high state (and interepisode interval is slightly shorter, too, because s has less to recover).

Finally, note that if we had used Eq. (4) and (5) instead of Eq. (1) and (3), that is if we had considered a cellular adaptation mechanism instead of a synaptic depression mechanism to drive the episodic behavior, we would obtain a similar dynamical behavior of the system. At this point, we do not see a qualitative distinction between these two mechanisms (cellular

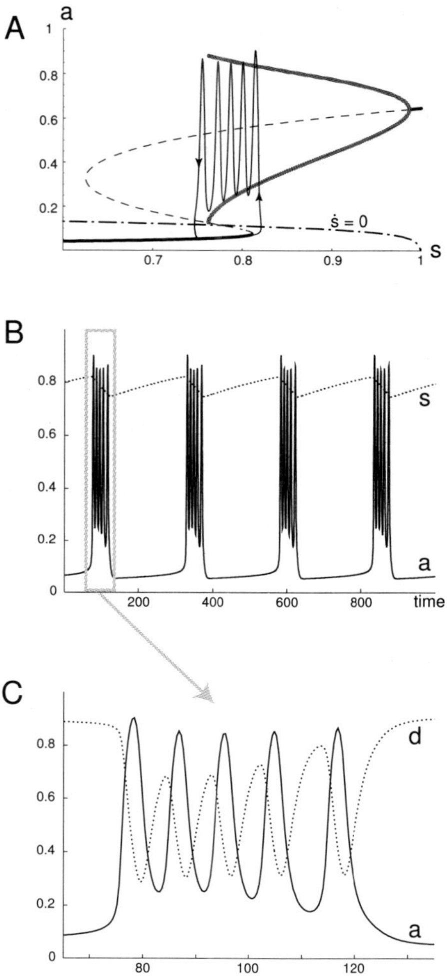

Fig. 11.5. Episodic and rhythmic behavior of the full system (Eqs. (1), (2) and (3)). A) Phase plane representation of the full system. Solid black line represents stable steady states; dashed line represents unstable setady states; gray lines delimit oscillatory states. Dot-dashed line is the s-nullcline. Thin black line shows the trajectory in the (s, a) plane. B) Time variations of a and s, showing the episodic behavior with fast oscillations. Note that episodes and intervals between episodes are shorter than in Fig. 11.4(A). This is mostly because episodes terminate at a higher value of s when the fast depression is present. C) Detail of an episode on a faster time scale, showing the fast oscillations of a and d that correspond to the cycling in Fig. 11.1.

or synaptic) of episode generation. In the next sections, we denote these models s-model (synaptic depression) and θ-model (cellular adaptation) and we will show particular parameter variations from which differences in their behaviors will emerge.

11.4.3. *Relationship between episode duration and inter-episode interval*

During an interval between episodes, can we trigger the network before synaptic strength (or firing threshold if we consider the θ-model) has fully recovered? We can answer this question directly by looking at Fig. 11.4(B). At any time during the inter-episode interval (while the system is tracking the lower branch of the S-curve), if we transiently "stimulate" the network so that activity increases above the middle branch (the network threshold), the phase point will move to the high state, initiating an episode. However, the episode will start from a lower value of s compared to a spontaneous episode, therefore the system will track a shorter segment of the upper branch before reaching the left knee and falling back to the low state. Therefore, the triggered episode is shorter than a spontaneous episode. More specifically, the longer we wait to artificially trigger an episode, the longer is the episode, as illustrated in Fig. 11.6(A), (B). Note, an implicit assumption here, while true for the model, is that whatever the value of s for which we may trigger an episode, the critical value of s at which the episode terminates is always the same. This model prediction is testable experimentally. Indeed, we have shown that it is possible to trigger episodes by stimulating sensory nerves afferent to the spinal cord, and that the duration of the stimulated episodes increases with the interval between the triggered episode and the end of the previous (spontaneous) episode, as shown in Fig. 11.6(C), (D) [42]. In other words, the longer we let the network excitability recover, the longer is the triggered episode. This suggests that in the experimental preparation, as in the model, there is a critical value of network excitability for which all triggered episodes terminate.

In Fig. 11.6(D) we have also plotted the durations of spontaneous episodes (gray dots) against the recovery interval that just preceded the episodes. Although their range is different, the relationship is the same as for stimulated episodes, suggesting again that all episodes (spontaneous or triggered) terminate at a fixed level of network excitability. To explore further this finding, we have also looked at the relationship between episode duration and the *following* inter-episode interval and found no correlation

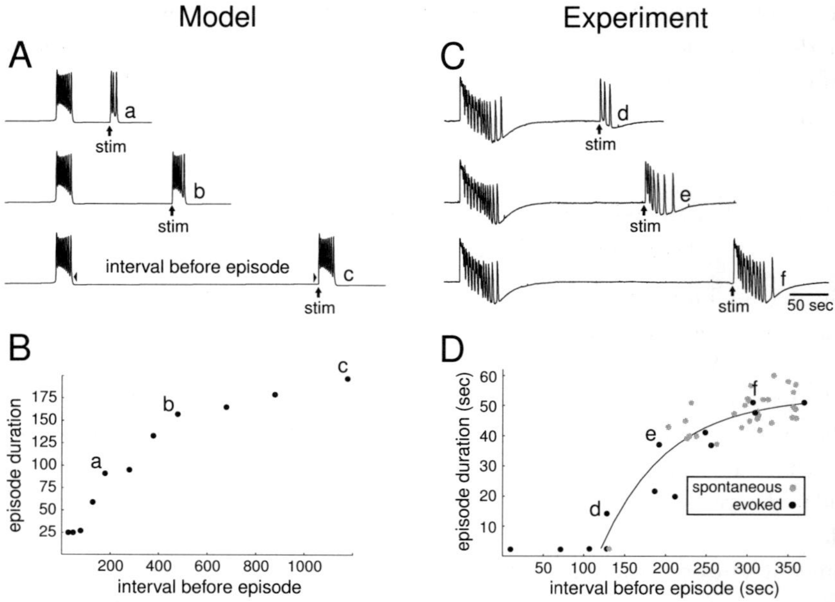

Fig. 11.6. Relationship between episode duration and interval preceding the episode. A) Time course of activity generated by the s-model, for different intervals between a spontaneous episode and a triggered (stim) episode. B) Plot of episode duration against preceding interval for the model; a, b, c correspond to the traces shown in A. C) Time course of activity generated by a spinal cord obtained from a 10 day old chick embryo. Stimulations (stim) were applied at different time intervals after a spontaneous episode. Traces were high pass filtered at 0.01 Hz. D) Plot of episode duration against preceding interval for evoked (black circles) and spontaneous episodes (gray circles); d, e, f correspond to the traces shown in C. Modified from [42].

[42]. This lack of correlation suggests that there is no "memory" of the system's state once an episode is terminated, supporting our finding that all episodes terminate at a fixed level of network excitability.

Fig. 11.6(D) shows that spontaneous episodes occur after various intervals. Unlike our simple model, episodes therefore can start at various levels of network excitability. Episode initiation is a stochastic event. Although a higher level of excitability means a higher probability of triggering an episode, the network needs a triggering event in order for an episode to start and this is where randomness plays a role. On the other hand, as our data suggest, all episodes terminate at the same value of network excitability; episode termination is a deterministic event. This seems to be a property of many developing or hyperexcitable systems that generate episodic activity, since similar relationships (positive correlation between episode duration and preceding - but not following - interval) were found in the developing retina [16], developing cortical networks [31], hippocampal slices [38] and disinhibited spinal networks [37, 40]. It is therefore tempting to suggest that similar qualitative mechanisms operate in the generation of periodic activity by all these different networks.

11.4.4. *Recovery of the activity after blockade of excitatory connections*

One of the most surprising features of the spontaneous activity is its robustness to pharmacological perturbation. When synaptic transmission mediated by the excitatory neurotransmitters glutamate and acetylcholine is blocked using pharmacological agents, the spontaneous activity stops for a long period of time (compared to the inter-episode intervals) but then recovers, as shown in Fig. 11.7(A) [8]. The activity is then thought to depend exclusively on GABAergic and glycinergic synapses, which have, early in development, functionally excitatory roles. It must be noted that the recovery is not gradual, as the new inter-episode intervals are not gradually decreasing to a new level but remain at a fixed level immediately after the activity has recovered (see Fig. 11.7(A), and note that after recovery the intervals are larger than in control conditions). We could imagine an additional process, through which the lack of activity is detected and compensated by slowly increasing network excitability until activity reaches its control level. However, this slow homeostatic process may cause a progressive - not abrupt - decrease of inter-episode intervals, unlike the experimental observation.

Surprisingly, the s-model can explain this recovery without introducing any additional variable in the model. If we decrease the connectivity parameter (w), in order to mimic the blockade of a fraction of the connections, the s-model reacts exactly like the chick spinal cord: activity first stops, then recovers with a fixed inter-episode interval (Fig. 11.7(B)). As for the experimental result, the new inter-episode intervals are larger than before the blockade. In addition, episode duration was only slightly affected, also in agreement with the experiments. On the other hand, the θ-model behaves in a different way: activity recovers quickly after the reduction in connectivity and the intervals are then slightly *lower* than in "control" (Fig. 11.7(B), "θ-model"). In addition, episode duration is markedly reduced for the recovered activity (not shown). This is an important qualitative difference

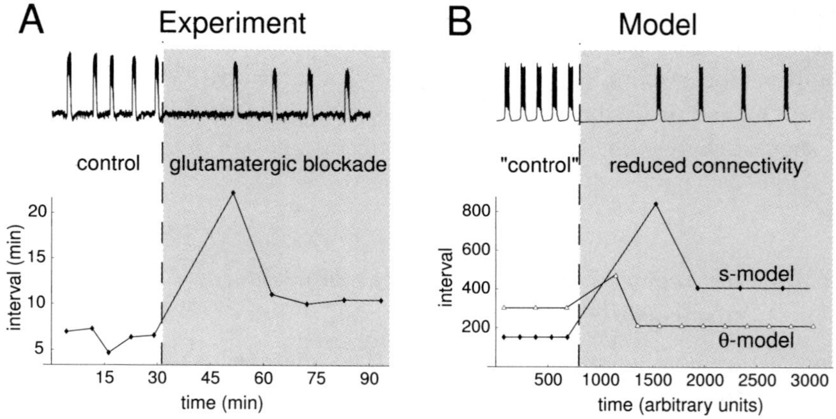

Fig. 11.7. Recovery of activity after partial block of excitatory connexions. A) results from a 10 day old chick, showing activity (upper trace) and inter-episode intervals in control and after blockade of some glutamatergic connexions (100 μM APV). B) model results before ("control") and after w was decreased from 1.2 to 0.9 (-25 %). The upper trace was obtained with the s-model. On the interval plot, results from both the s-model (filled diamonds) and θ-model (open triangles) are shown. Modified from [43].

between the s- and θ-models: in both cases activity can recover following a decrease in connectivity, but the s-model will have increased interepisode intervals, while the θ-model will have shorter episodes. This difference in how the models react to a decrease in connectivity suggests that the episodic nature of the spontaneous activity in the chick cord is due mostly to synaptic depression, not cellular adaptation.

In order to understand the recovery of activity, we plotted again the activity generated by the s-model in Fig. 11.8, together with the slow depression variable (s) and the effective connectivity ($w \cdot s$). As described previously, s and therefore $w{\cdot}s$ decrease during the episodes and increase during the inter-episode intervals. When the connectivity is suddenly decreased by 25% (from 1.2 to 0.9), this causes a corresponding decrease of $w \cdot s$, the effective connectivity in the network, i.e. the effective gain of the positive feedback due to excitatory connections. Activity is therefore blocked until this gain can reach back to its "control" value. This can happen because in the absence of activity, s keeps increasing towards its asymptotic value of one. As soon as $w \cdot s$ reaches its control value, episodes of activity reoccur. The intervals between episodes are somewhat longer than in control, because the exponential increase of s during the intervals is slower since s is now closer to its asymptotic value. Therefore, the activity can recover after a moderate decrease of connectivity because the system "automatically" compensates by decreasing the level of depression (increasing s). However, this would not be possible if the system were operating close to saturation.

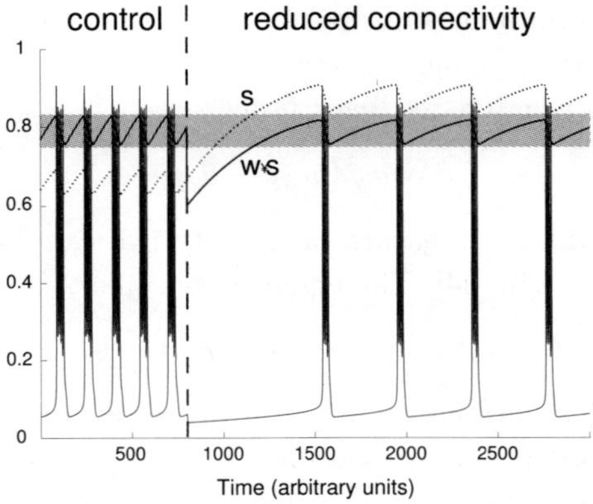

Fig. 11.8. Time course of activity, synaptic strength (s) and effective connectivity ($w \cdot s$) produced by the s-model before ("control") and after ("reduced connectivity") w was decreased by 25% (from 1.2 to 0.9). Activity stops after w was decreased, because the effective connectivity becomes too small to support network activity. This allows s to increase beyond its control level, until reaches its control level. Activity then reoccurs, although with larger inter-episode intervals. Modified [42].

This predicts that the synapses that were not blocked by the pharmacological agent see their availability or efficacy increase relative to their control level. To verify this prediction, we have stimulated a pathway (between adjacent ventral roots) that does not contain glutamatergic synapses. Indeed, we have shown that the strength of the response was increased after blockade of glutamatergic connections and subsequent recovery of the activity [42]. The developing spinal circuits are therefore able to approximately maintain their level of activity following the blockade of some of their connections. This is very important since the temporal pattern of activity may be important in the development of network and cellular properties [17, 39]. During development, some cells and connections may be lost, while other synapses may see their efficacy increased. Through the very mechanism that regulates its patterned activity (activity-dependent synaptic depression), the developing spinal cord is able to compensate for these changes and therefore maintain its activity level within a certain operating range.

11.5. Analogy between Network and Cellular Bursting

The bursting network activity that we have described above is called square wave bursting and is analogous, mathematically, to the models of cellular bursting presented in chapters 2, 8, 10, 12 and 13. Basically, a slow variable (here, s or θ) periodically switches a bistable fast subsystem between a low and a high state, the high state being oscillatory. To clarify the analogy between network and cellular bursters, we start from a simplified version of Eq. (1) with no negative feedback processes:

$$\tau_a \ \dot{a} = a_\infty(w \cdot a - \theta_0) - a.$$

Instead of a presynaptic measure of activity, we can use a postsynaptic measure, $V = w \cdot a - \theta_0$ [34]. The equation becomes:

$$\tau_a \dot{V} = -V + w \cdot a_\infty(V) - \theta_0$$

since both w and θ_0 are constant parameters. V represents the average "voltage" of the population of neurons (average over spikes and over the population). This equation is analogous to a membrane voltage equation:

$$\tau_m \dot{V} = -V + \bar{g}_{in} \cdot m_\infty(V) + I_{app}$$

where V is the intracellular membrane potential, τ_m is the membrane time constant, $\bar{g}_{in}$ the conductance of an inward current (sodium or calcium, for example) and m_∞ is the voltage-dependent activation curve of this current, and I_{app} is an applied current to the cell (due to tonic synaptic input or injected with a microelectrode). Here, the inward conductance provides excitatory feedback to the cell similarly as the excitatory connections provide positive feedback in our network model. The amount of positive feedback is controlled by $\bar{g}_{in}$ (the analog of connectivity, w) and the system can also be biased by applied current (the analog of $-\theta_0$ in the network model). For a range of parameter values, this voltage equation is bistable, and it can be slowly switched between high and low states by either modulating the inward current with an inactivating variable h:

$$\tau_m \dot{V} = -V + \bar{g}_{in} \cdot h \cdot m_\infty(V) + I_{app} \tag{6}$$

or by adding a slow outward current $\bar{g}_{out} \cdot n$:

$$\tau_m \dot{V} = -V + \bar{g}_{in} \cdot m_\infty(V) - \bar{g}_{out} \cdot n + I_{app}. \tag{7}$$

The inward current inactivation h is the analog of the synaptic depression variable s, as they both modulate the amount of positive feedback, while the outward current activation variable n is the analog of the cellular adaptation variable θ, as they both shift the input/output function of the systems. Equations (6) and (7) are equivalent to the network Eqs. (1) and (4) if the variables h and n (and their network equivalents) are very slow compared to V (and a).

We propose that Eqs. (6) and (7), together with differential equations for the gating variables h and n, capture the essence of square wave bursting. But these equations are extreme simplifications of the cellular burster models presented in other chapters. They do not include fast spiking processes, the time constants of h and n are not voltage-dependent, and we have ignored the driving force terms (i.e. these equations are current-based, not conductance-based, models). Nevertheless, these equations, i.e. the equations for the s-model and θ-model, behave similarly to sophisticated cellular burster models. For illustration, we refer to the models of mammalian respiratory pacemakers neurons presented in chapter 12 by Butera *et al.* In their Model 1, bursts are terminated by the inactivation h of a persistent sodium current, while in their Model 2 the bursts are terminated by the activation n of a potassium current [4]. Model 1 is the analog of our s-model, while Model 2 is the analog of our θ-model. We have ran simulations with both Model 1 and Model 2, during which we suddenly decreased the maximal persistent sodium conductance $\bar{g}_{N_aP}$. This manipulation of the cellular models is analogous to decreasing the connectivity w in our network models. The results of this manipulation are shown in Fig. 11.9(A). They show that Model 1 and 2 respond like the s-model and the θ-model, respectively. Furthermore, Fig. 11.9(B) shows that the recovery of bursting after a persistent sodium conductance decrease in Model 1 is identical to the recovery of activity in the s-model following a decrease in connectivity.

Interestingly, it has been shown that there are two types of respiratory bursters. One type, sensitive to riluzole (which blocks the persistent sodium current), seems to be described by Model 1. The other type, sensitive to cadmium (a calcium channel blocker), may correspond to Model 2 [33]. Norepinephrine (NE) modulates the rhythm generated by both types of neurons, possibly by increasing the conductance of calcium or sodium channel [45]. However, the effects depended on the type of bursters. Riluzole-sensitive neurons responded to NE by a decrease in the interburst interval (like Model 1 and the s-model) while cadmium-sensitive neurons responded with an increase in burst duration (like Model 2 and the θ-model).

Finally, our network models respond similarly to these cellular models following perturbations in cellular excitability (i.e., θ_0, I_{app}) (J. Tabak, unpublished results, and [4]).

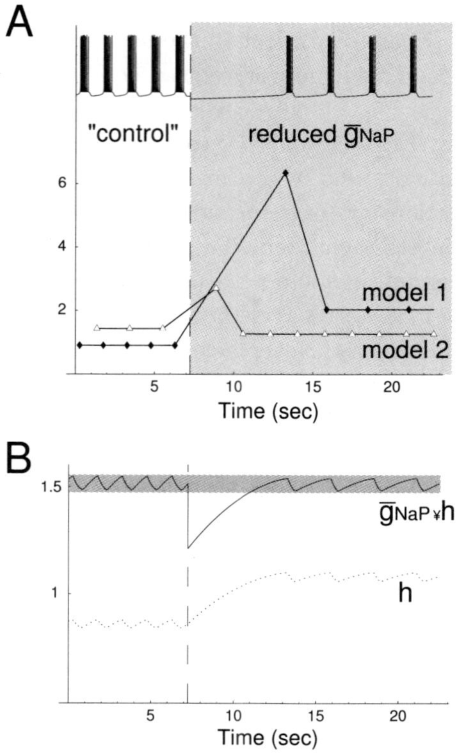

Fig. 11.9. Recovery of bursting following a decrease of the persistent sodium current in a model of respiratory pacemaker. A) Intracellular potential (upper trace, model 1) and interburst interval in control and after reduction of the persistent sodium conductance. $\bar{g}_{N_aP}$ was decreased from 3.5 to 2.8 nS for both model 1 and 2. Compare with Fig. 11.7(B). B) For model 1, variations of the sodium inactivation variable h (multiplied by 2 for clarity) and the product $\bar{g}_{N_aP} \cdot h$ (the "effective conductance"), before and after the reduction in conductance. Recovery of activity after decrease in conductance is achieved automatically by decreasing the level of inactivation of sodium current (increasing h). Compare with Fig. 11.8. The neurons were also excited by a tonic excitatory conductance of 0.35 nS for Model 1 and 0.75 nS for Model 2. All other common parameters were identical between Model 1 and 2.

11.6. Discussion

We have presented an idealized model of spontaneous bursting activity in developing neural networks. Despite its mean-field approach, the model captures the emergent nature of the phenomenon. Although we implicitly assumed that the network has a small amount of intrinsically firing cells (i.e., $a_{\infty}(0) \neq 0$), none of the cells need to have slow pacemaker capabilities. In our system the ensemble interactions are crucial for generating the episodic rhythm, not just for synchronizing cellular oscillators. Periodic activity is generated by the interaction of fast positive feedback and delayed negative feedback, as in many biological oscillators [15]. In the following, we discuss the generality of this type of mechanism, first in relation to other hyper excitable networks, then in relation to cellular oscillators.

11.6.1. *Bursting activity in neural networks*

The model presented in this chapter was developed to understand the spontaneous episodic activity in the developing spinal cord. However it is general enough to apply to spontaneous activity in other developing circuits. The developing circuits generating such spontaneous activity have been shown to be hyper excitable because the GABAergic connections that are inhibitory in the adult networks have excitatory effects early on. Further, other modeling and experimental studies have suggested that some activity-dependent depression of network excitability limit spontaneous bursts in the retina [5, 16, 28] and in cortical networks [31].

With maturation, networks acquire functional inhibitory connections and the spontaneous episodic activity stops. However, in some cases, the bursting activity can be uncovered by blocking inhibitory connections in these networks [3, 11, 50]. Furthermore, in some conditions, networks with functional inhibitory connections can generate bursting activity using the same type of mechanism as presented here. Examples include random networks in culture [23, 24, 41], hippocampus exhibiting epileptic-like activity [38] and cortical networks during sleep [10, 44]. This suggests that mature networks still have the potential to generate bursting activity reminiscent of the early spontaneous activity. This slow oscillatory activity can be evoked through the action of neuromodulators or pathological conditions that decrease synaptic inhibition and/or raise cellular excitability. It can be pathological (epilepsy) or physiologically useful (sleep). We note that, however, the time scales of episodic activity in the developing systems can be 1-2 orders of magnitude slower, and this poses interesting questions when one seeks specific biophysical mechanisms [26].

It will be particularly important to understand how network organization is changed as GABAergic synapses switch from excitatory to inhibitory during development. In some networks inhibitory connections play a primary role in coordinated rhythmogenesis, e.g. through post-inhibitory rebound mechanisms [36] or in synchronizing autonomously oscillating interneurons [46, 48]. However, in other networks it is possible that rhythmic bursting is still generated using excitatory connectivity and activity-dependent depression, with inhibition simply used to coordinate between different oscillatory subnetworks; this has been proposed for motor pattern generation in the spinal cord [19].

11.6.2. *Network vs cellular bursting*

The network model that we have presented is analogous to models of cellular bursting pacemakers (more precisely, square-wave bursters [47]). Some of the qualitative shared features can be seen by drawing analogies between a generalized Wilson-Cowan (WC) description for the activity of a single neuronal population [49] and the membrane potential equations of a Hodgkin-Huxley-type (HH) single compartment model [21]. Both formulations involve mean field descriptions and the genesis of excitability and oscillations reflect the interplay between fast regenerative processes and slower negative feedback.

In the mean field setting the units (neurons in networks and channels in membranes) loose their individual identities. In WC, the activity is assumed to affect all cells similarly, in a deterministic way, as does voltage affect all channels in the same way in HH models. In both cases, the "output variable" (activity, voltage) is an average over short space and time scales. The distributed nature of longer-range spatial interactions can be studied by using spatial integration kernels (for WC) or cable equations (for HH). To reconsider the effects of microscopic temporal fluctuations (individual spikes or synaptic events in WC or channel openings/closings in HH) in the mean field format is not clear in general, it is an active area of research [1].

Bistability in networks and cells is achieved in corresponding ways. In WC, excitatory cells provide positive feedback through recurrent excitatory connections; in HH the regenerative effect comes from voltage-activated inward current due to sodium or calcium channels. In both cases, this positive feedback is non-linear, represented by the sigmoidal input/output function a_∞ in network, and the gating activation curve m_∞ for conductance in single cells. These functions need to be relatively steep to allow bistability (Tabak *et al.*, unpublished).

In the network models that we presented, episodic activity is created by the switching between the high and low states. Bursts are terminated by a decrease in the efficacy of the excitatory connections (synaptic depression), or by a decrease in the neurons' ability to discharge (cellular adaptation). Synaptic depression directly decreases the amount of positive feedback as a multiplicative factor, while cellular adaptation affects the network's "transfer function." Similarly, in the cellular models, bursts can be terminated by inactivating inward currents (directly decreasing positive feedback), or by activating outward currents (decreasing the neuron's voltage and thus the ability of inputs to open sodium/calcium channels).

Although we have used cellular adaptation as a way to decrease neuronal firing in our network models, this could also be achieved using inhibitory connections. That is, inhibitory cells in WC models are analogous to potassium channels in HH. As discussed above, the presence of inhibitory cells may or may not fundamentally change network operations. This depends on the dynamics of the inhibitory cells and their connectivity. In the simplest cases, a tonic inhibitory population would simply shift network input/output function (subtractive effect, as θ_0) while inhibitory cells with diffuse connectivity and same dynamics as the excitatory cells would simply be similar to a reduction if excitatory connectivity (divisive effect, as s). But in other cases, inhibitory cells may fire with a delay, providing the network with another mechanism for generating oscillatory activity (similar to cellular adaptation). More interestingly, the maturation of inhibitory connections can segregate a network into several subnetworks, dramatically changing the structure of the network. Perhaps the distribution and dynamics of some potassium channels may affect the functional architecture of neurons in a similar way.

Acknowledgments

We thank Jay Demas for providing his data of mouse retinal activity.

References

[1] D. Amit and N. Brunel, Model of global spontaneous activity and local structured activity during delay periods in the cerebral cortex, *Cereb Cortex.* **7**, 237–252, (1997).

[2] Y. Ben-Ari, Excitatory actions of gaba during development: the nature of the nurture, *Nature Rev Neurosci.* **3**, 728–739, (2002).

[3] E. Bracci, L. Ballerini, and A. Nistri, Spontaneous bursts induced by pharmacological block of inhibition in lumbar motoneurons of the neonatal rat spinal cord, *J Neurophysiol.* **75**, 640–647, (1996).

[4] R. Butera, J. Rinzel, and J. Smith, Models of respiratory rhythm generation in the pre-Bötzinger complex: I. Bursting pacemaker neurons, *J Neurophysiol.* **82**, 382–397, (1999).
[5] D. Butts, M. Feller, C. Shatz, and D. Rokhsar, Retinal waves are governed by collective network properties, *J Neurosci.* **19**, 3580–3593, (1999).
[6] F. Chance, S. Nelson, and L. Abbott, Synaptic depression and the temporal response characteristics of V1 cells, *J Neurosci.* **18**, 4785–4799, (1998).
[7] E. Cherubini, J.-L. Gaiarsa, and Y. Ben-Ari, GABA: an excitatory transmitter in early postnatal life, *Trends Neurosci.* **14**, 515–519, (1991).
[8] N. Chub and M. O'Donovan, Blockade and recovery of spontaneous rhythmic activity after application of neurotransmitter antagonists to spinal networks of the chick embryo, *J Neurosci.* **18**, 294–306, (1998).
[9] N. Chub and M. O'Donovan, Post-episode depression of GABAergic transmission in spinal neurons of the chick embryo, *J Neurophysiol.* **85**, 2166–2176, (2001).
[10] A. Compte, M. Sanchez-Vives, D. McCormick, and X. Wang, Cellular and network mechanisms of slow oscillatory activity (< 1 Hz) and wave propagations in a cortical network model, *J Neurophysiol.* **89**, 2707–2725, (2003).
[11] P. Darbon, L. Scicluna, A. Tscherter, and J. Streit, Mechanisms controlling bursting activity induced by disinhibition in spinal cord networks, *Eur J Neurosci.* **15**, 671–683, (2002).
[12] B. Ermentrout, *Simulating, analyzing, and animating dynamical systems.* (SIAM, 2002).
[13] B. Fedirchuk, P. Wenner, P. Whelan, S. Ho, J. Tabak, and M. O'Donovan, Evoked synaptic potentials are transiently depressed following rhythmic activity in embryonic chick spinal neurons, *J Neurosci.* **19**, 2102–2112, (1999).
[14] R. Fitzhugh, Impulses and physiological states in theoretical models of nerve membrane, *Biophys J.* **1**, 445–466, (1961).
[15] W. Friesen and G. Block, What is a biological oscillator?, *Am J Physiol.* **246**, R847–853, (1984).
[16] N. Grzywacz and E. Sernagor, Spontaneous activity in developing turtle retinal ganglion cells: statistical analysis, *Vis Neurosci.* **17**, 229–241, (2000).
[17] X. Gu and N. Spitzer, Distinct aspects of neuronal differentiation en-

coded by frequency of spontaneous Ca^{2+} transients, *Nature.* **29**, 784–787, (1995).

[18] V. Hamburger and M. Balaban, Observations and experiments on spontaneous rhythmical behavior in the chick embryo, *Developmental Biology.* **7**, 533–545, (1963).

[19] J. Hellgren-Kotaleski, A. Lansner, and S. Grillner, Neural mechanisms potentially contributing to the intersegmental phase lag in lamprey.II. Hemisegmental oscillations produced by mutually coupled excitatory neurons, *Biol Cyber.* **81**, 299–315, (1999).

[20] S. Ho and M. O'Donovan, Regionalization and intersegmental coordination of rhythm-generating networks in the spinal networks of the chick embryo, *J Neurosci.* **13**, 1354–1371, (1993).

[21] A. Hodgkin and A. Huxley, A quantitative description of membrane current and its application to conduction and excitation in nerve, *J Physiol.* **117**, 500–544, (1952).

[22] L. Katz and C. Shatz, Synaptic activity and the construction of cortical circuits, *Science.* **274**, 1133–1138, (1996).

[23] P. Latham, B. Richmond, P. Nelson, and S. Nirenberg, Intrinsic dynamics in neuronal networks. I. Theory, *J Neurophysiol.* **83**, 808–827, (2000).

[24] P. Latham, B. Richmond, S. Nirenberg, and P. Nelson, Intrinsic dynamics in neuronal networks. II. Experiment, *J Neurophysiol.* **83**, 828–835, (2000).

[25] M. Li, M. Jia, R. Fields, and P. Nelson, Modulation of calcium currents by electrical activity, *J Neurophysiol.* **76**, 2595–2607, (1996).

[26] C. Marchetti, J. Tabak, N. Chub, M. O'Donovan, and J. Rinzel, Modeling spontaneous activity in the developing spinal cord using activity-dependent variations of intracellular chloride, *J Neurosci.* **25**, 3601–3612, (2005).

[27] E. Marder and R. Calabrese, Principles of rhythmic motor pattern generation, *Physiol Rev.* **76**, 687–717, (1996).

[28] M. Meister, R. Wong, D. Baylor, and C. Shatz, Synchronous bursts of action potentials in ganglion cells of the developing mammalian retina, *Science.* **252**, 939–943, (1991).

[29] M. O'Donovan, The origin of spontaneous activity in developing networks of the vertebrate nervous system, *Curr Opin Neurobiol.* **9**, 94–104, (1999).

[30] M. O'Donovan and L. Landmesser, The development of hindlimb motor activity studied in the isolated spinal cord of the chick embryo, *J*

Neurosci. **7**, 3256–3264, (1987).

[31] T. Opitz, A. De Lima, and T. Voigt, Spontaneous development of synchronous oscillatory activity during maturation of cortical networks in vitro, *J Neurophysiol.* **88**, 2196–2206, (2002).

[32] O. Paulsen and T. Sejnowski, Natural patterns of activity and long-term synaptic plasticity, *Curr Opin Neurobiol.* **10**, 172–179, (2000).

[33] F. Pena, M. Parkis, A. Tryba, and J.-M. Ramirez, Differential contribution of pacemaker properties to the generation of respiratory rhythms during normoxia and hypoxia, *Neuron.* **43**, 105–117, (2004).

[34] D. Pinto, J. Brumberg, D. Simons, and G. Ermentrout, A quantitative population model of whisker barrels: re-examining the wilson-cowan equations, *J Comput Neurosci.* **3**, 247–264, (1996).

[35] J. Rinzel and G. Ermentrout. Analysis of neural excitability and oscillations. In *Methods in Neuronal Modeling*, pp. 251–291. MIT Press, (1998).

[36] J. Rinzel, D. Terman, X. Wang, and G. Ermentrout, Propagating activity patterns in large-scale inhibitory neuronal networks, *Science.* **279**, 1351–1355, (1998).

[37] A. Rozzo, L. Ballerini, G. Abbate, and A. Nistri, Experimental and modeling studies of novel bursts induced by blocking Na^+ pump and synaptic inhibition in the rat spinal cord, *J Neurophysiol.* **88**, 676–691, (2002).

[38] K. Staley, M. Longacher, J. Bains, and A. Yee, Presynaptic modulation of CA3 network activity, *Nature Neurosci.* **1**, 201–209, (1998).

[39] D. Stellwagen and C. Shatz, An instructive role for retinal waves in the development of retinogeniculate connectivity, *Neuron.* **24**, 673–685, (2002).

[40] J. Streit, A. Tscherter, M. Heuschkel, and R. P, The generation of rhythmic activity in dissociated cultures of rat spinal cord, *Eur J Neurosci.* **14**, 191–202, (2001).

[41] J. Tabak and P. Latham, Analysis of spontaneous bursting activity in random neural networks, *Neuroreport.* **14**, 1445–1449, (2003).

[42] J. Tabak, J. Rinzel, and M. O'Donovan, The role of activity-dependent network depression in the expression and self-regulation of spontaneous activity in the developing spinal cord, *J Neurosci.* **21**, 8966–8978, (2001).

[43] J. Tabak, W. Senn, M. O'Donovan, and J. Rinzel, Modeling of spontaneous activity in the developing spinal cord using activity-dependent depression in an excitatory network, *J Neurosci.* **20**, 3041–3056, (2000).

[44] I. Timofeev, F. Grenier, M. Bazhenov, T. Sejnowski, and M. Steriade, Origin of slow cortical oscillations in deafferented cortical slabs, *Cereb Cortex.* **10**, 1185–1199, (2000).

[45] J.-C. Viemari and J.-M. Ramirez, Role of norepinephrine in respiratory rhythms generation, *Soc Neurosci Abs.* **755.1**, (2004).

[46] X. Wang and G. Buzsaki, Gamma oscillation by synaptic inhibition in a hippocampal interneuronal network model, *J Neurosci.* **16**, 6402–6413, (1996).

[47] X. Wang and J. Rinzel. Oscillatory and bursting properties of neurons. In ed. M. A. Arbib, *Handbook of Brain Theory and Neural Networks*, pp. 686–691. MIT Press, (1995).

[48] M. Whittington, R. Traub, and R. Jefferys, Synchronized oscillations in interneuron networks driven by metabotropic glutamate receptor activation, *Nature.* **373**, 612–615, (1995).

[49] H. Wilson and J. Cowan, Excitatory and inhibitory interactions in localized populations of model neurons, *Biophys J.* **12**, 1–24, (1972).

[50] R. Wong and R. Traub, Synchronized burst discharge in disinhibited hippocampal slice. I. Initiation in CA2-CA3 region, *J Neurophysiol.* **49**, 442–458, (1983).

[51] L. Zhang and M. Poo, Electrical activity and development of neural circuits, *Nature Neurosci.* **4 suppl**, 1207–1214, (2001).

CHAPTER 12

OSCILLATORY BURSTING MECHANISMS IN RESPIRATORY PACEMAKER NEURONS AND NETWORKS

Robert Butera

Laboratory for Neuroengineering, School of Electrical and Computer Engineering, Georgia Institute of Technology, Atlanta, GA 30332-0250 USA
e-mail: rbutera@ece.gatech.edu

Jonathan Rubin

Dept. of Mathematics, University of Pittsburgh, Pittsburgh, PA 15260 USA
e-mail: rubin@math.pitt.edu

David Terman

Dept. of Mathematics, The Ohio State University, Columbus, OH 43210-1174 USA
e-mail: terman@math.ohio-state.edu

Jeffrey Smith

Cellular and Systems Neurobiology Section, Laboratory of Neural Control, NINDS, National Institutes of Health, Bethesda, MD 20892-4455 USA
e-mail: jsmith@helix.nih.gov

An excitatory network of bursting neurons are postulated to be involved in generating the rhythm of breathing in the pre-Bötzinger complex of the mammalian brainstem. A subpopulation of these neurons exhibit complex voltage-dependent properties with multi-state behavior consisting of silence, oscillatory bursting and tonic spiking activity modes. In this chapter we review the development of single cell models, followed by simulation-based studies of population dynamics of a network of such model cells. In particular, we find that excitatory synaptic coupling increases the range of parameter space where bursting occurs, and that parameter heterogeneity of intrinsic and synaptic properties further increases this range, as well as the range of frequencies where bursting occurs at a network level. The mechanisms underlying these findings have been elucidated by recent mathematical analyses. We start with a geometric fast/slow approach to analyze bursting dynamics, including transitions to tonic spiking states in single model neurons as well as synaptically coupled pairs of model cells. Certain aspects of the increased dynamic range due to synaptic coupling can be understood from the effects of coupling strength on the bifurcation structure of a single, self-coupled cell. Additional complexity emerges when neuron pairs exhibit asynchrony of spikes within bursts. Here synaptic coupling changes the form of bursting from square-wave bursting to a bursting class known as fold/fold cycle or "top hat bursting". A two-variable slow averaged system analysis reveals the existence of, and transitions between, two subtypes of bursting. To conclude the chapter, we extend the fast/slow analysis to a larger cell population with heterogeneities, which further enhance the dynamic range of network bursting. We determine conditions for synchronized whole-population bursting, allowing for gradual jumps between the silent and active phases of each burst cycle. We conclude by highlighting unresolved problems in modeling and analyzing this system as well as considering limitations of our studies to date.

12.1. Introduction

In this chapter we discuss models of oscillatory bursting neurons and bursting neuron networks that are postulated to be involved in generating the rhythm of breathing in the mammalian brainstem. Breathing in mammals is an innate rhythmic motor behavior essential for life, and the nervous system mechanisms producing the respiratory rhythm have fascinated neuroscientists and physiologists for over a century and remain a subject of intense investigation. There is a rich tradition of both experimental and modeling work in this area, with modeling playing an increasingly important role for understanding the complex dynamics at cellular and neural network levels. Currently it is understood that the generation and control of the rhythm involves dynamic interactions between populations of neurons in networks distributed bilaterally in the ventrolateral medulla of the brainstem within a functionally-defined region called the ventral respiratory group (VRG). These networks constitute part of the respiratory central pattern generator, components of which generate the neural oscillation underling the rhythm [11, 26, 27]. A functionally specialized subregion of the VRG called the pre-Bötzinger complex (pre-BötC) [38] contains a local network of excitatory (glutamatergic) neurons [14, 20] that current experimental evidence indicates is an essential component of the oscillator. Our models focus on burst generation mechanisms operating specifically within the pre-BötC.

While the actual cellular and network mechanisms underlying rhythm generation are subject to some debate, the pre-BötC contains a heterogeneous population of excitatory neurons, some of which exhibit intrinsic oscillatory bursting properties. These bursting "pacemaker" neurons and synchronized activity in the pre-BötC network are postulated to contribute importantly to rhythm generation by initiating a pattern of rhythmic excitation in the VRG network that produces the inspiratory phase of the respiratory cycle. Indeed it is possible to isolate the pre-BötC experimentally in slices of the rodent medulla that maintain inspiratory rhythm generation *in vitro*, where it has been demonstrated experimentally that individual neurons [7, 20, 38] and the excitatory pre-BötC network as a whole [18] have autorhythmic properties. The models presented here are motivated by the experimental observations in this isolated *in vitro* system. In the more intact system *in vivo*, the local pre-BötC network is embedded in the larger VRG network, where inhibitory network interactions also contribute to the generation and control of the rhythm. This more intact system has been described as a "hybrid" of excitatory pacemaker network and inhibitory network mechanisms [39]. The mechanisms analyzed and discussed here for the pre-BötC excitatory network "kernel" therefore do not represent the complete set of cellular and network dynamics operating in the more intact system, but nevertheless represent an important component, giving rise to a rich set of dynamical behaviors that have proven amenable to analysis.

In the analysis, the critical issues to be resolved at the single-neuron level are:

- What are the essential biophysical mechanisms responsible for oscillatory bursting?
- What is the dynamic structure of the bursting mechanism(s)?
- How is the frequency of bursting regulated both by intrinsic and extrinsic mechanisms?

At the pre-BötC network level, key questions are:

- How does excitatory synaptic coupling affect the intrinsic bursting dynamics?
- How does synchrony arise in coupled populations of bursting cells?
- What higher order dynamics emerge as a result of synaptic coupling and heterogeneity of cellular properties within the network?

These questions, which are central to the analysis of many of the bursting systems considered in this volume, were originally addressed for the pre-BötC network by the modeling studies of Butera *et al.*, [2, 3] which should be consulted for reference. Extensions of these original studies, by Rubin and Terman [32] and Best *et al.*, [1] addressing analytical questions regarding dynamics of coupled bursting cells and heterogeneous networks, are also reviewed here. These analyses are providing general insights into the oscillatory dynamics of cellular and network bursting. In this chapter we first consider the experimental foundations and simulation results for our models of individual pre-BötC neurons (section 12.2), pairs of neurons (section 12.3), as well as network wide bursting (section 12.4). These simulation results suggest that both synaptic coupling and parameter heterogeneity play key roles in expanding the range of parameter space where bursting occurs as well as maintaining a broad range of frequencies at which the network can burst. The remainder of this chapter focuses on further analyses of these findings. In particular, we will examine the mechanism whereby synaptic coupling increases the parameter range of bursting (section 12.5), and in the process show that the mechanism for bursting is distinctly different for coupled cells than for individual cells. Finally, we consider large networks of bursting neurons and analyze mechanisms by which network excitability and heterogeneity of cellular parameters can promote synchronized network bursting (section 12.6).

12.2. Single Cell Dynamics: Evidence, Motivation, and Models

Our single cell models were motivated by a compelling body of experimental observations on the dynamics of respiratory neurons located within the pre-BötC. These observations include:

- *Capicity for endogenous rhythmic bursting.* A subpopulation of inspiratory neurons in the pre-BötC, when depolarized, will fire ectopically, i.e. firing bursts of action potentials at moments in time when an inspiratory discharge from the population is not occurring. When isolated pharmacologically, many of these pre-BötC neurons continue to demonstrate endogenous bursting [7, 17, 20, 38].
- *Voltage-dependent control of activity state and bursting frequency.* Neurons that burst during the inspiratory phase of the respiratory cycle and exhibit ectopic bursts in the intact network, have three intrinsic activity states after network activity is disrupted by experimentally removing network synaptic interactions: silence, oscillatory bursting, and tonic

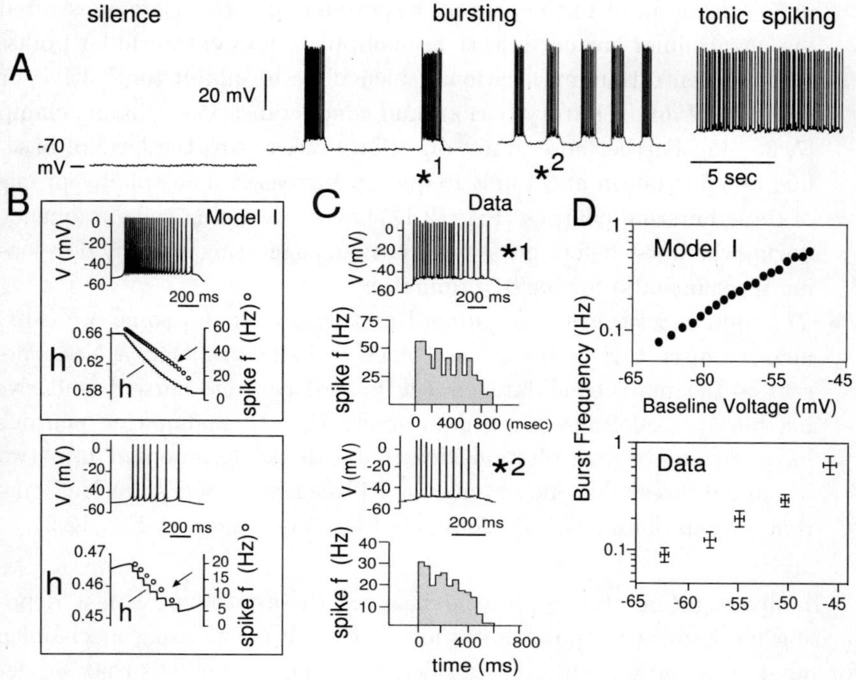

Fig. 12.1. Intrinsic electrophysiological behavior of pre-BötC bursting "pacemaker" neurons. A. Three main voltage-dependent activity states of a bursting neuron recorded *in vitro* (isolated from synaptic inputs): silence, voltage-dependent oscillatory bursting, and tonic spiking at depolarized voltage levels. Corresponding voltage-dependent control of activity state exhibited by Model I is shown in Fig. 12.3. In the bursting regime, burst frequency increases and burst duration decreases as the baseline level of voltage is depolarized by constant applied current (I_{app} in text). The spiking profile during bursts and the decrease in burst duration are illustrated for single bursts at two voltage levels from Model I simulations in B and from the recordings (indicated by *1 and *2 in A and C). Intraburst spike frequency (spike f) declines with time as shown by interspike intervals in B, and spike frequency histograms averaged over multiple recorded bursts in C. This profile results from progressive inactivation of I_{NaP}, as indicated by time course of inactivation parameter h (see also Fig. 12.4(A2)). Voltage-dependent control of bursting frequency is illustrated in D from Model I simulations and from a compilation of recordings. Model I reproduces the monotonic increase in frequency as baseline voltage is depolarized by either I_{app} or other tonic depolarizing input (e.g., current due to $g_{tonic-e}$ in Fig. 12.5).

spiking (Fig. 12.1). Experimentally, this is demonstrated by intracellular current injection (Fig. 12.1). Pacemaker neurons in the pre-BötC burst over an order of magnitude range of frequencies (from under 0.1 Hz to 1 Hz), and the frequency of bursting is controlled by the level of depolarizing input to the neuron. Experimentally, this is demonstrated via intracellular current injection, manipulation of extracellular potassium concentration, application of bicuculine to inhibit tonic drive, or addition of an excitatory background conductance via dynamic clamp [7, 38, 45]. Furthermore, burst duration decreases as the level of baseline depolarization and burst frequency increases. The spiking profile of these bursting neurons (Fig. 12.1) shows a declining spike frequency during the burst before burst termination, suggesting a slowly developing mechanism(s) for burst termination.

- *The ionic mechanism of bursting.* Bursting persists for some pre-BötC neurons after Ca^{2+} currents are blocked, indicating that a Na^+ current is the main candidate for the inward cationic current underlying bursting. Voltage-clamp data shows that these bursting neurons have current-voltage relationships that can be decomposed into two major subthreshold conductances: a TTX-sensitive persistent Na^+ current and an ohmic-like K^+-dominated leak conductance (Fig. 12.2).

In investigating the biophysical basis of these features, a fast depolarizing mechanism for burst initiation and a slower opposing mechanism for burst termination must be considered. In the two models that we developed [2], initiation occurs by the activation of a persistent Na^+ current (I_{NaP}). However, burst termination in the two models occurs by contrasting mechanisms. In Model I, burst termination occurs by the slow-inactivation of I_{NaP}, a persistent Na^+-current with slow inactivation. In Model II, a slowly-activating K^+-current (I_{KS}) is responsible for burst termination. This chapter will only consider Model I, as it is more consistent with experimental data, and subsequent experimental data focused on elucidating the ionic mechanism for bursting has provided strong confirmatory evidence for this mechanism [7, 8]. These models are minimalistic and are intended to focus solely on the proposed mechanism of bursting, and not the ionic currents mediating spiking activity. Recent investigations suggest that multiple types of bursting mechanisms may be present in pre-BötC neurons [24, 25].

The mechanism of single-cell bursting in Model I rests entirely on I_{NaP}. This subthreshold Na^+ current has a rapid voltage-dependent activation that initiates the burst. During bursting, a slow voltage-dependent inactivation term progressively decreases $\bar{g}_{NaP}$, until the burst ceases. The frequency of bursting increases with depolarization, and the baseline parameter set is capable of demonstrating burst frequencies from 0.1 Hz to

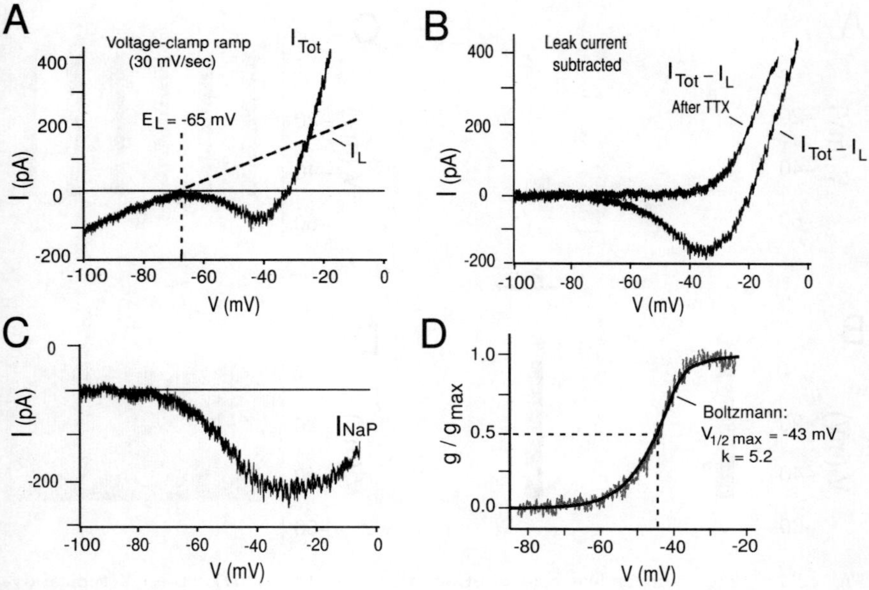

Fig. 12.2. Current-voltage (I-V) relationships of pre-BötC bursting neurons, illustrating decomposition of experimental I-V data into current components underlying bursting. A. Whole-cell I-V relationship obtained by voltage-clamp recording from a pre-BötC bursting neuron with behavior as in Fig. 12.1. The N-shaped I-V relationship obtained by a slow voltage-clamp ramp (30 mV/sec) represents the total membrane current (I_{Tot}) before decomposition. The I-V curve exhibits a linear region (< -65 mV) and an inward current (negative slope region) reaching peak current near -40 mV. This is followed by large voltage-activated outward currents (positive slope region) at more depolarized voltages. Linear region results from a non-voltage-activated K^+-dominated leak current (I_L), with 0 current intercept (E_L) near -65 mV. I_L is subtracted from I_{Tot} to yield voltage-activated current components in B. Inward, burst-generating current is blocked by Na^+ channel blockers (e.g. TTX), with resulting I-V curve consisting mainly of voltage-activated outward K^+ currents (positive slope regions in A and B). Burst-generating current (C) is extracted by subtracting curves before and after Na^+ current block, [8] yielding I_{NaP}. Boltzmann function (D) computed from the I_{NaP} curve, characterizes voltage-dependence of (quasi) steady-state activation, which in this example gives activation parameters of $V_{1/2max}$ = -43 mV with slope factor k = 5.2, which are similar to values used in Model I. (Data obtained by H. Koizumi and J. Smith.) I-V data indicates that the minimal representation of subthreshold currents by I_L and I_{NaP} in Model I is a useful approximation for analysis of burst generation mechanisms.

1 Hz. Furthermore, this bursting dynamic is robust to broad changes in $\bar{g}_{NaP}$[2]. Figure 12.3 illustrates the time-course of membrane potential for a range of values of I_{app}; similar results are obtained if E_K or $g_{tonic-e}$ are varied [3, 7].

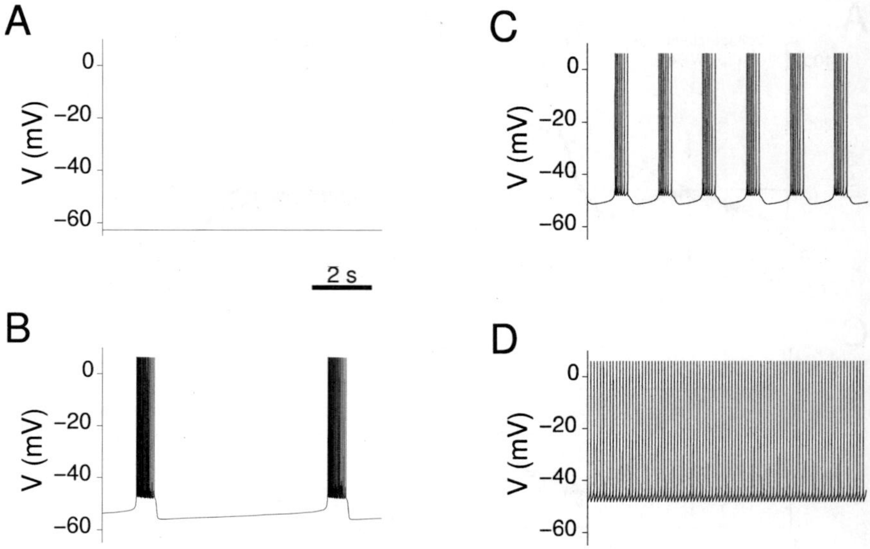

Fig. 12.3. Voltage-dependent control of bursting. Panels (A)-(D) represent typical dynamical activity of the model for different amounts of depolarizing input. Similar results are obtained if I_{app}, E_K, or a background level of excitatory input are increased.

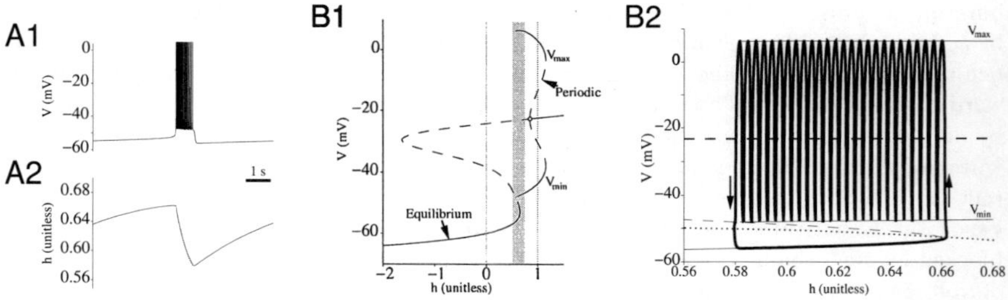

Fig. 12.4. Dynamics of bursting. (A1) and (A2) illustrate membrane potential and slow inactivation of I_{NaP}, respectively. (B1) illustrates bifurcation diagram of model when time-scales are separated and h is treated as a slow variable. Solid: stable equilibrium branch, dashed: unstable equilibrium branch, circle: Hopf bifurcation with periodic solution emanating from it, represented by the min and max of the oscillation. (B2): Closeup of shaded area in (B1). Trajectory during bursting is superimposed, and dotted line represents h nullcline.

Figure 12.4 illustrates the time-course of the membrane potential and h, the slow inactivation component of I_{NaP}. A bifurcation diagram of the system is also illustrated, and its general features are similar to other so-called "square-wave bursters" considered in this volume (see for example chapters 2, 8, 10, 11 and 13).

The model equations for our single cell model are listed below. It consists of four ionic currents: a fast Na^+ current I_{Na}, a delayed rectifier K^+ current I_K, a persistent Na^+ current with slow voltage-dependent inactivation I_{NaP}, and a leakage current I_L. I_{Na} is simplified through two assumptions: that the voltage-dependent activation is instantaneous and that the inactivation kinetics are approximately similar and inverse to the activation kinetics of I_K, i.e. they are approximated by $1 - n$, where n denotes the activation variable of I_K. These approximations are based on observations of Fitzhugh [12] of the original Hodgkin-Huxley model and have been studied systematically by others [21, 29].

The model, referred to below as Model I, takes the form

$$v' = (-I_{NaP} - I_{Na} - I_K - I_L - I_{tonic-e} - I_{syn-e} + I_{app})/C \tag{1}$$

$$n' = (n_\infty(v) - n_i)/\tau_n(v) \tag{2}$$

$$h' = \varepsilon(h_\infty(v) - h)/\tau_h(v) \tag{3}$$

where

$$I_{Na} = \bar{g}_{Na} m_\infty^3(v)(1-n)(v - E_{Na}) \tag{4}$$

$$I_K = \bar{g}_K n^4 (v - E_K) \tag{5}$$

$$I_{NaP} = \bar{g}_{NaP} m_\infty(v) h (v - E_{Na}) \tag{6}$$

$$I_L = \bar{g}_L (v - E_L). \tag{7}$$

The parameter ε is introduced in equation (3) to emphasize that h evolves on a slower timescale than v and n. Further, note that the $m_\infty(v)$ for I_{NaP} is distinct from the similarly named function in I_{Na} and is only indicated as such out of convention. All steady-state activation functions and time-constants are of the general form

$$x_\infty(v) = \frac{1}{1 + \exp((v - \theta_x)/d_x)} \tag{8}$$

$$\tau_x(v) = \frac{\bar{\tau}_x}{\cosh((v - \theta_x)/(2d_x))}. \tag{9}$$

External inputs consist of an applied stimulus current I_{app} and two synaptic input currents. Respiratory neurons receive a constant background level of synaptic input from a tonically firing population of neurons; in our thin brainstem slices this input is primarily excitatory. This background excitatory input is represented by $I_{tonic-e} = \bar{g}_{tonic-e}(v - E_{syn})$. Cells are also coupled amongst themselves by excitatory synaptic input [14, 20]. This input is represented by $I_{syn-e} = \bar{g}_{syn-e} s (v - E_{syn})$, with

$$s' = [(1-s)H(v_{pre} - \theta_s) - k_r s]/\tau_s, \tag{10}$$

where v_{pre} represents the membrane potential of a presynaptic neuron and $H(x)$ is a Heaviside function, which can alternatively be replaced by a steeply activating sigmoid. A complete list of model equations and parameters are specified in the papers of Butera *et al.* [2, 3].

12.3. Coupling Effects in Two Cells: A Pathway to Larger Populations

To study the effects of excitatory coupling on the dynamics of bursting, we initially consider the simple case of a pair of neurons. These neurons are reciprocally coupled by an excitatory synaptic current (I_{syn-e}). Each neuron in the pair also receives a mean level of tonic excitatory synaptic drive ($I_{tonic-e}$). We studied the dynamics of this pair of bursters as $\bar{g}_{syn-e}$ and $g_{tonic-e}$ were varied in order to assess the control of bursting frequency by excitatory tonic drive ($g_{tonic-e}$) and excitatory synaptic coupling ($\bar{g}_{syn-e}$). In all cases $g_{tonic-e}$ and $\bar{g}_{syn-e}$ were identical for each cell. The time course of the membrane potential oscillations for various values of $g_{tonic-e}$ and $\bar{g}_{syn-e}$ are illustrated in Fig. 12.5. An expanded version of this figure appears as Fig. 1, and a parametric analysis of burst frequency and duration as Fig. 2, in Butera *et al.* [3].

Both $g_{tonic-e}$ and $\bar{g}_{syn-e}$ activate excitatory currents, although $g_{tonic-e}$ may be described as constant and $\bar{g}_{syn-e}$ as phasic. Excluding the cases of weak coupling ($\bar{g}_{syn-e} < 2$ nS) and high tonic drive (large $g_{tonic-e}$), which are discussed separately below, several trends are evident in the rest of the ($g_{tonic-e}$, $\bar{g}_{syn-e}$) parameter space.

(1) At a given level of $g_{tonic-e}$, $\bar{g}_{syn-e}$ increases both the burst duration and the interburst interval, with a net effect of increasing the burst period. These effects are not independent: increasing excitatory coupling, which is triggered by the firing of action potentials, causes action potentials in each cell to further excite the other cell, with a net increase in intensity of firing in both cells. The higher spike frequency increases excitatory synaptic input during the active phase of a burst. In order for the burst to terminate, I_{NaP} must be inactivated further than it would in the absence of synaptic input. Thus the burst duration is extended. The additional inactivation of I_{NaP} prolongs recovery from inactivation as well, increasing the duration of the silent phase of the burst cycle. Thus the overall frequency of bursting is reduced.

(2) At a given level of $\bar{g}_{syn-e}$, burst duration increases with $g_{tonic-e}$. Through most of this range, the interburst interval decreases with

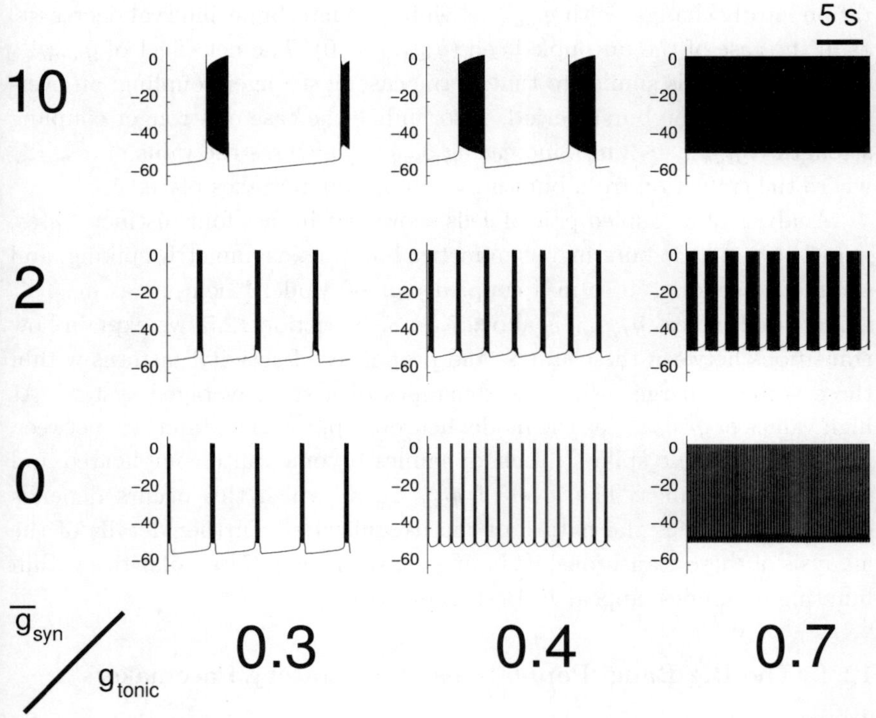

Fig. 12.5. Dynamics of a pair of synaptically coupled neurons as $\bar{g}_{syn}$ and g_{tonic} are varied. Only a single neuron is shown in each panel.

$g_{tonic-e}$. This decrease in interburst interval is the dominating effect and the overall burst period decreases. However, at higher values of $g_{tonic-e}$ in this parameter range, the interburst interval changes minimally or slightly increases, and the burst period increases.

(3) An important effect of synaptic coupling (except possibly for very strong $\bar{g}_{syn-e}$) is that it extends the range of values of $g_{tonic-e}$ over which bursting is supported, relative to the uncoupled case. This is partially evident for $\bar{g}_{syn-e}$=2 nS in Fig. 12.5 and more evident in Figs. 1 and 2 of Butera *et al.* [3] We will further consider this effect when we discuss the dynamics of a population of neurons below.

At low coupling strengths ($\bar{g}_{syn-e}$ < 2 nS), synaptic input during the firing of action potentials synchronizes the bursts of the two cells but does not significantly alter the dynamics of each cell (compared to the uncoupled state). In this case the bursts of the two cells synchronize but the burst duration hardly changes with $g_{tonic-e}$, while the interburst interval decreases, as in the case of the uncoupled cell ($\bar{g}_{syn-e} = 0$). The net effect of $g_{tonic-e}$ on burst period is similar to that in the case of stronger coupling: an overall decrease in the burst period. Also, unlike the case of stronger coupling strengths ($\bar{g}_{syn-e} > 2$ nS), increasing $\bar{g}_{syn-e}$ *increases* the value of $g_{tonic-e}$ where the transition from bursting to tonic spiking takes place.

Analysis of a coupled pair of cells show that in fact four distinct states, namely symmetric bursting, asymmetric bursting, asymmetric spiking, and symmetric spiking, arise in a coupled pair of Model I neurons as $g_{tonic-e}$ is increased, unless $\bar{g}_{syn-e}$ is above 7.5 nS. In section 12.5, we explain how transitions between these states, and properties of activity patterns within these states, emerge, using the dynamics of a slow averaged system. At high values of $g_{tonic-e}$, as the model neurons approach an interface between bursting and tonic spiking, their dynamics become quite complicated and sometimes irregular. The level of $g_{tonic-e}$ at which this occurs depends on $\bar{g}_{syn-e}$, as does the nature of the irregularities. Further details of the analysis of these transitions, including consideration of irregularities within bursting dynamics, appear in Best *et al.* [1].

12.4. The Big Bang: Populations of Excitatory Pacemakers

The two-cell network is ideal for analysis of synaptic interactions among pacemaking pre-BötC neurons. However, larger scale network simulations are necessary to consider population dynamics, especially when parameter heterogeneity is present. We modeled the pacemaker pre-BötC population by a network of 50 neurons where the subthreshold conductances ($\bar{g}_{NaP}$ and g_L) as well as synaptic conductances were randomly distributed via a normal distribution with a particular mean and variance. We found that 50 cells was the smallest possible population that generally preserved dynamics observed for larger population sizes, and that randomly distributing additional parameters (like $\bar{g}_{Na}$ and $\bar{g}_K$) produced similar results but complicated our analyses.

12.4.1. *Synchronized bursting in a heterogeneous population*

The net effect of this heterogeneous population is that, in isolation, some cells are silent, some are intrinsically bursting, and other are tonically spiking (Fig. 12.6(A)). When coupled together by a sufficient amount of excitatory synaptic coupling, they will burst in synchrony (Fig. 12.6(B)). For lower amounts of coupling or more extreme intrinsic parameter heterogene-

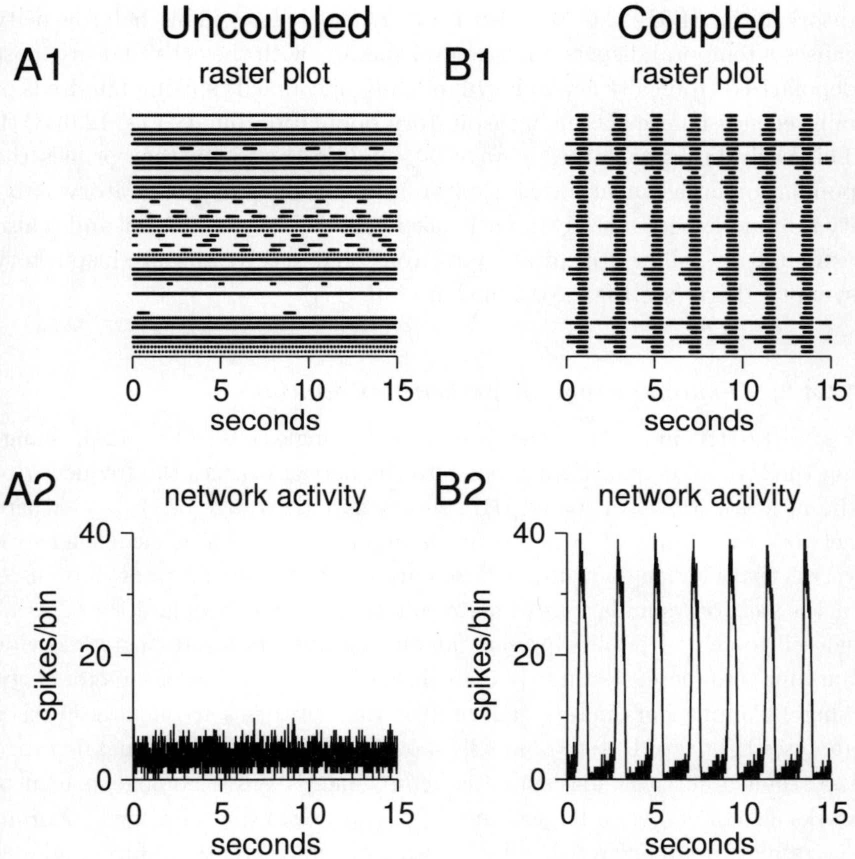

Fig. 12.6. Typical heterogeneous network simulations. (A1)/(B1). Raster plots of 50 neurons with randomly distributed properties when uncoupled (A1) and after excitatory synaptic coupling (B1). (A2)/(B2) measures of network activity for uncoupled (A2) and coupled (B2) data by binning raster data into 10 ms bins. Modified from Fig. 3 of Butera *et al.* [3]

ity, unstable as well as subharmonic rhythms are possible (see Fig. 4 of Butera *et al.* [3] and Fig. 10 of Del Negro *et al.* [7]).

In the nominal case of network-wide synchronous bursting, excitatory synaptic interactions, coupled with I_{NaP} activation, readily synchronize the initiation of the burst. I_{NaP} inactivation during bursting causes a relatively synchronous termination of inspiratory activity. Only a fraction of the pacemaker population need to be in the oscillatory bursting regime for the synaptic coupling to generate a synchronized, population-level inspiratory burst (Fig. 12.6, see also Fig. 12.7(B) below). This heterogeneity causes a temporal dispersion of neuron spiking, with the cells that are most depolarized (tonically active if synaptically uncoupled) spiking hundreds of milliseconds before the main inspiratory population burst (Fig. 12.6(B1)). This early firing generates a wave of synaptic excitation that primes the population for a synchronized inspiratory burst. Such pre-inspiratory activity is found experimentally in pacemaker cells *in vitro* [15, 17, 20] and is also exhibited by follower inspiratory neurons that receive the pre-inspiratory synaptic drive (see Fig. 2 of Johnson *et al.* [17]).

12.4.2. *Dynamic range of network oscillations*

Figure 12.7(A) illustrates that, just as in the single cells in Fig. 12.3, changing the level of depolarizing input into the network biases the frequency of the network. However, panel (B1) shows that the range of $g_{tonic-e}$ where network wide bursting occurs is much larger for the heterogeneous network versus that of a single neuron whose parameters are the mean of those used in the network simulations. This result leads us to speculate that intrinsic cell-to-cell variability present among neurons promotes network-wide bursting and increases the "dynamic range" - the range of parameter space whereby input parameters can control the network's frequency. Further analyses (Fig. 8 of Butera *et al.* [3]) show that this extended dynamic range is a result of intrinsic and synaptic heterogeneity. While homogeneous networks also burst over a larger range of $g_{tonic-e}$ than that of a single neuron, the range of frequencies whereby bursting occurs is greatly reduced; adding heterogeneity restores the range of frequencies where bursting occurs to even beyond that of the mean single neuron and also further extends the dynamic range of input parameter space. Panel (B2) of Fig. 12.7 illustrates the range of $g_{tonic-e}$ where each neuron in the simulations of (A1)-(A7) is intrinsically bursting in the absence of synaptic input. Panel (B3) further summarizes this data by highlighting the number of neurons intrinsically silent, bursting, or spiking at each value of $g_{tonic-e}$. While this data does not directly identify a mechanism for increased dynamic range, it does highlight the fact that at all values of $g_{tonic-e}$ where network bursting occurs, at least some neurons in the network are intrinsically bursting. A more throrough investigation into the relationship between synaptic coupling and dynamic range is presented in section 12.5, and the relationshionship between heterogeneity and coupled cell bursting is analyzed in section 12.6.

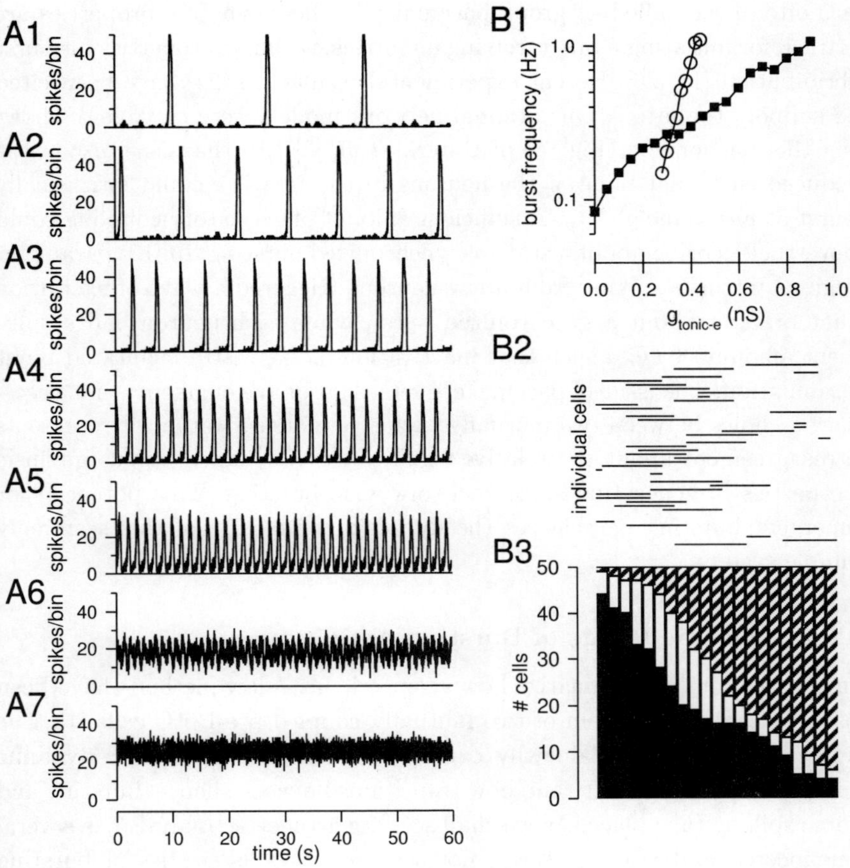

Fig. 12.7. Heterogeneous network simulations as a function of background level of depolarization. (A1)-(A7). Network activity for steadily increasing values of $g_{tonic-e}$ (0, 0.05, 0.2, 0.4, 0.55, 0.7, 0.9 nS). (B1). Frequency of the same heterogeneous network (black squares) and for a single cell with parameter values that are the mean of those used in the heterogeneous network simulation (open circles). (B2). Each bar indicates the range of $g_{tonic-e}$ where bursting occurred when each neuron in the simulations of (A1)-(A7) was decoupled from the network. (B3). Stacked bar chart illustrating number of neurons intrinsically silent (black), bursting (white), or spiking (hatched) when decoupled from the network at a particular value of $g_{tonic-e}$. Modified from Figs. 7 and 9 of Butera *et al.* [3]

12.4.3. *Emergent rhythms: Pacemakers vs. group pacemakers*

There has been a debate between the notion of a pacemaker-based rhythm, where pacemaking properties are essential for rhythm-generation, and what has often been called a "group-pacemaker", where synaptic properties are critical for initiating a burst, relying on intrinsic cellular properties for burst termination [11, 26]. Recent experimental results [23, 24] have been cited to support the latter. Our original network models were capable of showing this phenomena (Fig. 10 of Butera *et al.* [3]). In that case, $\bar{g}_{NaP}$ was reduced such that none of the neurons in the network could intrinsically burst at *any* value of I_{app}. A sufficient amount of excitatory coupling could nevertheless bring about a state of synchronized bursting. In this parameter regime, intrinsic spiking from a few neurons triggered a wave of excitation that brought about a synchronized burst, while each neuron had a sufficient amount of I_{NaP} such that inactivation of I_{NaP} still facilitated burst termination. The issue of pacemakers versus group pacemakers is not necessary a choice between two mutually exclusive models. Rather, it represents a disagreement about the relative significance of synaptic versus intrinsic properties in generating stable network-wide bursting. This potential for emergent bursting emphasizes the dynamic complexity of this seemingly simple system.

12.5. Dynamic Range of Bursting Activity

In this section, we summarize how geometric fast/slow methods have been used to analyze a system of two mutually coupled pre-BötC cells [1]. The analysis will help explain why coupling of cells increases their dynamic range of bursting activity and how transitions between silence, bursting and tonic spiking take place. As we shall see, the geometric analysis has several unexpected and novel features, not seen in previous studies of bursting oscillators. In the next section, we extend this analysis to the study of larger networks and explore the role of heterogeneities in shaping synchronized burst activity [32].

12.5.1. *Fast/slow analysis of a single cell*

To begin the analysis, we describe the fast/slow decomposition of a single self-coupled cell. This corresponds to a network in which the cells are completely synchronous. A single self-coupled Model I cell satisfies equations (1), (2), (3) and (10), with $v_{pre} = v$ in the synaptic equation.

Suppose, for example, that $(g_{tonic-e}, \bar{g}_{syn-e}) = (.2, 0)$, corresponding to no coupling. Then system (1), (2), (3) exhibits square-wave bursting, and this can be analyzed using standard fast/slow analysis [28, 30, 31]. That is, we set $\varepsilon = 0$ in (3) and treat the slow variable h as a bifurcation parameter in the fast subsystem (1), (2). The bifurcation diagram of the fast subsystem, projected onto (h, v)–space, is shown in Fig. 12.8. Note that the set of fixed points of the fast subsystem forms an S-shaped curve, denoted by $\mathcal{S}$. The lower branch of $\mathcal{S}$ consists of stable fixed points of the fast subsystem. There is a subcritical Hopf bifurcation along the upper branch of $\mathcal{S}$ and a family of unstable periodic orbits emanates from this bifurcation. This family meets with a second, outer family of stable periodic orbits; the outer family, denoted as $\mathcal{P}$ in Fig. 12.8, terminates in a homoclinic bifurcation.

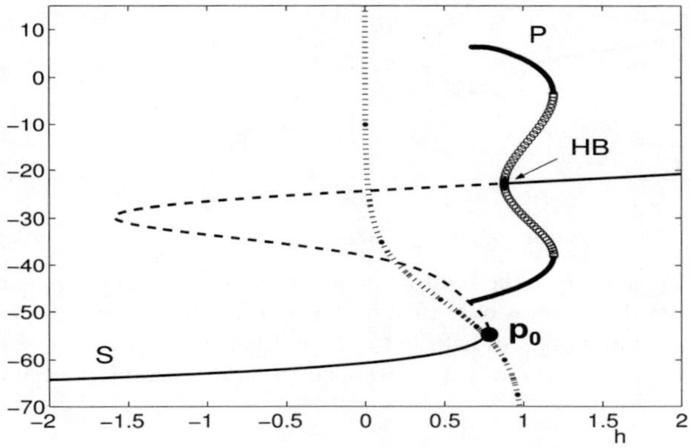

Fig. 12.8. The bifurcation diagram for the fast subsystem (1), (2) projected into (h, v)-space, along with the h-nullcline (thin dashed). The solid (dashed) curve is the curve $\mathcal{S}$ of stable (unstable) critical points of (1), (2). A family of unstable periodic orbits, labeled by open circles, emanates from $\mathcal{S}$ in a Hopf bifurcation at the point marked HB. This family coalesces with the family of stable periodic orbits $\mathcal{P}$, labeled by dark, thick curves, in a saddle-node bifurcation at h near 1.2.

The h–nullsurface is also shown in Fig. 12.8. Note that this intersects $\mathcal{S}$ at three points; these are all fixed points of the full system. The only fixed point relevant for our analysis is the one labeled p_0. When this fixed point lies along the middle branch of $\mathcal{S}$, below the homoclinic point, (1)-(3) exhibits bursting oscillations, consisting of active phases spent near $\mathcal{P}$ and silent phases spent near the lower branch of $\mathcal{S}$. If p_0 lies along the lower branch of $\mathcal{S}$, then p_0 is attracting and (1)-(3) exhibits quiescent behavior, while if p_0 lies above the homoclinic point, then we expect (1)-(3) to exhibit tonic spiking. These cases can all be realized if parameters are varied. First we first describe the effect of varying $g_{tonic-e}$ and then we consider changes in $\bar{g}_{syn-e}$.

As $g_{tonic-e}$ increases, it has three effects on the bifurcation diagram for the fast subsystem. Increasing $g_{tonic-e}$ causes the lower part of $\mathcal{S}$ to move to smaller h values, causes $\mathcal{P}$ to move to smaller h values, and causes the homoclinic point to move toward the lower knee of $\mathcal{S}$. These effects can be seen for the case of $\bar{g}_{syn-e}$=0 in Fig. 12.9(A).

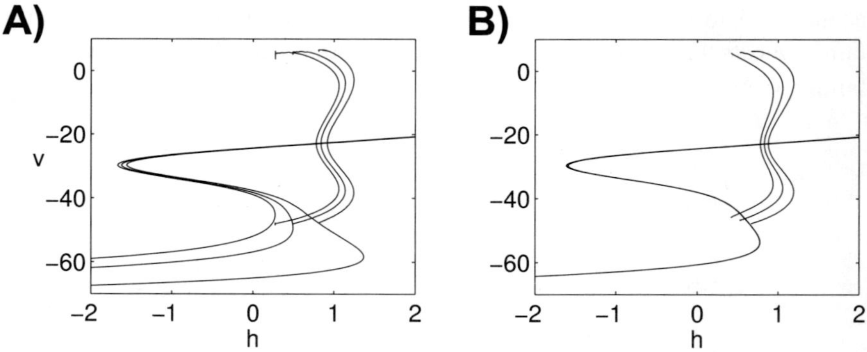

Fig. 12.9. Dependence of the bifurcation structure of (1), (2) on $g_{tonic-e}$ and $\bar{g}_{syn-e}$. The upper plots show curves of critical points and families of periodic orbits for varying values of $g_{tonic-e}$ and $\bar{g}_{syn-e}$. Left: $g_{tonic-e} = 0, 0.4, 0.7, \bar{g}_{syn-e} = 0$. Right: $g_{tonic-e} = 0.2, \bar{g}_{syn-e} = 0, 4, 8$. Larger values correspond to more leftward structures.

Examples of voltage traces derived from the evolution of equations (1)-(3), with no synaptic input, are shown in Fig. 12.10. Observe that as $g_{tonic-e}$ increases, the cell switches from quiescence to bursting to tonic spiking. In the quiescent case, the trajectory is attracted to the stable fixed point p_0 lying along the lower branch of $\mathcal{S}$ (Fig. 12.10(A)). As $g_{tonic-e}$ increases, p_0 moves to the middle branch of $\mathcal{S}$ and (1)-(3) exhibits square-wave bursting oscillations (Fig. 12.10(B), (C)). Note that for those values of $g_{tonic-e}$ for which (1)-(3) exhibits square-wave bursting, there is an interval of h-values for which the dynamics of the fast subsystem are bistable. Specifically, for each h in this range, there are a stable critical point on the lower branch of $\mathcal{S}$ and a stable periodic orbit from $\mathcal{P}$. As $g_{tonic-e}$ increases, the homoclinic point approaches the lower knee of $\mathcal{S}$ and the range of bistable h shrinks, leading to shorter bursts (Fig. 12.10(C)). For still larger values of $g_{tonic-e}$, p_0 moves past the homoclinic point along the middle branch of $\mathcal{S}$, yielding the transition to tonic spiking dynamics in (1)-(3) [42, 43]. This is evident in particular in Fig. 12.11, which shows how the h-value of p_0 switches from above that of the homoclinic point to below it, as $g_{tonic-e}$ increases. For $g_{tonic-e}$ sufficiently large, there is no region of bistability, and the trajectory is pinned in the vicinity of $\mathcal{P}$, such that tonic spiking results. This is the case shown in Fig. 12.10(D).

We now keep $g_{tonic-e}$ fixed and consider the effect of varying $\bar{g}_{syn-e}$ on the bifurcation structure of the fast subsystem. Because of the influence of equation (10), changes in $\bar{g}_{syn-e}$ are not equivalent to changes in $g_{tonic-e}$. In particular, $s = 0$ along the lower branch of the fast nullcline, while $(v - E_{syn})$ is near zero along the upper branch of the fast nullcline. Thus, increasing $\bar{g}_{syn-e}$ leaves the projection of $\mathcal{S}$ to (h, v)-space largely unchanged, as seen in Fig. 12.9(B). Increasing $\bar{g}_{syn-e}$ does cause $\mathcal{P}$ to move to smaller h values, however, which widens the range of h values for which bistability occurs in the fast subsystem.

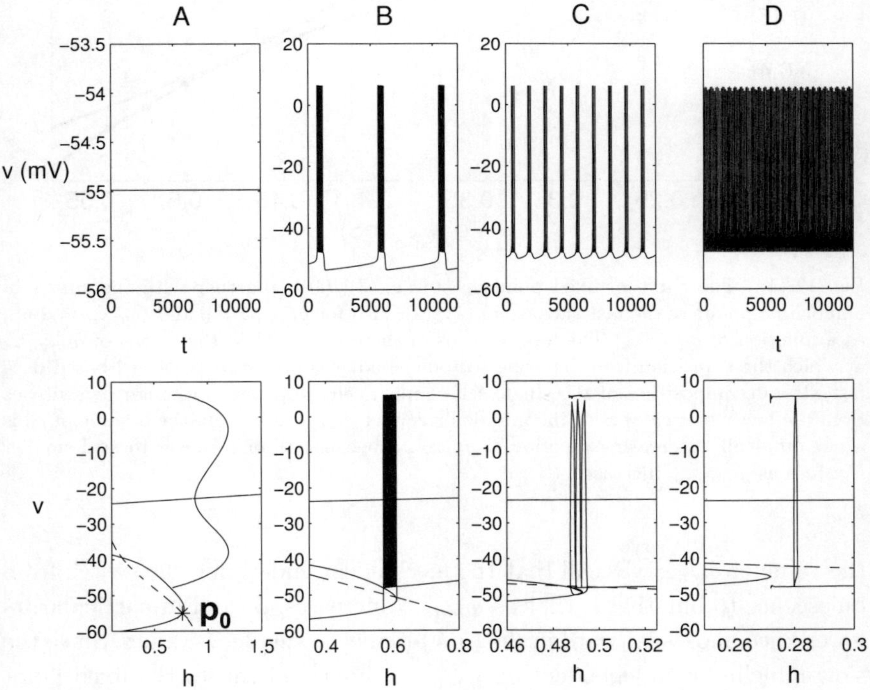

Fig. 12.10. Voltage traces (top row) and bifurcation diagrams with superimposed trajectories (bottom row). In all panels, $\bar{g}_{syn-e} = 0$. The parameter $g_{tonic-e}$ takes values (in nS) 0.2 (A - quiescence; stable critical point on the lower branch of $\mathcal{S}$ denoted by p_0), 0.3 (B - bursting), 0.4 (C - bursting), and 0.7 (D - tonic spiking). Note the different scales in each panel in the bottom row.

We note that the value of $g_{tonic-e}$ at which the switch from quiescence to bursting occurs, namely $g_{tonic-e} \approx 0.26$, depends only very weakly on

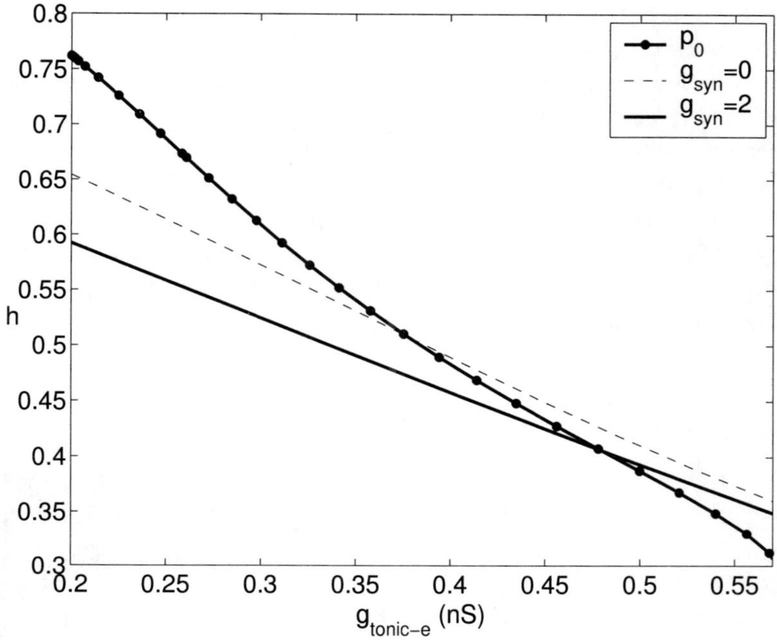

Fig. 12.11. The curve of fixed points p_0 of (1)-(3), (10), together with the curves of homoclinic points of the fast subsystem (1), (2), (10) for $\bar{g}_{syn-e} = 0$ and $\bar{g}_{syn-e} = 2$ nS, as a function of $g_{tonic-e}$. The intersections of these curves yield the values of $g_{tonic-e}$ at which the transition from bursting to tonic spiking is predicted to occur, based on a fast/slow decomposition of the single self-coupled cell. Note that although p_0 switches from the lower branch of $\mathcal{S}$ to the middle branch at $g_{tonic-e} \approx 0.26$, the h-value of p_0 is a monotonically decreasing function of $g_{tonic-e}$, because all of $\mathcal{S}$ moves toward smaller h values as $g_{tonic-e}$ increases.

the value of $\bar{g}_{syn-e}$. Recall that the mechanism underlying the switch from quiescence to bursting is that as $g_{tonic-e}$ increases, $\mathcal{S}$, and in particular its lower knee, moves leftward in the (h, v)-plane, to smaller h-values. Since the slow nullcline is independent of $g_{tonic-e}$, this trend causes the fixed point p_0 to transition from lying on the lower branch of $\mathcal{S}$ to lying on the middle branch of $\mathcal{S}$, by passing through the lower knee of $\mathcal{S}$. Bursting, rather than tonic spiking, results from the transition for the parameter values of interest due to a combination of two factors: there is always bistability between the lower branch and $\mathcal{P}$ when this transition occurs, and there is a net leftward drift in h during the active phase. This transition is relatively independent of $\bar{g}_{syn-e}$ because, as noted above, $\bar{g}_{syn-e}$ has little impact on the position of $\mathcal{S}$.

It remains to consider why the transition from bursting to tonic spiking occurs at larger $g_{tonic-e}$ for a self-coupled cell than for an uncoupled cell. As described earlier, the transition to tonic spiking takes place when the h-nullsurface crosses a homoclinic point at p_0 as $g_{tonic-e}$ is increased. As illustrated in the examples in Fig. 12.9(B) and particularly in Fig. 12.11, the homoclinic point for the self-coupled cell lies at smaller h than that for the uncoupled cell. Thus, $g_{tonic-e}$ must be increased more for the h-nullsurface to cross the curve of homoclinic points in the self-coupled case, and the transition to tonic spiking occurs at a higher value of $g_{tonic-e}$ for a self-coupled cell than for an uncoupled cell; that is, a self-coupled cell has a larger dynamic range of bursting oscillations than has an uncoupled cell. The curve of homoclinic-fixed point intersections can be plotted in $(g_{tonic-e},\bar{g}_{syn-e})$ parameter space, showing that the predicted transition value of $g_{tonic-e}$ increases as $\bar{g}_{syn-e}$ increases from 0 to about 2 nS and then decreases again as $\bar{g}_{syn-e}$ increases further, remaining above the $\bar{g}_{syn-e} = 0$ value except possibly for very large $\bar{g}_{syn-e}$ [1]. We note, however, that this single-cell analysis does not fully explain why coupling of cells increases their dynamic range of bursting activity. Indeed, the full, coupled system has a significantly larger dynamic range than that predicted by the analysis of a single, self-coupled cell. As we shall see, the reason for this is that solutions of the full system are not completely synchronized. This will be discussed, in detail, in the following sections.

12.5.2. *The transition from bursting to spiking in coupled cells with $h_1 = h_2$*

In the previous section, we assumed that the cells were completely synchronized and concluded that this does *not* accurately predict the full increase of dynamic range for the coupled system. The reason for this is that while the cells appear to burst together, their spikes fire out-of-phase. We must, therefore, extend the fast/slow analysis to the case in which we consider asynchronous spiking. This will be done in two steps. In this section, we suppose that the fast variables (v_i, n_i, s_i) for each cell $(i = 1, 2)$ are governed by equations (1), (2), (10), with $v_{pre} = v_j$ for $j = 3-i$, but we assume that the slow variables h_1 and h_2 are equal. Under this assumption, we can perform the fast/slow analysis with a single slow variable, $h = h_1 = h_2$. This simplification leads to an accurate prediction for the transition to tonic spiking for large values of $\bar{g}_{syn-e}$. Moreover, the resulting bifurcation structure has some rather novel features not seen in the analysis of the self-coupled cell. For moderate and low values of $\bar{g}_{syn-e}$, we can no longer assume that $h_1 = h_2$; these must be considered as separate slow variables. The two slow-variable analysis will be carried out in section 12.5.3.

Consider two sets of equations (1), (2), (10), indexed by $i = 1$ and $i = 2$, with $h_1 = h_2 \equiv h$ assumed to be a single slow variable in these equations. Figure 12.12(A) shows an example of the associated bifurcation diagram for h treated as a bifurcation parameter in (1), (2), (10) with $i = 1, 2$, which we henceforth refer to as the fast subsystem. This diagram is projected onto the (h, v_1)-plane. There is a family of periodic orbits that emanates from the curve of equilibria $\mathcal{S}$ at a subcritical Hopf bifurcation. This family corresponds to anti-phase oscillations. We note that there are one or more additional branches of periodic orbits that emanate from S at additional Hopf points. These other periodic orbit families correspond to in-phase oscillations; these are unstable with respect to the fast subsystem and are not shown in Fig. 12.12. A similar splitting into anti-phase and in-phase families of periodic orbits is seen when diffusive coupling is introduced between square-wave bursters derived from a model for bursting in pancreatic β-cells [6, 36].

The family of antiphase periodics consists of three branches. The branch that emanates from the subcritical Hopf consists of unstable limit cycles. This branch terminates at a saddle-node of periodic orbits where it coalesces with a second branch of *stable* periodic orbits. This second branch will be very important in the analysis and we label it as $\mathcal{AP}$. This branch terminates in another saddle-node bifurcation of periodic orbits where it coalesces with a third family of unstable periodics. The third family terminates in an orbit homoclinic to the middle branch of $\mathcal{S}$.

Figure 12.12(B) shows the projection of the corresponding bursting solution to the full two-cell system onto this bifurcation diagram. As usual, the silent phase lies along the lower branch of $\mathcal{S}$ and the active spiking phase begins when the trajectory reaches the lower knee of $\mathcal{S}$. During the active phase, the trajectory lies close to $\mathcal{AP}$ and the active phase ends when the trajectory reaches the saddle-node of periodics. Note that this bifurcation structure no longer corresponds to square-wave bursting, where spiking ends at a homoclinic orbit, but rather represents a different bursting class [16, 37] which we refer to as *top hat bursting*. We have, therefore, demonstrated the rather surprising result that coupling of cells leads to a change in the class of bursting activity (see also [6]). As we demonstrate below, this will partially explain why the coupled system has an increased dynamic range.

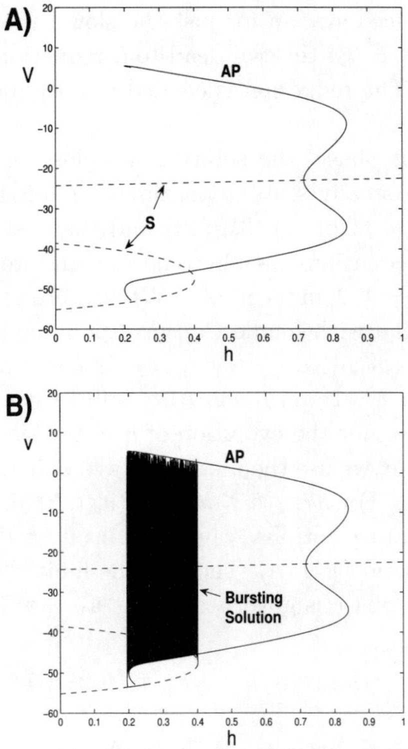

Fig. 12.12. Bifurcation structure of the fast subsystem. Here, $h = h_1 = h_2$ is the bifurcation parameter. A branch of antiphase periodic orbits, labeled $\mathcal{AP}$, emanates from $\mathcal{S}$, the curve of fixed points. The projection of the bursting solution onto this plane is shown in the right panel.

Top hat bursters have several important features that distinguish them from square-wave bursters. The active phase of a square-wave bursters ends at a homoclinic orbit. For this reason, the spike frequency becomes small at the end of each burst. For top hat bursters, the active phase ends at a saddle-node of limit cycles. Hence, the spike frequency approaches some fixed value, bounded away from zero, at the termination of burst activity.

A second difference between square-wave and top hat bursting is related to the transition to tonic spiking as a parameter, such as $g_{tonic-e}$, is varied. Recall that for a square-wave burster, this transition takes place as the homoclinic point crosses the slow nullsurface. For top hat bursters, this transition arises from a very different mechanism. To understand this new mechanism, we use singular perturbation methods to reduce the full system of equations to a reduced system for just the slow variables. Since we are now assuming that $h_1 = h_2$, this will lead to a reduction of the full model to a single equation. The reduction is carried out separately for the silent and active phases.

While in the silent phase, the solution lies close to the lower branch of $\mathcal{S}$ and we invoke a steady state approximation. That is, introduce the slow time variable $\tau = \varepsilon t$ in (1)-(3), (10) and then set $\varepsilon = 0$. The right hand sides of the fast equations then become zero and we may solve for fast variables (v_i, n_i, s_i), $i = 1, 2$, in terms of h. While there are multiple possible solutions, we choose that with smallest v, corresponding to the silent phase, and of course we find $(v_1, n_1, s_1) = (v_2, n_2, s_2)$ since we assume the same h value when solving for $i = 1$ and $i = 2$. After substituting this into (3), we obtain a single equation for the evolution of h in the silent phase.

For the active phase, we use the method of averaging. Suppose that $\mathcal{AP}$ exists for $h_L \leq h \leq h_R$. For $h_L \leq h \leq h_R$, let $(v_i(t,h), n_i(t,h), s_i(t,h)), i = 1, 2$, be the corresponding antiphase periodic orbit of the fast subsystem and assume that its period is $T(h)$. Then, in the limit $\varepsilon \to 0$, the evolution of h during the active phase is governed by the averaged equation

$$\dot{h} = \frac{1}{T(h)} \int_0^{T(h)} (h_\infty(v_i(t,h)) - h)/\tau_h(v_i(t,h))dt \equiv a(h). \tag{11}$$

Here, differentiation is respect to τ. We may choose v_1 or v_2, since we are assuming that $h_1 = h_2$ and we are therefore integrating over a common periodic orbit for $i = 1$ and $i = 2$ (although the cells may be out-of-phase along the orbit).

Now the system exhibits bursting if $a(h) < 0$ for all $h \in (h_L, h_R)$. In this case, the solution drifts to the left while oscillating along $\mathcal{AP}$. Tonic spiking, on the other hand, corresponds to a stable fixed point of (11). Such a fixed point will exist if $a(h_L) > 0 > a(h_R)$; that is, solutions drift to the left for h near h_R and solutions drift to the right near h_R. We therefore expect that the transition from bursting to tonic spiking takes place when $a(h_L) = 0$. Recall that h_L corresponds to the saddle-node of periodic orbits as shown in Fig. 12.12(A).

We have numerically computed the values of $(g_{tonic-e}, \bar{g}_{syn-e})$ where $a(h_L) = 0$ [1]. This generates a curve that accurately predicts the transition from bursting to tonic spiking for large values of $\bar{g}_{syn-e}$. For small and moderate values of $\bar{g}_{syn-e}$, this curve does not match the actual transition; it severely underestimates the increase in dynamic range of bursting activity. The reason for this discrepancy is that for small and moderate values of $\bar{g}_{syn-e}$, it is incorrect to assume that $h_1 = h_2$. We must, therefore, extend our fast/slow analysis to the case of two slow variables.

12.5.3. *The transition from bursting to tonic spiking in the full model for two coupled cells*

The previous subsections demonstrate that to capture the full picture of the dynamic range of bursting for two coupled pre-BötC cells, it is necessary to consider the full four-equation model (1)-(3), (10) for each cell. Again, there is a natural fast-slow decomposition, achieved by taking h_1, h_2 as slow variables; below, we refer to the *fast subsystem* to mean the other six equations with h_1, h_2 frozen. Rather than visualizing fast subsystem bifurcation structures, we will now consider dynamics projected to the (h_1, h_2)-plane.

To start, fix $(g_{tonic-e}, \bar{g}_{syn-e})$ and note that for some pairs (h_1, h_2), the fast subsystem will support sustained oscillations, while for others, stable oscillations will not exist. We can use direct simulation of the fast subsystem (e.g., fixing h_2, varying h_1 systematically, and then repeating for a different h_2), to estimate a boundary curve for the *oscillation region* $\mathcal{O}$ in (h_1, h_2)-space, such that for (h_1, h_2) values below this curve, stable oscillations do not exist for the fast subsystem.

We use averaging to reduce the full system to a system of two equations for just the slow variables. The reduced system can be written as

$$\begin{aligned} \dot{h_1} &= \tfrac{1}{T(h_1,h_2)} \int_0^{T(h_1,h_2)} g(v_{1_p}(h_1, h_2; t), h_1)\, dt \ \equiv a_1(h_1, h_2), \\ \dot{h_2} &= \tfrac{1}{T(h_1,h_2)} \int_0^{T(h_1,h_2)} g(v_{2_p}(h_1, h_2; t), h_2)\, dt \ \equiv a_2(h_1, h_2) \end{aligned} \tag{12}$$

where $(h_1, h_2) \in \mathcal{O}$, $T(h_1, h_2)$ is the period of the fast subsystem periodic orbit for this choice of (h_1, h_2), and v_{1_p}, v_{2_p} are the time courses of v_1, v_2 around the orbit, which both depend on both h_1 and h_2, since the orbit itself does. Note that tonic spiking corresponds to a stable fixed point of (12) in $\mathcal{O}$. In fact, the complete transition from bursting to tonic spiking for the full system can be understood by analyzing the phase planes generated by (12) [1].

For the purposes of exposition, we fix $\bar{g}_{syn-e} = 3$ and consider the phase plane of (12) for increasing values of $g_{tonic-e}$. If $g_{tonic-e} = .57$ nS, as in Fig. 12.13(A), then there are no fixed points of (12) in $\mathcal{O}$ and in fact every solution of the slow averaged equations (12) eventually leaves $\mathcal{O}$, such that the full system exhibits bursting. The termination of the active phase of bursting corresponds to when the solution of the slow equations (12) crosses the boundary of $\mathcal{O}$, and hence we refer to the boundary of $\mathcal{O}$ as the jump-down curve (Fig. 12.13).

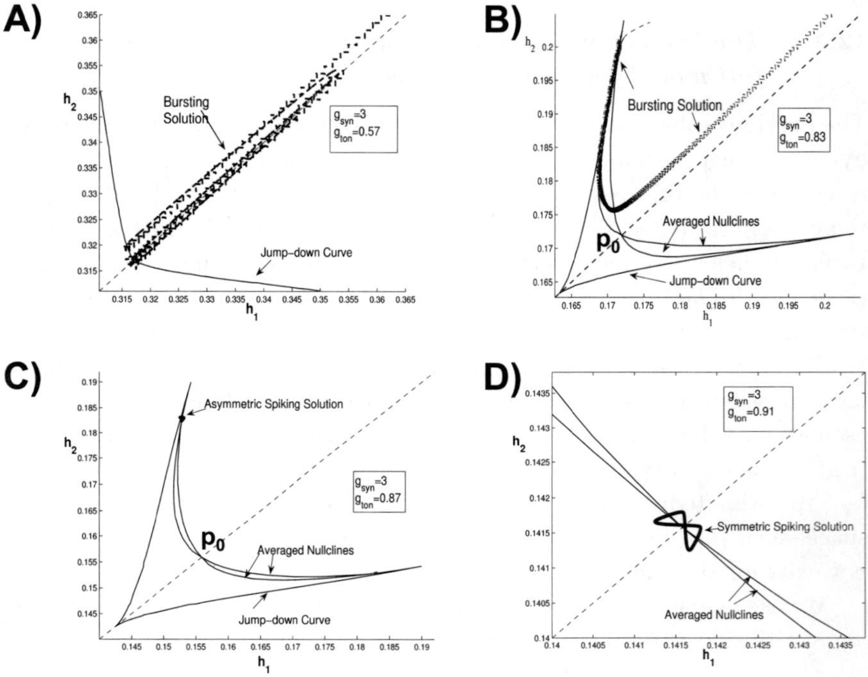

Fig. 12.13. Averaged phase planes. A) Every solution of the averaged equations leaves the oscillatory region through the jump-down curve and the system exhibits symmetric bursting. B) There is an unstable fixed point p_0 where the averaged nullclines intersect. The system exhibits asymmetric bursting. C) The averaged nullclines intersect at three fixed points, two of which are stable (while p_0 is unstable). The system exhibits asymmetric tonic spiking. D) p_0 is now a stable fixed point and the system exhibits symmetric spiking.

Next, suppose that $g_{tonic-e} = .83$ nS. Then the full system still exhibits bursting; however, the slow system (12) now has a fixed point, which will be referred to as p_0, in $\mathcal{O}$. This corresponds to (unstable) tonic spiking. To better understand the phase space of (12), we have numerically computed the averaged nullclines, $\mathcal{A}_1 = \{(h_1, h_2) : a_1(h_1, h_2) = 0\}$ and $\mathcal{A}_2 = \{(h_1, h_2) : a_2(h_1, h_2) = 0\}$. Note in Fig. 12.13(B) that these nullclines intersect at the fixed point p_0. From the configuration of these nullclines, we find that p_0 is an unstable saddle and the tonic spiking solution of the full system is unstable. By symmetry, the stable manifold of p_0 is precisely the line $\mathcal{L} \equiv \{(h_1, h_2) : h_1 = h_2\}$. Since (12) does not have any stable fixed points, every solution of (12) not lying on $\mathcal{L}$ must eventually leave $\mathcal{O}$, and bursting results. We note that if we had only considered solutions of (1), (2), (10) with $i = 1, 2$ and with $h_1 = h_2$, then we would have predicted that tonic spiking would occur here. That is, p_0 is stable if we restrict ourselves to solutions of (1), (2), (10), $i = 1, 2$, that lie on $\mathcal{L}$. This explains why the analysis in the preceding section did not accurately predict the full dynamic range of rhythmic bursting oscillations for low/moderate values of $\bar{g}_{syn-e}$.

Next suppose that $g_{tonic-e} = .87$ nS and consider the slow averaged phase plane shown in Fig. 12.13(C). There is still a fixed point p_0 along $\mathcal{L}$ that is an unstable saddle. However, the averaged nullclines $\mathcal{A}_1$ and $\mathcal{A}_2$ now intersect at two new fixed points in the oscillatory region $\mathcal{O}$. These are stable fixed points, as can be seen from the configuration of the nullclines, and the full system exhibits (stable) tonic spiking. We say that the tonic spiking is asymmetric because $h_1 \neq h_2$ at the stable fixed points.

Finally, suppose that $g_{tonic-e} = .91$ nS. In this case, p_0 is a stable fixed point of (12) and the full system exhibits symmetric tonic spiking. As we increase $g_{tonic-e}$ from .87 nS to .91 nS, there is a pitchfork bifurcation in which the stable asymmetric fixed points come together at p_0. At this bifurcation point, p_0 switches from a saddle to a stable node, and the full system switches from exhibiting asymmetric spiking to exhibiting symmetric spiking.

In summary, as $g_{tonic-e}$ is increased for $\bar{g}_{syn-e} = 3$, our fast/slow analysis predicts a transition from quiescence sequentially through symmetric bursting, asymmetric bursting, asymmetric spiking, and finally symmetric spiking, based on changes induced in the average nullclines $\mathcal{A}_1$, $\mathcal{A}_2$ of system (12). Further details on transitions between activity modes, how they vary with $\bar{g}_{syn-e}$, and their implications for burst frequency and other burst characteristics are presented elsewhere [1].

12.6. Effects of Heterogeneity

12.6.1. *Motivation and introduction to modeling approach*

An important point raised and explored by Butera *et al.* [3] is that synchronized bursting of pre-BötC cells is actually enhanced by heterogeneities in intrinsic cellular parameters and in coupling strengths within the population. That is, within the pre-BötC, when coupling among cells is blocked, there are silent cells, cells that spike repeatedly, and intrinsically bursting cells (Fig. 12.6(A1)), although cells in all groups seem to be capable of bursting if given appropriate inputs. Further, burst frequencies vary across bursting cells. With sufficiently strong coupling, however, this intrinsically heterogeneous population engages in bursting oscillations that may be characterized as synchronized. More precisely, recruitment of cells into the active phase may be somewhat gradual, but all cells do enter the active phase during each cycle and they exit the active phase together (Fig. 12.6(B1)). This robustness of oscillatory behavior in the presence of network heterogeneities would certainly represent an attractive property for any network serving as a rhythmic pacemaker.

In section 12.4, we saw that for a simulated network of Model I pre-BötC cells, with heterogeneity in $\bar{g}_{syn-e}$, $\bar{g}_{NaP}$, and/or E_L, the range of $g_{tonic-e}$ over which the full population engages in bursts is broader than that for a homogeneous network, with a wider range of burst frequencies achieved. The predominant effect of the introduction of heterogeneity is that it allows bursting to occur for much smaller levels of $g_{tonic-e}$ than it would occur at without heterogeneity (Fig. 12.7).

We have mathematically analyzed several aspects of bursting in a heterogeneous network of Model I pre-BötC cells [32]. We simplified the cells in the model network by omitting the spike-generating currents I_{Na} and I_K, and hence the variable n, from system (1)-(3). With this modification, the dynamics of each uncoupled cell can be represented in a 2-dimensional phase plane, corresponding to v and h; the specific model studied is presented in subsection 12.6.3. With N cells in a network, the overall phase space is $2N$-dimensional. However, an idea that is useful for a network of identical cells is to consider each cell as a different particle in the same 2-d phase plane, rather than attempting to analyze a flow in a $2N$-d space. Synaptic coupling does introduce a third variable for each cell, yet we can still project dynamics to the 2-d (v, h)-phase plane as long as we keep track of how the evolution of synaptic inputs to each cell modulates its trajectory. Recent work, including our study of the pre-BötC network, has extended this approach to a heterogeneous population [31, 32, 44]. Before considering a large population in subsection 12.6.3, however, we present a relevant mechanism in a two-cell network in subsection 12.6.2.

12.6.2. *The role of fast threshold modulation*

Using the approach described above, one can show that, assuming that v is a fast variable and h is a slow variable and considering the singular limit, a pair of identical cells coupled by synaptic excitation can stably synchronize through an effect known as *fast threshold modulation* (FTM) [40, 44]. This mechanism can work whether the cells are oscillatory or excitable (i.e., with a stable critical point on the left branch of the v-nullcline), under appropriate conditions. To consider the key to FTM in brief, assume that the onset of synaptic excitation is instantaneous and that the cells are oscillatory, with

$$\begin{aligned} v_i' &= F(v_i, h_i, \sigma_i) \equiv f(v_i, h_i) - g_{syn}\sigma_i(v - v_{syn}) \\ h_i' &= \varepsilon g(v_i, h_i) \\ s_i' &= \alpha H(v_j - \theta_s)(1 - s_i) - \beta s_i,\ j \neq i \end{aligned} \tag{13}$$

for $i = 1, 2$, where $0 < \varepsilon \ll 1$, $H(x)$ is the Heaviside step function, and σ_i can be either s_i or $s_1 + s_2$. Let $\mathcal{N}_v(\sigma)$ denote the family of v-nullclines for a cell, parameterized by σ, each of which is assumed to be cubic, with $F(v, h, \sigma) < 0$ (> 0) below (above) $\mathcal{N}_v(\sigma)$. Select θ_s to lie at a value intersected by the middle branches of the relevant v-nullclines. For excitatory coupling, we have $v - v_{syn} < 0$, so increases in σ_i lower the v-nullcline; see Fig. 12.14. Let $(v_{LK}(\sigma), h_{LK}(\sigma))$ denote the curve of left knees of $\mathcal{N}_v(\sigma)$, and assume that $\mathcal{N}_v(0)$ intersects $\{(v, h) : g(v, h) = 0\}$ in one point on the middle branch of $\mathcal{N}_v(0)$, such that both cells are oscillatory without coupling. Singular solutions to (13) consist of trajectories on the left (silent phase) and right (active phase) branches of members of $\mathcal{N}_v(\sigma)$, which evolve on the slow timescale $\tau = \varepsilon t$, connected by fast jumps between branches. Moreover, in the singular limit, each cell jumps up to the active phase when it reaches the left knee of any cubic. For concreteness, suppose that cell 1 reaches $(v_{LK}(0), h_{LK}(0))$ at a time at which cell 2 lies on the left branch of $\mathcal{N}_v(0)$. Then v_1 jumps up and crosses θ_s, and s_2 jumps to $\sigma_{max} := \alpha/(\alpha+\beta)$, instantaneously with respect to τ. The relevant nullcline for cell 2 therefore becomes $\mathcal{N}_v(\sigma_{max})$, and if $h_2 > h_{LK}(\sigma_{max})$, then cell 2 will instantaneously join cell 1 in the active phase, as shown in Fig. 12.14.

With heterogeneity between the cells, a similar effect can occur. For example, if one cell is oscillatory and the other is excitable, then the jump-up of the oscillatory cell can pull the excitable cell into the active phase as well via FTM. In fact, this is the essence of how heterogeneities extend the bursting range to lower values of $g_{tonic-e}$: at small values of $g_{tonic-e}$, for which typical cells will be quiescent, some cells with parameters away from the mean will still be able to fire intrinsically, and these will recruit the silent cells. With just two heterogeneous 2-dimensional model cells, one can

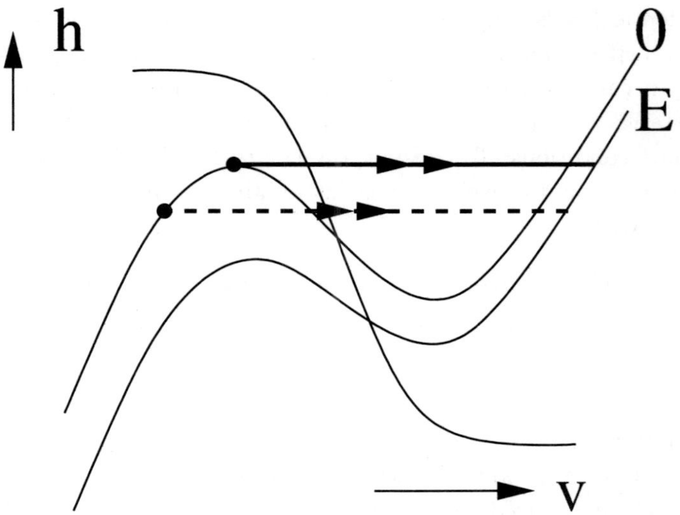

Fig. 12.14. Instantaneous onset of synaptic excitation can pull a cell up to the active phase, in the singular limit. The v-nullcline labelled '0' corresponds to $\sigma = 0$ and the v-nullcline labelled 'E' corrsponds to $\sigma = \sigma_{max}$; the other solid curve is the h-nullcline. The solid circles show the initial positions of two identical cells. The upper cell jumps up to the active phase, and due to instantaneous synaptic excitation, the lower cell immediately follows via FTM. In this case both cells are oscillatory, but a similar result occurs if one cell is excitable.

still visualize them both as diferent points in the same phase plane, each with its own set of nullclines, even when both receive the same inputs. For the complete version of Model I, a similar idea applies. As seen in the previous section (Fig. 12.9(A)), as $g_{tonic-e}$ is lowered, for a fixed set of intrinsic parameter values, the family $\mathcal{S}$ of critical points of the fast subsystem (1), (2) moves rightward in the (h, v)-plane. Since the slow h-nullcline is independent of $g_{tonic-e}$ this causes the lowest-v intersection of the nullclines to pass through the lower knee of $\mathcal{S}$ to the lowest branch of $\mathcal{S}$, becoming stable via a Hopf bifurcation for the full system. With heterogeneity, this bifurcation occurs at different $g_{tonic-e}$ for different cells. The mechanism by which heterogeneities extend the bursting range of $g_{tonic-e}$ to smaller values is that cells that are still above their bifurcations, and thus able to oscillate, are able to pull up silent cells to the active phase via synaptic coupling through a generalized form of FTM.

An example of this effect is illustrated in Fig. 12.15. To generate this figure, we simulated a network of two Model I pre-BötC cells with $g_{tonic-e} = 0.24$, cell 1 with $I_{app} = 0$ and cell 2 with I_{app}=5 pA. When the two were uncoupled, cell 1 was silent, while cell 2 bursted periodically (Fig. 12.15(A)). When $\bar{g}_{syn-e}$ was increased from 0 to 4 nS, the cells bursted synchronously (Fig. 12.15(B)). Figure 12.15(C) shows the bifurcation diagram for cell 1, similar to those in the previous section, with the S-shaped curves of critical points and emanating families of periodic orbits for $\bar{g}_{syn-e}$= 0 and $\bar{g}_{syn-e}s$ = 0.68. Note that the case of $\bar{g}_{syn-e}s$ = 0.68 here is different from that of the single self-coupled cell, since $\bar{g}_{syn-e}s$ here is held constant, independent of v. The value 0.68 is chosen since the maximal value of the synaptic input variable s generated by the bursting oscillations of cell 2 with $\bar{g}_{syn-e}$ = 4 nS was observed numerically to be approximately 0.17. The introduction of synaptic input from cell 2 to cell 1 shifts the critical point curve for cell 1 leftward, enabling cell 1 to jump up to the active phase via FTM, as evident in the superimposed trajectory from cell 1 in the coupled simulation, also shown in Fig. 12.15(C). In the next section, we discuss a more detailed analysis of conditions under which synchronized bursting will occur, and of how cells behave in synchronized bursting solutions, using a larger heterogeneous population of reduced model pre-BötC cells.

12.6.3. *Analysis of a synchronized bursting in a heterogeneous population*

To address mathematically the complication of heterogeneities in a population of cells, we introduced the idea of the *curve of effective knees* [32]. This idea allows us to continue to visualize the dynamics of a population of cells and analyze their behavior using a two-dimensional phase plane. For a single cell within a network, consider the reduced model

$$\begin{aligned} C_m v' &= g_{NaP-h} m_\infty(v) h(v - E_{Na}) - g_L(v - E_L) - I_{syn} + I_{app} \\ h' &= (h_\infty(v) - h)/\tau_h(v), \end{aligned} \tag{14}$$

where h_∞, m_∞ are monotone decreasing and increasing sigmoidal functions, respectively. This model is derived by blocking the sodium and potassium spiking currents from Model I [2, 3, 32]. In the first equation in (14), $I_{syn} = g_{syn} s_{tot}(v - E_{syn})$ and I_{app} denote input currents. Note that s_{tot} denotes the total synaptic input to the cell, which is excitatory here ($v < E_{syn}$ for all relevant v). Also, we use the constant I_{app} as a simplified representation for $I_{tonic-e}$ for convenience; a single cell will oscillate if I_{app} is sufficiently large and otherwise will be excitable, remaining silent without additional inputs. The second equation in (14) describes the slow inactivation of the persistent sodium current. For biophysically relevant parameter values, (14)

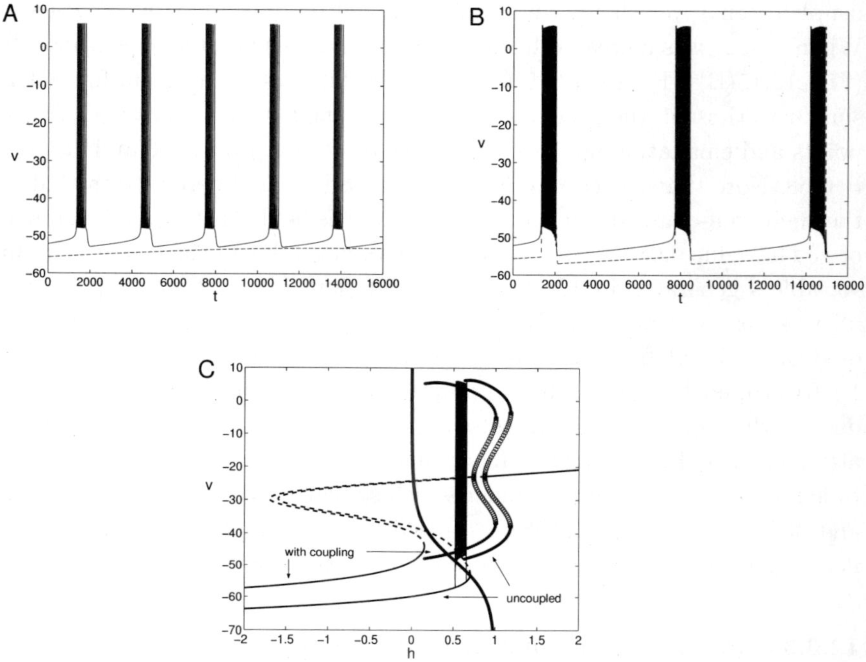

Fig. 12.15. (A) Time courses of two uncoupled pre-BötC cells, with $I_{app} = 5$ pA (solid) and $I_{app} = 0$ pA (dashed). Over much longer simulations, the latter cell remains silent (not shown here). (B) Time courses of the same two cells, with $\bar{g}_{syn-e} = 4$ nS introduced, showing synchronized bursting. (C) Bifurcation diagram for the cell with $I_{app} = 0$, for the uncoupled and coupled cases, with the trajectory of a burst from (B) superimposed. Note that the synaptic coupling shifts the structures in the diagram to the left (in fact, for $\bar{g}_{syn-e} = 4$ nS, p_0 no longer exists).

can be considered as singularly perturbed, since h evolves much more slowly than v.

Importantly, we assume all-to-all coupling. Thus, for a discrete population of N cells, each characterized by variables (v_i, h_i) governed by (14), $s_{tot} = g_{syn} \sum_{k=1}^{N} s_\infty(v_k)/N$, where we take $s_\infty(v) = 1/(1+\exp((v-\theta_s)/\sigma_s))$ for threshold parameter θ_s and slope parameter σ_s, corresponding to instantaneous synaptic dynamics. For purposes of analysis, we also consider the continuum limit of infinitely many cells on a spatially continuous domain, say $D \subset \mathbb{R}^3$. In this case, the dependent variables from (14) become $v(x,t)$ and $h(x,t)$, with $x \in D$, and $I_{syn} = I_{syn}(x,t)$ for $s_{tot}(x,t) = (g_{syn}/Vol) \int_D s_\infty(v(x,t))\, dx$, with $Vol = \int_D dx$.

Butera *et al.* [3] considered heterogeneity in $\bar{g}_{syn-e}$, $\bar{g}_{NaP}$, and E_L. For simplicity, we focus on E_L. Note that $-g_L(v-E_L) = \tilde{I} - g_L v$ for $\tilde{I} = g_L E_L$. Let $I = I_{app} + \tilde{I}$, which we define as the heterogeneity parameter. Rewrite (14) as

$$\begin{aligned} v' &= f(v,h) + I - I_{syn} \\ h' &= \varepsilon g(v,h), \end{aligned} \tag{15}$$

where we have factored out a small, positive parameter ε from the h-equation as in equation (3) and where I_{syn} is defined as above. In this notation, the v-nullclines, which we assume maintain a cubic shape for all I of interest, are the solutions to

$$f(v,h) + I - I_{syn} = 0, \tag{16}$$

parametrized by I. As previously, increasing I_{syn} or I will lower the v-nullcline; see Figs. 12.16(A) and 12.16(B). The dependence on I_{app} noted in (14) carries over to a similar dependence on I in (15); in particular, Fig. 12.16 shows that the dynamics of (15) are excitable for $I = I_1$ and oscillatory for $I = I_2 > I_1$. As in section 12.5, to work in the singular limit, we define a slow flow

$$\dot{h} = g(v,h) \tag{17}$$

with differentiation with respect to $\tau = \varepsilon t$, where $v = v(h)$ in equation (17) solves (16). In the singular limit, solutions are concatenations of trajectories of (17) that follow the left ($v = v_L(h)$) and right ($v = v_R(h)$) branches of the v-nullcline, respectively, together with fast jumps between the branches, governed by the v-equation of (15) with h constant. These jumps take place at the knees of the v-nullclines. In addition to equation (16), the left knees $(v_{LK}(I), h_{LK}(I))$ of these nullclines, at which jumps up occur, also satisfy $\partial(f - I_{syn})/\partial v = 0$.

Now, consider a continuous population of cells with each value $I(x)$ drawn from some distribution on the interval $[I_{min}, I_{max}]$, such that cells are excitable if $I < I_c$ and oscillatory if $I > I_c$ for some $I_c \in [I_{min}, I_{max}]$. Assume that all cells with the same I-value are synchronized, which allows us to characterize cells by $(v(I,t), h(I,t))$, rather than $(v(x,t), h(x,t))$. Suppose that cells with $I = I_{max}$ jump up at some time t^{up}. This may induce other cells to jump up at that same moment as well, if the coupling strength is strong enough and the cells are appropriately positioned in phase space. Assume that any other cells that jump up do so in order of decreasing I and consider a cell with $I = I^* \in [I_{min}, I_{max})$. This cell will jump up instantaneously if and only if its h-value lies above the

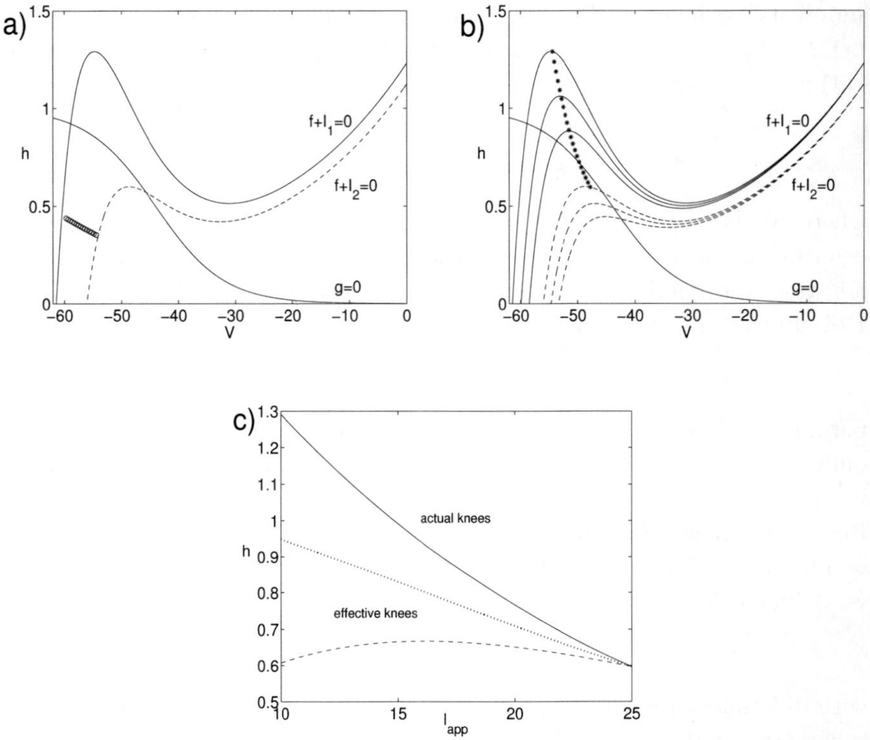

Fig. 12.16. Nullclines for (14) in the (v, h)-phase plane, generated numerically with XPPAUT [10]. (a) Increasing $I > 0$ (from $I_1 = 10$ pA to $I_2 = 25$ pA) lowers the v-nullcline (here $I_{syn} = 0$). Cells with a range of I values can all be visualized in the same phase plane; an example representing the position of 15 cells is shown by the thick curve. Note that cells with $I = I_1$ are excitable while those with $I = I_2$ are oscillatory. (b) Excitatory synaptic inputs further lower nullclines for $v < E_{syn}$, as shown here for 3 different levels of $g_{syn}s_{tot}$ for each of $I = I_1$ (solid) and $I = I_2$ (dashed). The dark dotted curve gives a numerical approximation to the left curve of knees for $I_{syn} = 0$ and for I ranging in discrete steps from I_1 up to I_2. (c) Uncoupled and effective left knees. The solid curve shows the left knee curve from part (b), corresponding to the absence of synaptic coupling. The other curves show *effective knees* computed numerically for $g_{syn}/N = .005$ nS (dotted) and $g_{syn}/N = .01$ nS (dashed) with I_{syn} computed by assuming that cells jump up to the active phase in order of decreasing I. Larger g_{syn} lowers the effective knees, promoting synchrony. This figure has been published previously, together with relevant animated simulations [32].

left knee of the appropriate nullcline, which we call the *effective left knee.* The relevant nullcline is the solution to equation (16) with $I = I^*$ and with $I_{syn} = I_{syn}^{up}(v, I^*)$, defined to be the amount of synaptic input generated when exactly those cells with $I > I^*$ lie in the active phase. In the continuum limit, this corresponds to $v(I,t) > \theta_s$ if and only if $I > I^*$, with $I^{up}_{syn}(v, I^*) = (g_{syn}/Vol)(v - v_{syn})\mu\{x : I(x) > I^*\}$, where μ denotes Lebesgue measure. Finally, the *effective left knee* for $I = I^*$ is obtained by solving $\partial(f - I^{up}_{syn}(v, I^*))/\partial v = 0$ simultaneously with (16); we denote this by $(v^{eff}_{LK}(I^*), h^{eff}_{LK}(I^*))$.

Proceeding as above, we can define $I^{up}_{syn}(v, I)$ for each $I \in [I_{min}, I_{max}]$, with a corresponding v-nullcline satisfying $f(v,h) + I - I^{up}_{syn}(v, I) = 0$ and having a left knee $(v^{eff}_{LK}(I), h^{eff}_{LK}(I))$. Examples are illustrated in Fig. 12.16(C). With this notation, the condition for the full population to jump up together becomes $h(I,t) > h^{eff}_{LK}(I)$ for all $I \in [I_{min}, I_{max})$, at the time t^{up} when cells with $I = I_{max}$ jump up. Animated simulations showing examples of population behavior, together with relevant curves of left and right knees, can be viewed online [32].

We have derived consistency conditions under which synchronized, full-population oscillations will occur [32]. Different conditions are derived from different assumptions. If we assume that all cells jump up and jump down at the same moment (*full synchrony*) and simplify the h-dynamics somewhat, then the relevant consistency conditions yield a functional map, which can be solved for a unique linear fixed point curve $h_{FP}(I) = h_{LK}(I_{max}) + \alpha(I_{max} - I)$ for $I \in [I_{min}, I_{max}]$. Here, $\alpha > 0$ is directly related to the parameters in (14). The fixed point curve represents an initial configuration of a continuum of reduced model pre-BötC cells, with I_{max} cells located at the jump-up point (that is, $h_{FP}(I_{max}) = h_{LK}(I_{max})$) and all other cells in the silent phase, from which the population will display periodic bursting oscillations with fully synchronized jumps. Importantly, the fixed point is shown to be stable within the class of linear functions, and more technical conditions for stability to arbitrary perturbations, based on a contraction argument and stated in terms of parameters in (14), can be derived [32]. Finally, consistency conditions that ensure that jumps are fully synchronized and are led by cells with $I = I_{max}$, also stated in terms of model parameters, can be obtained as well [32]. Not surprisingly, large g_{syn} promotes this strong synchrony, while a steep curve of left knees ensures that I_{max} cells lead the jump up.

While sufficiently strong synaptic coupling promotes fully synchronized jumps, it is more biologically relevant to consider weaker coupling, for which all cells jump up on each cycle, but their jump times differ (Fig. 12.6(B)). In this situation, let $h(I, \tau)$ denote a curve, parameterized by I, specifying cell positions at the slow time $\tau = \varepsilon t$. The approximate initial configuration $h_0(I) \equiv h(I, 0)$, corresponding to a periodic, synchronized solution at the moment when all cells jump down, can be obtained as the solution of a nonlinear boundary value problem. This boundary value problem can be obtained by deriving a system of three equations for the three unknown functions $h_0(I)$, $h_\mu(I) \equiv h(I, T_S)$, and $\Delta(I)$, where T_S is the minimum positive time (again on the slow timescale) at which cells with $I = I_{max}$ jump up and $\Delta(I)$ for each I is the slow timescale delay from time T_S to the times when cells with that I-value jump up (in particular, $\Delta(I_{max}) = 0$). The first equation in this system relates $h_0(I)$ and $h_\mu(I)$ based on the fact that in time T_S, $h_0(I)$ evolves to $h_\mu(I)$. The second equation comes from the evolution of $h_\mu(I)$ to its jump-up position in the additional time $\Delta(I)$ for each I. This involves an integral, because cells with different I values are in the active phase at different times between T_S and $\Delta(I_{min})$; thus, the system of three equations is nonlocal. Note that in the notation introduced above, the condition for jump up is $h(\Delta(I)) = h_{LK}^{eff}(I)$. The third equation comes from noting that, assuming a completely synchronized jump down, cells evolve from $h_{LK}^{eff}(I)$ to $h_0(I)$ in time $T_A - \Delta(I)$, where T_A is the time spent in the active phase by cells with $I = I_{max}$, which can be approximated. Finally, the boundary condition is given by $h_0(I_{max}) = h_{RK}(I_{max})$. This system, although complicated, can be solved numerically using XPPAUT [10] for a periodic, synchronized solution with gradual jumps up, after some manipulation [32]. Further, a similar approach applies with gradual jumps down in addition to gradual jumps up, although that case may be biologically less relevant.

12.7. Contemporary Issues and Unresolved Problems

The excitatory pre-BötC network has rich dynamics that arise from interactions of intrinsic cellular properties, synaptic coupling, and heterogeneities of bursting behavior. There are many opportunities for extending the modeling and analyses at both single neuron and network levels, several of which are highlighted here along with our current perspectives on the major issues addressed in the chapter.

12.7.1. *Single neuron properties and models*

At the single cell level, we have used biophysically minimal, conductance-based models with subthreshold burst-generating currents represented by I_{NaP} and I_L. High voltage-activated, spike-generating currents are represented by I_{Na} and I_K. These initial model formulations were reinforced by the experimentally observed current-voltage profile of pre-BötC neurons, indicating that this reduced formulation is a useful approximation. Model I can in fact reproduce main features of the voltage-dependent bursting behavior observed experimentally, and heterogeneous networks of Model I neurons replicate data on pre-BötC network behavior [7]. A particularly interesting feature of these models is that the oscillatory bursting dynamics are controlled by the kinetic (inactivation) properties of I_{NaP}. This conductance is emerging as an important cellular mechanism generating bursting and persistent activity (sustained tonic spiking) in many different types of neurons, including neocortical, hippocampal , cerebellar, and spinal neurons [5, 13, 19, 22, 41]. The models and analyses discussed here apply to this general problem of I_{NaP}-dependent neuronal and network activity. Our analyses emphasize that this conductance mechanism, in combination with I_L, endows neurons with a number of important properties: multiple activity modes including oscillatory bursting, rebound bursting [2], and synchronized bursting promoted through interaction with depolarizing synaptic currents (synaptic "current amplification") in the excitatory network. It remains an important experimental problem to fully characterize the inactivation time constants of I_{NaP} in pre-BötC neurons, since this is the key subthreshold voltage-dependent kinetic parameter in Model I. In this regard it is of interest that inactivation time constants in the range of many seconds, originally predicted by Model I to account for oscillatory bursting dynamics of pre-BötC cells, have subsequently been measured in neocortical neurons [22].

The general features of bursting behavior given by Model I appear robust with respect to I_{NaP} parameter values, and reformations of Model I that have incorporated newer data [35] on steady-state activation properties of I_{NaP} and I_{Na} exhibit the basic features of voltage-dependent bursting given by the original Model I, which was constructed before data was available for pre-BötC neurons. So far, a major reformulation regarding I_{NaP} involves the steady-state activation parameters, where $V_{1/2max}$ of the activation Boltzmann function is shifted to more hyperpolarized potentials and the slope factor k is slightly smaller, in agreement with our recent data (Fig. 2; Koizumi and Smith, in preparation). There is considerable cell-cell variability with some neurons exhibiting voltage-dependence of activation similar to Model I parameter values [8]. This variability emphasizes the heterogeneity of cellular parameters, which have important consequences on network dynamics as discussed in the chapter. As newer data becomes available, particularly on inactivation kinetics, further quantitative revision of Model I parameters are likely to be required, although the fundamental features of voltage-dependent bursting and multiple activity states would not be expected to change.

Pre-BötC neurons unquestionably have additional voltage-activated conductances, particularly calcium currents [20], which may contribute importantly to bursting dynamics, especially above spiking threshold, and could be included in the models. There is also recent evidence for calcium-activated, non-specific cationic current (CAN) in some pre-BötC cells [24, 25]. The picture emerging, although still incomplete, is that some neurons may have a heterogeneous mixture of inward currents that collectively promote bursting. Available data does however indicate that bursting in many of the pre-BötC oscillatory neurons depends largely on I_{NaP} with Model I-type dynamics. CAN currents are interesting because they activate following spike-dependent Ca^{2+} influx (i.e., they activate on a slower time scale than I_{NaP}), promote plateau-like bursting, and thus can sustain the active burst phase. This may require additional conductances for burst termination (e.g., slowly activating K^+ currents as in the original Model II). Including these other conductance mechanisms to account for behavior of cells with CAN currents would clearly introduce novel dynamics. Pre-BötC neurons also have a complicated somato-dendritic structure. Other important extensions of our single compartment models would therefore be to consider multi-compartment neurons and analyze bursting dynamics when I_{NaP} and other currents are distributed on dendrites. There is data from other neurons for dendritic localization of I_{NaP}[4]. Synaptic current interactions with I_{NaP} may actually occur in dendrites, so the analysis of coupled cell dynamics could also fruitfully be extended to multi-compartment cells.

12.7.2. *Analysis of coupled cells and networks*

Our analysis of the transitions between bursting and tonic spiking activity patterns is based on consideration of a slow averaged system for a pair of coupled cells, derived from a fast/slow decomposition. In the asymmetric bursting and asymmetric spiking regions of parameter space, the synchronized state is unstable with respect to the flow of this system, leading to a prediction of asynchrony of spikes. A fully rigorous analysis of why the stable state features anti-phase spiking in these regions has not been performed, nor has a full analysis of why the cells synchronize, or come close to synchrony, outside of these regions.

Application of the dynamic clamp, to obtain a hybrid network of a

Model I neuron and a real neuron with I_{NaP}-mediated bursting, may represent a fruitful approach to experimentally address these issues. The effects of $\bar{g}_{syn-e}$ and $g_{tonic-e}$ on burst duration, duty cycle, and other burst properties can be shown to relate to their influence on the slow averaged dynamics [1], yet unresolved details remain. Further, this analysis has not yet been extended to larger populations of cells.

While results have been obtained on the influence of heterogeneities on synchronized bursting in the pre-BötC network with reduced dynamics [32], a more complete understanding will arise from introducing heterogeneity in the setting of the full version of Model I, extending the analysis in section 12.5. As discussed in subsection 12.6.2, the mechanism by which heterogeneity extends bursts to lower $g_{tonic-e}$ is clear, but additional details remain to be elucidated. For example, heterogeneity appears to increase the frequency range of bursting solutions and to extend bursting to slightly larger $g_{tonic-e}$ values as well [3], relative to the homogeneous coupled case. It is likely that at least some aspects of these numerical findings could be better understood using the approaches presented in section 12.5.

Numerical studies have considered heterogeneities in $\bar{g}_{NaP}$ from equation (6) and $\bar{g}_{syn-e}$[3]. The reduced model approach used for heterogeneities in g_L may be useful for analyzing the effects of such heterogeneities, which we currently understand are an important property that influences overall network dynamics (see below). Further, the analysis performed on the reduced model considered all-to-all coupling, and for biological relevance, it will be important to explore the robustness of synchronized bursting to changes in connectivity patterns. Finally, through decreases in $\bar{g}_{syn-e}$, increases in external potassium concentration, or other modifications in I_K, clustered periodic solutions may become stable or aperiodic behavior may result [9, 32, 33]. Since various quasiperiodic and mixed-mode oscillations have been observed in spontaneous breathing of human infants and neonatal rodents, even in the absence of sensorimotor feedback [9], it will be important to analyze transitions away from full-population bursting to achieve a complete understanding of pacemaker network dynamics.

In the original analysis of population bursting dynamics [3], an important finding was that heterogeneous networks can still exhibit oscillatory bursting when parameter values for $\bar{g}_{NaP}$ and g_L fall within the range where there are no network neurons with intrinsic bursting properties (when isolated from synaptic inputs). These emergent network oscillations (section 12.4.3) arise when synaptic coupling strengths are sufficient to promote synchronized bursting through dynamic interaction of synaptic currents with

I_{NaP}, provided that tonically spiking cells are present in the network. The general issue that requires further analysis is that excitatory networks with features, such as I_{NaP}, that promote individual neuronal bursting have multiple dynamic states (see discussions in Butera *et al.*, [3] and Smith *et al.* [39]). Indeed, as discussed in section 12.4.3, there continues to be debate from experimental studies regarding the role of "pacemaker-driven" oscillations vs. "emergent" network oscillations that could occur in different states of network excitability [23, 24, 39]. It is likely that the pre-BötC network operates differently under various excitability conditions that produce different combinations of $\bar{g}_{NaP}$ and g_L and thus different network compositions of intrinsically bursting, tonically spiking, and silent neurons. The network dynamics with different heterogeneous distributions of $\bar{g}_{NaP}$ and g_L, as well as different synaptic coupling patterns, requires further exploration.

Finally, there is an important set of problems related to the dynamic regulation of the pre-BötC excitatory network by phasic synaptic inhibition, which occurs when the network is embedded in the larger respiratory central pattern generating network in the brainstem. Conceptual and computational models have now been formulated to address this problem [34, 39]. Rigorous analysis of basic problems such as frequency control that we have addressed here for the simpler pre-BötC network, however, has not yet been undertaken for these larger networks. Clearly the respiratory oscillator has challenging dynamical complexity at both cellular and network levels that will keep experimentalists and modelers working together and occupied for many decades.

Acknowledgments

We would like to thank the many collaborators who have contributed to the work discussed here. This work was supported by the National Science Foundation (DMS-0414057 to DT, DMS-0414023 to JR) and National Institutes of Health (R01-MH62057 to RB, and intramural research program for JS).

References

[1] J. Best, A. Borisyuk, J. Rubin, D. Terman, and M. Wechselberger. The dynamic range of bursting in a model respiratory pacemaker network, (2005). Preprint.

[2] R. J. Butera, J. Rinzel, and J. C. Smith, Models of respiratory rhythm

generation in the pre-Bötzinger complex: I. Bursting pacemaker neurons, *J. Neurophysiol.* **82**, 382–397, (1999).

[3] R. J. Butera, J. Rinzel, and J. C. Smith, Models of respiratory rhythm generation in the pre-Bötzinger complex: II. Populations of coupled pacemakers., *J. Neurophysiol.* **82**, 398–415, (1999).

[4] W. E. Crill, Persistent sodium current in mammalian central neurons, *Ann. Rev. Physiol.* **58**, 349–362, (1996).

[5] P. Darbon, C. Yvon, J. C. Legrand, and J. Streit, I_{NaP} underlies intrinsic spiking and rhythm generation in networks of cultured rat spinal cord neurons, *Eur. J. Neurosci.* **20**, 976–88, (2004).

[6] G. de Vries and A. Sherman. Beyond synchronization: modulatory and emergent effects of coupling in square-wave bursting. In eds. S. Coombes and P. Bressloff, *Bursting: The Genesis of Rhythm in the Nervous System.* World Scientific, Singapore, (2005). This volume, chapter 10.

[7] C. A. DelNegro, S. M. Johnson, R. J. Butera, and J. C. Smith, Models of respiratory rhythm generation in the pre-Bötzinger complex. III. Experimental tests of model predictions, *J. Neurophysiol.* **86**, 59—74, (2001).

[8] C. A. DelNegro, N. Koshiya, R. J. Butera, and J. C. Smith, Persistent sodium current, membrane properties and bursting behavior of pre-botzinger complex inspiratory neurons in vitro, *J. Neurophysiol.* **88**, 2242–2250, (2002).

[9] C. A. DelNegro, C. G. Wilson, R. J. Butera, H. Rigatto, and J. C. Smith, Periodicity, mixed-mode oscillations, and quasiperiodicity in a rhythm-generating neural network, *Biophys. J.* **82**, 206–214, (2002).

[10] B. Ermentrout, *Simulating, Analyzing, and Animating Dynamical Systems.* (SIAM, Philadelphia, 2002).

[11] J. L. Feldman and D. R. McCrimmon. Neural control of breathing. In *Fundamental Neuroscience*, chapter 37. Academic Press, (2002).

[12] R. A. Fitzhugh, Impulses and physiological states in theoretical models of nerve membrane, *Biophys. J.* **1**, 445–466, (1961).

[13] I. A. Fleidervish, A. Friedman, and M. J. Gutnick, Slow inactivation of Na+ current and slow cumulative spike adaptation in mouse and guinea-pig neocortical neurones in slices, *J. Physiol. (London).* **493**, 83–97, (1996).

[14] G. Funk, J. C. Smith, and J. L. Feldman, Generation and transmission of respiratory oscillations in medullary slices: Role of excitatory amino acids, *J. Neurophysiol.* **70**, 1497–1515, (1993).

[15] P. A. Gray, J. C. Rekling, C. M. Bocchiaro, and J. L. Feldman, Modulation of respiratory frequency by peptidergic input to rhythmogenic neurons in the prebtzinger complex, *Science.* **286**, 1566–1568, (1999).
[16] E. Izhikevich, Neural excitability, spiking and bursting, *Int. J. Bif. Chaos.* **10**, 1171–1266, (2000).
[17] S. Johnson, J. Smith, G. Funk, and J. Feldman, Pacemaker behavior of respiratory neurons in medullary slices from neonatal rat, *J. Neurophysiol.* **72**, 2598–2608, (1994).
[18] S. M. Johnson, N. Koshiya, and J. C. Smith, Isolation of the kernel for respiratory rhythm generation in a novel preparation: the pre-Bötzinger complex "island", *J Neurophysiol.* **85**(4), 1772–6, (2001).
[19] A. R. Kay, M. Sugimori, and R. Llinas, Kinetic and stochastic properties of a persistent sodium current in mature guinea pig cerebellar purkinje cells, *J. Neurophysiol.* **80**, 1167–79, (1998).
[20] N. Koshiya and J. Smith, Neuronal pacemaker for breathing visualized *in vitro*, *Nature.* **400**, 360–363, (1999).
[21] V. I. Krinskii and Y. M. Kokoz, Analysis of equations of excitable membranes – I. Reduction of the Hodgkin-Huxley equations to a second-order system, *Biofizika.* **18**, 506–511, (1973).
[22] J. Magistretti and A. Alonso, Biophysical properties and slow voltage-dependent inactivation of a sustained sodium current in entorhinal cortex layer-ii principal neurons: a whole-cell and single-channel study, *J. Gen. Physiol.* **114**, 491–509, (1999).
[23] C. A. D. Negro, C. Morgado-Valle, and J. L. Feldman, Respiratory rhythm: An emergent network property?, *Neuron.* **34**, 821–830, (2002).
[24] C. A. D. Negro, C. Morgado-Valle, J. A. Hayes, D. D. Mackay, R. W. Pace, E. A. Crowder, and J. L. Feldman, Sodium and calcium current-mediated pacemaker neurons and respiratory rhythm generation, *J. Neurosci.* **25**, 446–453, (2005).
[25] F. Pena, M. A. Parkis, A. K. Tryba, and J. M. Ramirez, Differential contributions of pacemaker properties to the generation of respiratory rhythms during normoxia and hypoxia, *Neuron.* **8**(1), 105–117, (2004).
[26] J. C. Rekling and J. L. Feldman, Pre-Bötzinger complex and pacemaker neurons: Hypothesized site and kernel for respiratory rhythm generation, *Ann. Rev. Physiol.* **60**, 385–405, (1998).
[27] D. W. Richter and K. M. Spyer, Studying rhythmogenesis of breathing: comparison of in vivo and in vitro models, *Trends Neurosci.* **24**(8), 464–72, (2001).
[28] J. Rinzel. Bursting oscillations in an excitable membrane model. In eds.

B. Sleeman and R. Jarvis, *Ordinary and Partial Differential Equations.* Springer-Verlag, New York, (1985).
[29] J. Rinzel, Excitation dynamics: Insights from simplified membrane models, *Federation Proc.* **44**, 2944–2946, (1985).
[30] J. Rinzel. A formal classification of bursting mechanisms in excitable systems. In ed. A. Gleason, *Proceedings of the International Congress of Mathematicians*, pp. 1578–1594. American Mathematical Society, Providence, RI, (1987).
[31] J. Rubin and D. Terman. Geometric singular perturbation analysis of neuronal dynamics. In ed. B. Fiedler, *Handbook of Dynamical Systems, vol. 2: Towards Applications.* Elsevier, (2002).
[32] J. Rubin and D. Terman, Synchronized bursts and loss of synchrony among heterogeneous conditional oscillators, *SIAM J. Appl. Dyn. Sys.* **1**, 146–174, (2002).
[33] I. Rybak, N. Shevtsova, W. St-John, J. Paton, and O. Pierrefiche, Endogeneous rhythm generation in the pre-Bötzinger complex and ionic currents: modeling and *in vitro* studies, *Eur. J. Neurosci.* **18**, 239–257, (2003).
[34] I. A. Rybak, N. A. Shevtsova, J. F. Paton, T. E. Dick, W. M. St-John, M. Morschel, and M. Dutschmann, Modeling the ponto-medullary respiratory network, *Respir. Physiol. Neurobiol.* **143**, 307–19, (2004).
[35] I. A. Rybak, N. A. Shevtsova, K. Ptak, and D. R. McCrimmon, Intrinsic bursting activity in the pre-botzinger complex: role of persistent sodium and potassium currents, *Biol. Cybern.* **90**, 59–74, (2004).
[36] A. Sherman, Anti-phase, asymmetric, and aperiodic oscillations in excitable cells. I. Coupled bursters, *Bull. Math. Biol.* **56**, 811–835, (1994).
[37] A. Shilnikov and G. Cymbaluyk, Transition between tonic-spiking and bursting in a neuron model via the blue-sky catastrophe, *Phys. Rev. Lett.* **94**, 048101–01–04, (2005).
[38] J. Smith, H. Ellengerger, K. Ballanyi, D. Richter, and J. Feldman, Pre-Bötzinger complex: a brainstem region that may generate respiratory rhythm in mammals, *Science.* **254**, 726–729, (1991).
[39] J. C. Smith, R. J. Butera, N. Koshiya, C. Del Negro, C. G. Wilson, and S. M. Johnson, Respiratory rhythm generation in neonatal and adult mammals: the hybrid pacemaker-network model, *Respir Physiol.* **122** (2-3), 131–47, (2000).
[40] D. Somers and N. Kopell, Rapid synchronization through fast threshold modulation, *Biol. Cybern.* **68**, 393–407, (1993).
[41] A. Taddese and B. P. Bean, Subthreshold sodium current from rapidly

inactivating sodium channels drives spontaneous firing of tuberomammillary neurons, *Neuron.* **33**, 587–600, (2002).
[42] D. Terman, Chaotic spikes arising from a model for bursting in excitable membranes, *SIAM J. Appl. Math.* **51**, 1418–1450, (1991).
[43] D. Terman, The transition from bursting to continuous spiking in an excitable membrane model, *J. Nonlinear Sci.* **2**, 133–182, (1992).
[44] D. Terman and D. L. Wang, Global competition and local cooperation in a network of neural oscillators, *Physica D.* **81**, 148–176, (1995).
[45] C. G. Wilson, R. J. Butera, C. A. DelNegro, and J. C. Smith, Interfacing computer models with real neurons: Respiratory 'cyberneurons' created with the dynamic clamp, *Adv. Exp. Biol. Med.* **499**, 120–124, (2001).

CHAPTER 13

GEOMETRIC ANALYSIS OF BURSTING NETWORKS

Janet Best

Mathematical Biosciences Institute,
The Ohio State University, Columbus, Ohio 43210 USA
e-mail: jbest@mbi.osu.edu

David Terman

Department of Mathematics & Mathematical Biosciences Institute,
The Ohio State University, Columbus, Ohio 43210 USA
e-mail: terman@math.ohio-state.edu

Three examples in which geometric singular perturbation methods have been used to analyze firing patterns in models of bursting oscillators are discussed. In the first example, we consider a single square-wave burster and review rigorous results concerned with the existence, uniqueness and stability of the bursting oscillation. The analysis demonstrates that the bursting solution may not be uniquely determined for arbitrarily small values of the singular perturbation parameter. In the second example, we consider wave-propagation in a one-dimensional array of neuronal oscillators arising in models of thalamic networks. This network may generate two types of waves: smoothly propagating waves and lurching waves which propagate in a saltatory fashion. Geometric singular perturbation methods are used to derive explicit formulas for when a particular wave exists and for how the velocity of the wave depends on parameters. Finally, in the third example, we consider transitions between activity patterns in an excitatory-inhibitory network; this network was first introduced as a model for neuronal activity within the basal ganglia. Geometric methods are used to uncover mechanisms both for generating irregular firing and for synchronizing subsets of cells into regularly bursting clusters.

13.1. Introduction

Mathematical models for bursting oscillations often display a rich structure of dynamic behavior [3, 17, 18]. Besides periodic bursting oscillations, these systems may exhibit other types of periodic solutions, such as continuous spiking, as well as more exotic behavior including chaotic dynamics. Networks of bursting oscillators can generate complex population rhythms; these including propagating waves, synchronous or clustered rhythms and irregular, uncorrelated firing patterns [2, 14–16]. Models for bursting activity usually contain multiple time scales and geometric, singular perturbation methods have been extremely useful in understanding the mathematical, as well as biological, mechanisms underlying these firing patterns [13, 14, 17, 18]. In fact, most classification schemes of bursting oscillations are in terms of geometric properties or the bifurcation structure of the fast subsystem [7, 12].

In this chapter, we discuss three examples in which geometric singular perturbation methods have been used to analyze firing patterns in models of bursting oscillators. In the first example, we consider a single square-wave burster and review rigorous results concerned with the existence, uniqueness and stability of the bursting oscillation [9]. An interesting feature of these models is that the bursting solution need not always be unique or stable. For example, the number of spikes per burst will increase as the singular perturbation parameter ε decreases. The analysis in Terman [17] demonstrated that these transitions can be quite complicated. In particular, the bursting solution may not be uniquely determined for those values of ε for which the transitions take place. For each positive integer n there corresponds a range of values for ε during which the model makes a transition from n to $n+1$ spikes per burst. These ranges of parameter values accumulate onto $\varepsilon = 0$ as $n \to \infty$. Hence, there is an infinite collection of parameter ranges for which the model may exhibit chaotic bursting behavior. Here we characterize the set of parameters for which the bursting solution is uniquely determined; in this case the solutions must also be stable.

In the second example, we consider wave-propagation in a one-dimensional array of neuronal oscillators. We review results where singular perturbation methods were used to construct traveling waves for models of thalamic networks [16]. These models were originally developed in order to study mechanisms that underlie delta and spindle sleep rhythms [6, 11]. Here we consider a single layer of mutually connected inhibitory neurons, each of which has the ability to rebound after hyperpolarization. This network may generate two types of waves: smoothly propagating waves and lurching waves which propagate in a saltatory fashion [6, 16]. Using geometric singular perturbation methods, we derive explicit formulas for when a particular wave exists. These formulas also determine how the velocity of the waves depends on network parameters. Moreover, each type of wave may leave a variety of different sorts of activity patterns in its wake [16]. The geometric methods are very useful in understanding the mechanisms responsible for these different patterns.

In the third example, we consider transitions between activity patterns in an excitatory-inhibitory network. While the network is capable of a rich variety of firing patterns, we focus on two of these: uncorrelated, irregular firing and synchronous bursting rhythms. The model was developed to explore mechanisms underlying alterations in firing patterns that accompany Parkinson's disease [15], where a transition from irregular to clustered firing has been shown to accompany the development of pathology. The cells form a network consisting of a layer of inhibitory neurons and a layer of excitatory neurons that can rebound after hyperpolarization. We review results where geometric singular perturbation methods were used to uncover mechanisms both for generating irregular firing and for synchronizing subsets of cells into regularly bursting clusters [2]. These methods reveal how the interaction between the excitatory and inhibitory cells can lead to irregular firing both at the cellular and at the network level and how changing significant parameters in the model can shift the network to clustered firing. Furthermore, these methods show that the transition to clustering can occur via multiple mechanisms depending on the parameter regime.

13.2. Existence, Uniqueness and Stability of Square-Wave Bursters

In this section, we consider a general model for square-wave bursting and characterize the set of parameters for which the bursting solution is uniquely determined; in this case the solutions must also be stable. Our approach is straightforward; we determine when a certain flow-defined map gives rise to a uniform contraction. However, in order to analyze the return map, we must carefully follow trajectories as they pass through different regions of phase space. These regions correspond to different types of solutions to the fast subsystem in which the singular perturbation parameter is set equal to zero. The analysis becomes especially delicate at the termination of the spiking activity when the bursting trajectory passes close to a homoclinic orbit of the fast subsystem. It is at this point that many standard singular perturbation theories break down, so more delicate analysis is required. In fact, the homoclinic orbits are often directly responsible for the generation of chaotic dynamics.

13.2.1. *Assumptions on the geometric model*

Here we describe the precise assumptions needed for the theorem. The analytic framework is quite general, so instead of restricting our attention to one specific model, we consider a general system of the form

$$\begin{aligned} v' &= f_1(v, w, y) \\ w' &= f_2(v, w, y) \\ y' &= \varepsilon g(v, w, y). \end{aligned} \tag{1}$$

Here f_1, f_2, and g are sufficiently smooth (say C^3) functions and ε is a small singular perturbation parameter. If $\varepsilon = 0$, then y is constant, and we can consider y to be a parameter in the first two equations of (1). We refer to these equations (with y constant) as the fast system (FS). We refer to the last equation in (1) as the slow equation.

The assumptions on the nonlinear functions in (1) are geometric in the sense that we make assumptions on the nature of the fixed points, periodic and other bounded solutions of (FS) and the slow equation. Most of these conditions are straightforward to verify for a specific model using numerics. Some conditions are technical; however, all of the more technical assumptions are quite natural. Examples of a specific set of equations which satisfy these assumptions can be found in Rubin and Terman [13].

We assume that the set of fixed points of (FS) consists of an 'S-shaped' curve, denoted by $\mathcal{S}$, as shown in Fig. 13.1. That is, there exist $y_\lambda < y_\rho$ such that if $y < y_\lambda$ or $y > y_\rho$, then (FS) has exactly one fixed point, while if $y_\lambda < y < y_\rho$ then (FS) has precisely three fixed points. We assume that the lower branch, denoted by $\mathcal{L}$, consists of fixed points which are stable as solutions of (FS) and the middle branch consists of fixed points which are saddles. See also Fig. 13.2.

We further assume that there exists a one-parameter family of periodic solutions of (FS) as shown in Fig. 13.1. This branch, denoted by $\mathcal{P}$, surrounds a portion of the upper branch of fixed points and terminates at a solution which is homoclinic to one of the fixed points on the middle branch. We denote this homoclinic point by $p_h = (v_h, w_h, y_h)$.

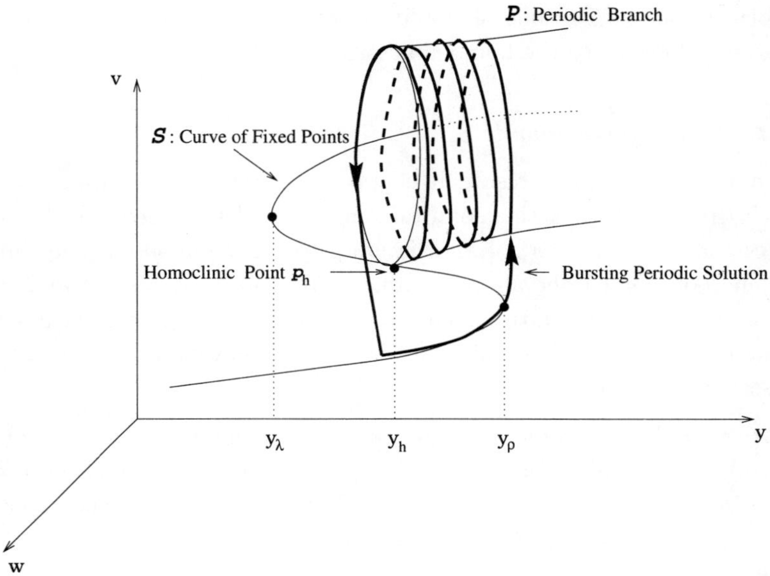

Fig. 13.1. Geometric model for bursting. The fast system has an S-shaped curve of fixed points and a branch of stable periodic solutions. The bursting solution passes near the lower branch of fixed points in the silent phase and passes near the periodic branch in the active phase.

Our next assumption is concerned with the $y-$nullsurface, $\mathcal{N} \equiv \{g = 0\}$. We assume that this defines a smooth surface which intersects the curve $\mathcal{S}$ at a unique point which lies below p_h. We further assume that $g > 0$ below $\mathcal{N}$, $g < 0$ above $\mathcal{N}$, and $\mathcal{N} \cap \mathcal{P} = \emptyset$.

We now state the more technical assumptions required for our analysis. The first technical assumption is that the homoclinic orbit arises from the transverse intersection of the two manifolds formed by taking the unions of the stable and unstable trajectories to the fixed points along the middle branch. The second technical assumption is concerned with the right knee. We assume that this knee is nondegenerate in some (obvious) sense. We next consider the lower branch of fixed points. We have already assumed that each of these fixed points is stable as a solution of (FS). We further assume that each is hyperbolic; that is, the linearization of (FS) about each fixed point has both eigenvalues with strictly negative real parts. We also need to assume that the manifold $\mathcal{P}$ is normally hyperbolic [5]. The final assumption is that the set of solutions of (FS) considered so far represents all the bounded solutions of (FS). That is, every solution of (FS) approaches in forward time either one of the fixed points along $\mathcal{S}$, one of the periodic solutions along $\mathcal{P}$, or the homoclinic orbit.

13.2.2. *The main result*

We now state our main result. It characterizes the range of values of ε for which the periodic bursting solution is uniquely determined. The Theorem states that the bursting solution is unique except for possibly an infinite sequence of small intervals of ε values. We note that results in Terman [17] imply that the bursting solution may not be uniquely determined for values of ε in these narrow intervals; in fact, (1) may exhibit chaotic, Smale horseshoe dynamics.

Theorem: The periodic bursting solution is uniquely determined and asymptotically stable for all values of $\varepsilon > 0$ sufficiently small except for those in a set of the form $\cup_{i=1}^{\infty} (\varepsilon_i - \delta_i, \varepsilon_i + \delta_i)$. The ε_i and δ_i can be chosen so that $\lim_{i\to\infty} \varepsilon_i = 0$. Moreover,

$$\varepsilon_i - \varepsilon_{i+1} > C_1\varepsilon_i^2 \qquad \text{and} \qquad \delta_i \leq C_2 e^{-k/\varepsilon_i}$$

for some positive constants C_1, C_2 and k.

The Theorem is proved in Lee and Terman [9]. Here we outline some of the main ideas in the proof.

13.2.3. *Bursting solution*

Before outlining the proof of the Theorem, we describe why one expects (1) to exhibit bursting oscillations. We then explain, in the next subsection, what difficulties may arise for some values of ε.

It is easy to understand why the system (1) will give rise to a bursting solution. Here we give a heuristic description of how this solution behaves in phase space. Our description follows Rinzel [12] and the trajectory is shown in Fig. 13.1.

Assume that ε is small, but positive. We start the trajectory near the lower branch. Because the lower branch consists of stable fixed points of (FS), the trajectory will quickly approach a small neighborhood of the lower branch. Now $g > 0$ near the lower branch. The solution must therefore track near the lower branch moving towards the right knee. This continues until the slow dynamics push the trajectory past the right knee. The trajectory is then attracted to near one of the periodic solutions along $\mathcal{P}$. This corresponds to the jump-up from the silent phase to the active phase. The fast spike-like oscillations of the bursting solution corresponds to the trajectory passing near and around $\mathcal{P}$. The slow dynamics now force the orbit to move slowly to the left. This continues until the trajectory passes near the homoclinic orbit of (FS). Once past this homoclinic orbit, the trajectory must eventually fall back to the silent phase. This completes one cycle of the bursting solution.

As we shall see, this informal description for the bursting solution can be easily justified, except for the portion of the trajectory near the homoclinic orbit. It requires delicate analysis in order to fully understand the passage near the homoclinic orbit and the mechanism for jumping down to the silent phase. This will turn out to be the key to understanding when the bursting solution is uniquely determined. In the next subsection we consider this in detail.

13.2.4. *When do trajectories jump down?*

In order to understand when the bursting solution jumps down to the silent phase, we need to consider the stable and unstable manifolds of the fixed points of (FS) along the middle branch. Note that there are two trajectories in the unstable manifold of each of these fixed points. See Fig. 13.2. One of these evolves towards the active phase, looping around the upper branch. If $y > y_h$, then this trajectory approaches one of the periodic solutions along $\mathcal{P}$, while if $y < y_h$, then it ultimately approaches a stable fixed point along the lower branch. The other unstable trajectory evolves directly towards the silent phase and approaches the stable fixed points along the lower branch.

Now the stable manifolds to the fixed points along the middle branch separate the two unstable manifolds. Hence, if a trajectory lies close to the middle branch, it will either give rise to a spike or jump down to the silent phase depending on which side of the stable manifold it lies on.

What we have described so far holds for $\varepsilon = 0$, however this all carries over for small $\varepsilon > 0$. To make this more precise, let W_0^s and W_0^u be the union of all the stable and unstable manifolds to the fixed points along the middle branch when $\varepsilon = 0$. (We must actually exclude small neighborhoods of the left and right knees.) These are both smooth, two-dimensional, invariant manifolds. For $\varepsilon > 0$, these manifolds perturb to manifolds W_ε^s and W_ε^u (see Fenichel [5]). These manifolds are both smooth, two-dimensional, invariant, and lie a C^1-distance $O(\varepsilon)$ close to W_0^s and W_0^u near the middle branch. If we let $W_\varepsilon^c = W_\varepsilon^s \cap W_\varepsilon^u$, then W_ε^c, W_ε^s, and W_ε^u are the center, center-stable, and center-unstable manifolds corresponding to the middle branch,

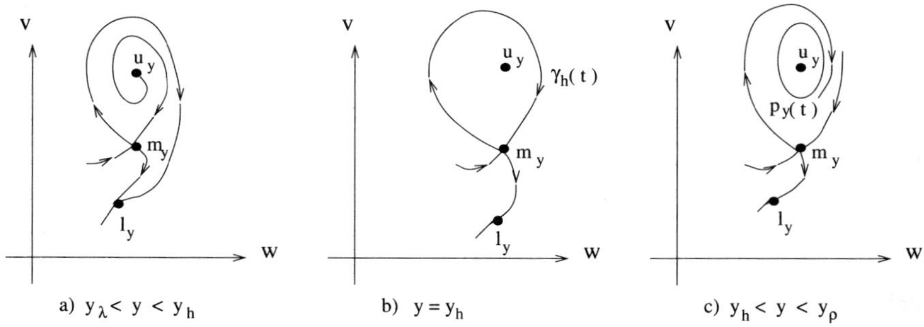

Fig. 13.2. The phase plane of (FS) for different values of y. For each $y \in (y_\lambda, y_\rho)$, one of the two trajectories in the unstable manifold of the fixed point along the middle branch approaches the stable fixed point on the lower branch. If $y > y_h$, then the other trajectory approaches the periodic solution; while, if $y < y_h$, then it ultimately approaches the lower stable fixed point.

respectively.

As before, W^s_ε divides W^u_ε into two pieces; one piece 'points' towards the active phase, while the other piece 'points' towards the silent phase. Hence, a trajectory near the middle branch may give rise to another spike or may jump down depending on which side of W^s_ε it lies on.

We now discuss the significance of this to the bursting solutions. We start the bursting solution in the active phase near the branch of periodic orbits $\mathcal{P}$. It will then give rise to spikes as it tracks near $\mathcal{P}$ moving slowly to the left. As the orbit approaches the homoclinic orbit, it passes closer to the middle branch. As long as it keeps spiking, the orbit must lie on the 'jump-up' side of W^s_ε. Eventually, however, the orbit will cross to the other side of W^s_ε. It is then that the orbit must jump down to the silent phase.

It is possible for the orbit to actually lie precisely on W^s_ε and it is important to understand the fate of these trajectories. As shown in Fig. 13.3, these orbits must track close to the middle branch (actually W^c_ε) slowly moving to the left. The orbit eventually jumps down near the left knee. Note that if we start very close to W^s_ε, then the trajectory will track close to the middle branch for some finite distance before it either jumps up or jumps down. If the bursting solution behaves in this way, then it will not behave like the 'typical' bursting solution, as described in section 13.2.3. It is precisely this mechanism (lying close to W^s_ε) which can destroy the uniqueness and stability of the bursting solution. Hence, in order to determine whether the bursting solution is uniquely determined, we must estimate how close it passes to W^s_ε.

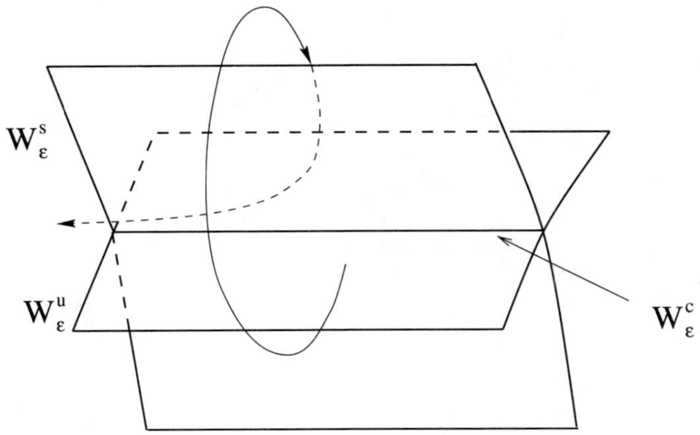

Fig. 13.3. The mechanism explaining why the uniqueness of bursting solutions may be destroyed. If an orbit lies very close to W_ε^s, then it tracks close to the middle branch for some finite distance.

13.2.5. *Return map and outline of the proof*

We will now outline the proof of the Theorem. The Theorem is proved by constructing a two-dimensional section Σ transverse to the flow defined by (1) and then considering the return map from Σ back into Σ. We denote this map by π_ε. Existence, uniqueness and stability of a bursting solution follows once we demonstrate that this map is a uniform contraction. We choose Σ so that it lies just above the right knee, as shown in Fig. 13.4. Hence, trajectories cross Σ transversely as they jump up to the active phase. The distance from Σ to the right knee is assumed to be small, but still independent of ε.

In order to determine when the return map is a contraction, we write it as the composition of several other maps; these maps correspond to the different pieces of the trajectories as they move around in phase space. The different pieces are:

(P1) the jump up

(P2) tracking near the branch of periodic solutions $\mathcal{P}$

(P3) motion near the homoclinic orbit and interaction with the middle branch

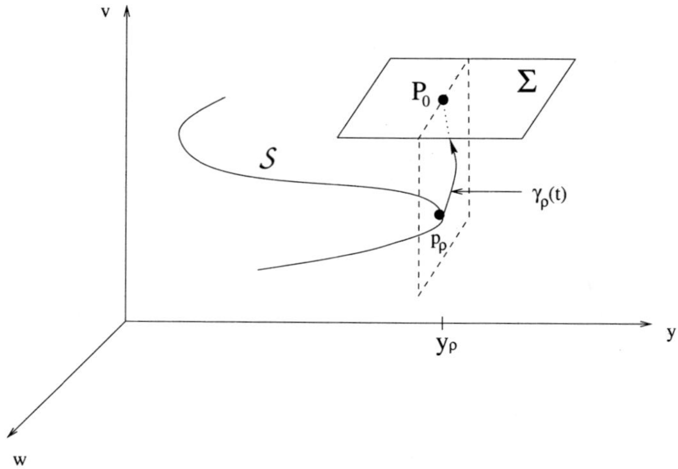

Fig. 13.4. The two-dimensional section Σ above the right knee. The Poincare return map π_ε is from Σ back to itself.

(P4) the jump down

(P5) tracking near the lower branch

(P6) passing near the right knee.

We need to estimate the amount of expansion or contraction induced by each of these pieces of the flow. We note that there will be a huge amount of contraction as trajectories pass near the lower branch. This contraction is so large that trajectories will enter an $O(e^{-k_0/\varepsilon})$ neighborhood of the lower branch. This contraction will easily dominate any possible expansion that can occur over the pieces (P1), (P2), (P4) or (P6). Hence, the only possible expansion that can ultimately destroy the uniform contraction of the entire map π_ε must occur during the piece labeled (P3). It will, in fact, be possible for exponential expansion to occur as the trajectories pass near the middle branch, just before they jump down to the silent phase. This is of course consistent with the discussion in the preceding section.

In order to obtain uniqueness, we must somehow avoid W_ε^s, the center-stable manifold of the middle branch. If it were true that Σ had empty intersection with a small neighborhood of W_ε^s, then there would be no problem with proving uniform contraction; however, as we shall see, this can never be the case. What may be true, however, is that W_ε^s has empty intersection with the range of the return map π_ε. We denote this range as $\Sigma_1^\varepsilon \equiv \pi_\varepsilon(\Sigma)$. If this intersection is empty, then we will be able to obtain uniform contraction by restricting π_ε to Σ_1^ε.

We can now outline our strategy for proving the theorem. We consider two subsets of Σ. The first one is Σ_1^ε, the range of π_ε. For the second subset, we consider W_ε^s and follow it backwards by the flow until it intersects Σ. Denote this set by $\hat{\Sigma}_2^\varepsilon$. The analysis in Lee and Terman [9] demonstrates that this set consists of a large number of curves in Σ as shown in Fig. 13.5. The number of such curves is asymptotically $O(1/\varepsilon)$. We then let Σ_2^ε be a small neighborhood of $\hat{\Sigma}_2^\varepsilon$. This is a (large) number of narrow strips. Uniform contraction will follow if we can show that $\Sigma_1^\varepsilon \cap \Sigma_2^\varepsilon = \emptyset$.

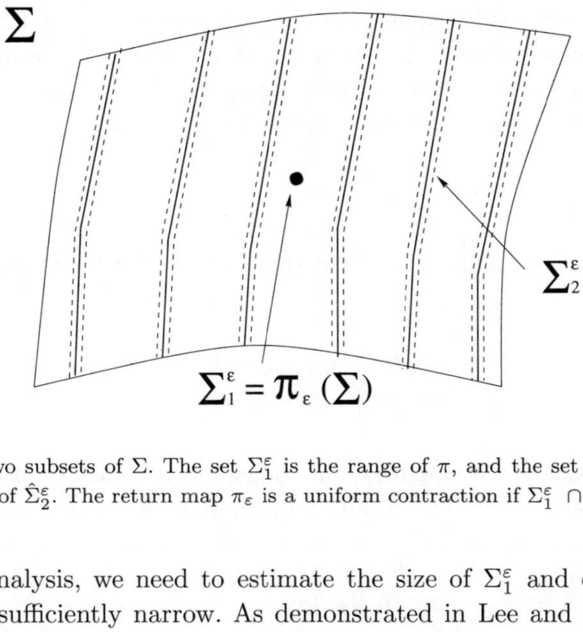

Fig. 13.5. Two subsets of Σ. The set Σ_1^ε is the range of π, and the set Σ_2^ε is a small neighborhood of $\hat{\Sigma}_2^\varepsilon$. The return map π_ε is a uniform contraction if $\Sigma_1^\varepsilon \cap \Sigma_2^\varepsilon = \emptyset$.

In the analysis, we need to estimate the size of Σ_1^ε and choose each strip in Σ_2^ε sufficiently narrow. As demonstrated in Lee and Terman [9], the size of Σ_1^ε is $O(e^{-k_0/\varepsilon})$ for some constant k_0 and we need to choose the width of each strip to be $O(e^{-k_1/\varepsilon})$ for some constant k_1. Since the distance between the strips is $O(\varepsilon)$ it does not seem very likely that Σ_1^ε and the strips will intersect. To prove this, however we need to consider how these sets change with respect to ε. A key ingredient in the analysis is that both of these sets change their positions as ε is varied, but the speed at which they move is different. For most values of ε, Σ_1^ε and Σ_2^ε have empty intersection. However, as ε varies, Σ_1^ε 'passes through' Σ_2^ε. This corresponds to the bursting solution either gaining or losing a spike in each of its bursts. For these values of the parameters, the bursting solution may not be uniquely determined. Details of the analysis can be found in Lee and Terman [9].

13.3. Propagating Activity Patterns

We now consider wave-propagation in a one-dimensional array of mutually inhibitory neuronal oscillators. This system is motivated by models of thalamic sleep rhythms [6, 11]. These models may exhibit different types of propagating activity patterns including smoothly propagating waves and lurching waves which propagate in a saltatory fashion [11, 16]. Each type of wave may leave a variety of different sorts of activity patterns in its wake. Here we review results where singular perturbation methods were used to construct both of these types of waves [16]. These methods were also used to derive explicit formulas for when a particular wave exists and how the velocity of the waves depends on network parameters.

13.3.1. *The model*

In the numerical simulations, individual cells satisfy differential equations of the form

$$\begin{aligned} C_m v' &= -g_L(v - v_L) - g_{Ca} m_\infty(v) h(v - v_{Ca}) \\ h' &= \varepsilon(h_\infty(v) - h)/\tau_h(v). \end{aligned} \tag{2}$$

The definitions of the nonlinear functions and parameters in (2) are given in Terman *et al.* [16]. The results do not, however, depend on the precise details of the equations. For this reason, we usually write (2) as

$$\begin{aligned} v' &= f(v, h) \\ h' &= \varepsilon(h_\infty(v) - h)/\tau_h(v). \end{aligned} \tag{3}$$

The following assumptions on the nonlinear functions in (3) will be needed for the analysis: We assume that the v-nullcline $\{f = 0\}$ represents a cubic-shaped curve, denoted by C, as in Fig. 13.6. We further assume that $v' > 0$ (< 0) above (below) C. The h-nullcline $\{h = h_\infty(v)\}$ is taken to be a nonincreasing curve that intersects C at a unique point, which we denote by $p_0 = (v_0, h_0)$. Moreover, $\tau_h(v)$ is assumed to be positive and nonincreasing; it then follows that $h' > 0$ (< 0) below (above) the h-nullcline.

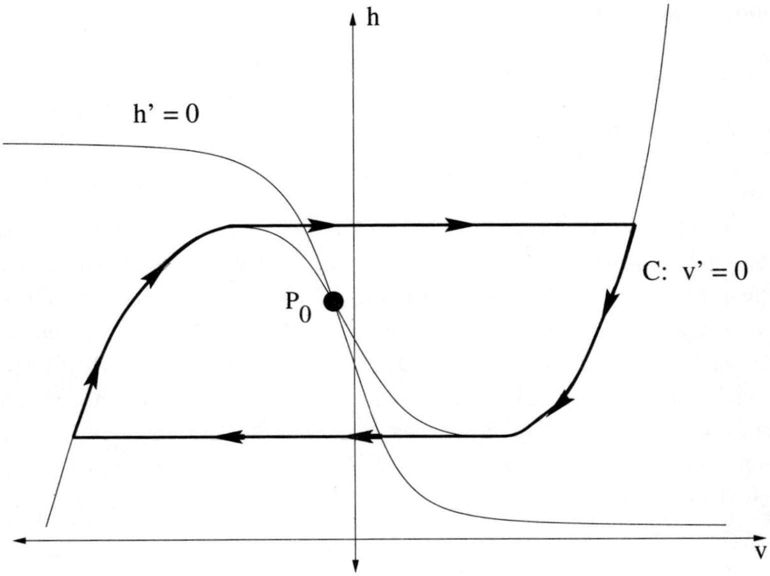

Fig. 13.6. Nullclines corresponding to a single oscillatory cell. The bold curve represents the singular periodic solution.

We model two mutually-coupled cells as

$$\begin{aligned} v_i' &= f(v_i, h_i) - g_{syn} s_j (v_i - v_{syn}) \\ h_i' &= \varepsilon (h_\infty(v_i) - h_i)/\tau_h(v_i) \\ s_i' &= \alpha(1 - s_i) H(v_i - \theta) - \varepsilon \beta s_i. \end{aligned}$$

Here, $i, j = 1, 2$ and $i \neq j$. The constants α, β and g_{syn} are all positive and H is the Heaviside step function. Hence, θ is a threshold above which the presynaptic cell j must be to activate the synaptic variable s_j. If $v_j < \theta$, then s_j decays slowly to 0 (deactivates) at the rate $\varepsilon\beta$. On the other hand, if $v_j > \theta$, then s_j activates at the rate $\alpha + \varepsilon\beta$ which is $O(1)$ with respect to ε. Our choice of synaptic turn on and turn off rates is motivated by models for thalamic sleep rhythms. The synapses are said to be *excitatory* if the reversal potential v_{syn} satisfies $v_{syn} > v_0$, and *inhibitory* if $v_{syn} < v_0$. Here we will only consider inhibitory synapses.

Here we consider one-dimensional arrays of cells. Some results for two-layered networks are given in Terman *et al.* [16]. A single-layered network is modeled as

$$\begin{aligned} v_i' &= f(v_i, h_i) - \frac{g_{syn}}{N}(v_i - v_{syn}) \sum_j W_{ij} s_j \\ h_i' &= \varepsilon(h_\infty(v_i) - h_i)/\tau_h(v_i) \\ s_i' &= \alpha(1 - s_i)H(v_i - \theta) - \varepsilon\beta s_i. \end{aligned} \tag{4}$$

Here, N is the total number of cells in the network, the sum is over all the cells in the network and W_{ij} represents a synaptic weight; it can be viewed as the probability that there is a synaptic connection between cell j and cell i. We assume that W_{ij} is of the form $W_{ij} = W(i - j)$ where $W(x)$ is a positive, even function, often referred to as the 'synaptic footprint'. Fig. 13.7 shows two possible choices for $W(x)$. In Fig. 13.7(A), $W(x)$ has a maximum at $x = 0$ and is decreasing for $x > 0$. This is referred to as *on-centered* connectivity. In Fig. 13.7(B), the connectivity is *off-centered*, where $W(x)$ is small for x small and has a maximum at some $x_0 > 0$.

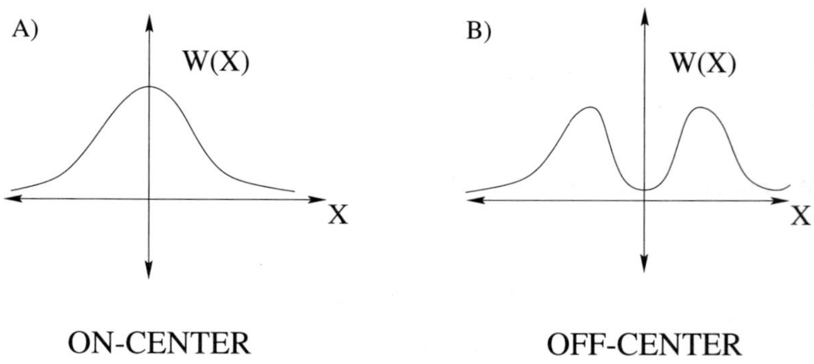

Fig. 13.7. Examples of two different types of synaptic footprint: A) on-centered and B) off-centered.

For the analysis it will be convenient to consider a continuum limit as the number of cells becomes unbounded. We are then led to consider the integral-differential equation:

$$\begin{aligned} v_t &= f(v, h) - g_{syn}(v - v_{syn}) \int_{-\infty}^{\infty} W(x - y)s(y, t)dy \\ h_t &= \varepsilon(h_\infty(v) - h)/\tau_h(v) \\ s_t &= \alpha(1 - s)H(v - \theta) - \varepsilon\beta s \end{aligned} \tag{5}$$

where (v, h, s) are functions of (x, t).

13.3.2. *Numerical results*

To illustrate the numerous types of propagating patterns, here we describe some results obtained from numerical simulations of a full two-layered network. Two general classes of waves are observed, referred to as *smooth waves* and *lurching waves*. A smooth wave corresponds to a fixed profile moving with constant velocity, much like a single action potential traveling down a nerve axon. If we keep track of where the leading edge of the membrane potential is some fixed value, then this defines a straight line of the form $x - \mu t =$ constant, where the slope μ corresponds to the wave speed.

Several types of smooth waves are shown in Fig. 13.8. Parameter values are given in Terman *et al.* [16]. A solitary pulse is illustrated in Fig. 13.8(A). Multiple pulses may also exist and a double pulse is shown in Fig. 13.8(B). There may also exist periodic smooth wave trains. Finally, a more exotic smooth wave is shown in Fig. 13.8(C); three bursts at a frequency of about 6-7 Hz are followed by a silent period of about 200 ms, and this is then followed by another sequence of three bursts.

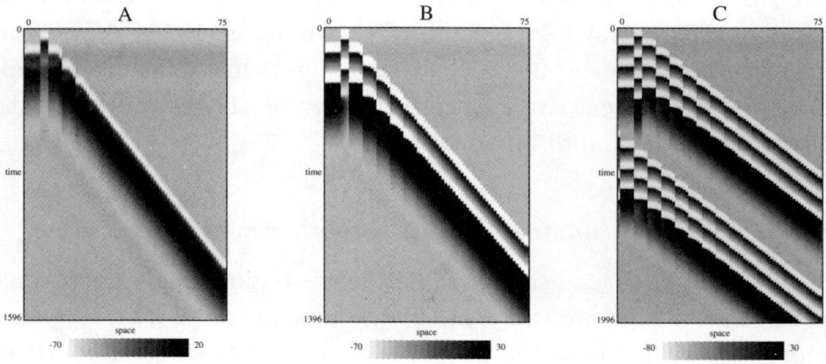

Fig. 13.8. Smooth waves for a two-layered network: A) a solitary pulse, B) a double pulse, C) a multiple pulse solution.

A lurching wave does not propagate with constant velocity. Instead, the propagating wave recruits groups or clusters of cells in discrete steps. The leading edge of active cells inhibits some cluster of cells ahead of it; the size of this cluster depends on the synaptic footprint. Inhibited cells must wait until the active cells fall back to the silent phase, and then for inhibition to wear off, before they are able to jump up to the active phase.

Several types of lurching waves are illustrated in Fig. 13.9. There may

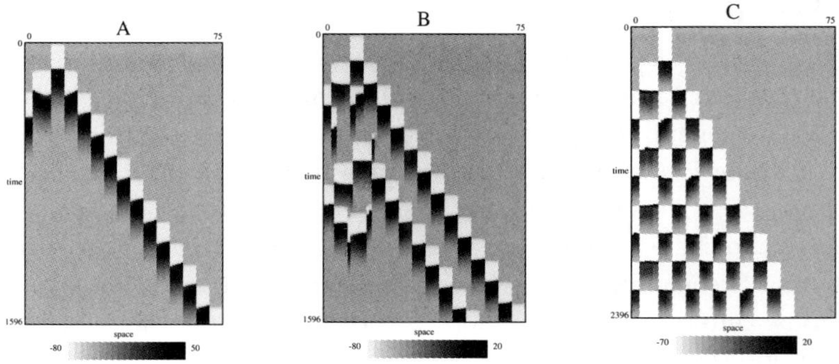

Fig. 13.9. Lurching waves for a two-layered network: A) a solitary lurcher, B) a double lurcher, C) a lurching wave with periodic clustering in the wake.

exist single and multiple lurching pulses as shown in Figs. 13.9(A) and (B). For each of these solutions, the network eventually returns to rest in the wake of the propagating wave. The network may, however, also exhibit sustained oscillations. Cells in the wake of the wave may oscillate synchronously, or may form clusters as shown in Fig. 13.9(C). The firing of cells within each cluster is nearly synchronous, while different clusters are desynchronized. The activity patterns in the wake of the wave may also be quite complicated and disorganized.

13.3.3. *Singular construction of smooth waves*

We will now use geometric singular perturbation methods to analyze smooth waves. First we will demonstrate how to construct a singular trajectory corresponding to the wave. We then use the singular construction to derive *a priori* estimates for the wave speed.

Consider a one-dimensional continuous array of cells coupled through mutual inhibition. A smooth wave corresponds to a traveling wave solution of (5); that is, it is a solution of (5) of the form

$$(v(x,t), h(x,t), s(x,t)) \;=\; (v(\xi), h(\xi), s(\xi)), \qquad \xi \;=\; x + \varepsilon ct.$$

Plugging the above into (5), we find that (v, h, s) satisfy the system

$$\begin{aligned} \varepsilon cv' &= f(v,h) - g_{syn} S_{tot}(\xi)(v - v_{syn}) \\ \varepsilon ch' &= \varepsilon(h_\infty(v) - h)/\tau_h(v) \\ \varepsilon cs' &= \alpha(1-s)H(v-\theta) - \varepsilon\beta s \end{aligned} \tag{6}$$

where the derivative is with respect to ξ and

$$S_{tot}(\xi) = \int_{-\infty}^{\infty} W(\xi - y)s(y)\, dy. \tag{7}$$

A smooth wave is then a solution of (6) that satisfies the boundary conditions

$$(v, h, s)(\pm\infty) \;=\; (v_0, h_0, 0).$$

We will consider $c > 0$; that is, waves moving to the left. Note, also, that the velocity of the wave is taken to be $O(\varepsilon)$.

We can reduce this integral-differential equation to a system of ordinary differential equations as follows. Consider a solitary (single-peaked) pulse and assume that $v(\xi) > \theta$ if and only if $0 < \xi < a$ where the constant a is yet to be determined. Once c and a are known, we can solve the third equation in (6) for $s(\xi)$. In the limit $\varepsilon \to 0$, we find that

$$s(\xi) \;=\; \begin{cases} 0 & \text{if} \quad \xi < 0 \\ 1 & \text{if} \quad 0 < \xi < a \\ \exp\left\{-\frac{\beta}{c}(\xi - a)\right\} & \text{if} \quad \xi > a. \end{cases} \tag{8}$$

Now plug this formula for $s(\xi)$ into (7) to obtain an expression for $S_{tot}(\xi)$. Since this depends on the unknown constants c and a, we will sometimes write $S_{tot}(\xi; c, a)$. The first two equations in (6) can then be treated as a system of nonautonomous ordinary differential equations.

We construct a singular solution of (6) by dissecting the trajectory into different pieces corresponding to either the silent or active phases or to a transition between these phases. Over each piece, the solution satisfies reduced equations in either the fast or slow variables. We begin our construction at $\xi = -\infty$ and increase ξ, describing the singular trajectory in the (v, h) phase plane along the way.

We will assume a footprint of unit length; that is, $W(\xi) = 0$ for $|\xi| \geq 1$. The translation of the wave is chosen so that the initial jump up to the active phase occurs at $\xi = 0$. It then follows that for $\xi < -1$, $S_{tot}(\xi) = 0$ and $(v(\xi), h(\xi))$ lie at the rest point (v_0, h_0) on the left branch of the $S_{tot} = 0$ cubic.

For $-1 < \xi < 0$, the cells lie in the silent phase along the left branch of the cubic associated with $S_{tot}(\xi)$, which we write as $v = v_L(h, S_{tot})(\xi)$. The variable $h(\xi)$ evolves according to the second equation in (6), a nonautonomous ODE in which $v = v_L(h, S_{tot})(\xi)$. We view $h(\xi)$ and $S_{tot}(\xi)$ as the slow variables. Note that they depend on the unknown constants a and

c. These constants should be chosen so that $(h(0), S_{tot}(0))$ lies on the curve of knees $h = h_{LK}(S)$ in the slow phase plane (since the jump-up to the active phase is supposed to occur at $\xi = 0$). Such a choice may not be possible, in which case the smooth wave will not exist.

For example, take a square on-center synaptic footprint, without gaps. In this case, $S_{tot}(\xi)$ is nearly constant while in the silent phase; so, given that the cells are excitable for all levels of synaptic input, $(v(\xi), h(\xi))$ must approach the fixed point along the left branch of the cubic associated with this constant S_{tot} level. A smooth wave is therefore not possible. In contrast, if there is a gap in the synaptic footprint, then $S_{tot}(\xi)$ will achieve a maximum at some point $\xi_0 \in (-1, 0)$ and then begin to decrease. For simplicity of calculation, we work with a synaptic footprint of unit length that has rectangular peaks and a gap of length 2γ between them, as described in the Appendix. We see that S_{tot} reaches a maximum at $\xi = -\gamma$, after which it decreases as $\xi \to 0$. In this case $(h(\xi), S_{tot}(\xi))$ is able to evolve to the curve of knees, thus escaping the silent phase and making possible the existence of a smooth wave. We will denote the jump-up point on the curve of knees by (h_J, S_J).

A reduced equation for the fast jump up can be derived by introducing the fast variable $\eta = \xi/\varepsilon$ into the first two equations of (6) and then letting $\varepsilon = 0$. This yields the fast equations $cv' f(v, h) - g_{syn} S_{tot}(0)(v - v_{syn})$ and $h' = 0$, where differentiation is now with respect to η. Along the jump up, both h and S_{tot} are constant; that is, $(h, S_{tot}) = (h_J, S_J)$. During the active phase, when $0 < \xi < a$, $(v(\xi), h(\xi))$ travels along the right branch of the cubic determined by $S_{tot}(\xi)$. There is then a jump down at $\xi = a$. As with the jump up, we can obtain a reduced equation for v with both h and S_{tot} constant. This is as far as we'll take the description of the singular solution for now.

13.3.4. *Estimating the wave speed*

The singular construction allows us to obtain estimates on the wave speed. This is based on reducing the integral-differential system (6) to a two-point boundary value problem involving the unknown parameters a and c. The boundary value problem can then be solved using the numerical continuation package AUTO [4].

Consider (6) for $-1 \leq \xi \leq 0$; recall that this corresponds to the silent phase of the singular solution. We begin by writing the first two equations of (6) as the autonomous system

$$\begin{aligned} \varepsilon c v' &= f(v,h) - g_{syn} S_{tot}(x)(v - v_{syn}) \\ c h' &= (h_\infty(v) - h)/\tau_h(v) \\ x' &= 1. \end{aligned} \tag{9}$$

Note that there are three dependent variables along with two unknown parameters a and c. In order to have a unique solution, we need to specify boundary conditions.

Since, as stated earlier, $(v(\xi), h(\xi))(v_0, h_0)$ for $\xi < -1$, a natural condition at $\xi = -1$ is

$$v(-1)v_0, \quad h(-1) = h_0 \quad \text{and} \quad x(-1) = -1. \tag{10}$$

For a boundary condition at $\xi = 0$, we use the fact that this is when the jump up takes place, and that $(v(0), h(0))$ must lie on the curve of left knees. We assume that this curve is linear, i.e., $h_{LK}(S) = h_{LK}(0) + \lambda S$ for some constant λ whose value can be estimated from plots of nullclines. Hence, we have the boundary condition

$$h(0) = h_{LK}(0) + \lambda S_{tot}(0; c, a) \tag{11}$$

where $S_{tot}(0; c, a)$ is calculated from (8) and (7).

To complete the system, one more condition relating the parameters is needed. This arises by considering the active phase of the singular solution. During the active phase, when $0 < \xi < a$, reasonable simplifying assumptions are that $h_\infty(v) = 0$ and $\tau(v) = \tau_R$ for some positive constant τ_R. These imply that $h(\xi)$ satisfies $ch' = -h/\tau_R$, and hence $h(\xi)h(0)e^{-\xi/c\tau_R}$. We will further assume that $S_{tot} = 0$ at the jump down. This is not quite correct; however, provided β is not too small, it will be a reasonable approximation as numerical simulations will show. It then follows that $h_{RK}(0) = h(0)e^{-a/c\tau_R}$, or

$$a = c\tau_R \ln\left(\frac{h(0)}{h_{RK}(0)}\right) = c\tau_R \ln\left(\frac{h_{LK}(0) + \lambda S_{tot}(0)}{h_{RK}(0)}\right). \tag{12}$$

Note that $S_{tot}(0)$ depends on a so this is a nonlinear implicitly defined condition on a. Our boundary value problem therefore consists of the ODEs (9) together with the boundary conditions (10), (11), and (12). There are five conditions for this three-dimensional system. However, we have two free parameters, the pulse width, a and the velocity, c, so there is a possibility for finding solutions.

We now demonstrate how one can derive analytical estimates on the wave speed. We also present estimates on how large the gap in the synaptic footprint should be for there to exist a singular smooth wave. Our calculations here are done using a rectangular footprint and cells are assumed to be excitable for all levels of synaptic input. First, we need the following lemmas.

Lemma 1: Let a be the width of the singular smooth pulse; then $0 < a < 1$.

Proof: If $a \geq 1$, then $S_{tot}(\xi) = 1/2$ for $-\gamma \leq \xi \leq 0$. That is, $(v(\xi), h(\xi))$ lies on the left branch of the $S_{tot} = 1/2$ cubic for $-\gamma \leq \xi \leq 0$. It is then impossible for (v, h) to lie along the curve of knees at $\xi = 0$ in order to jump up to the active phase. Hence, a smooth wave cannot exist.

Lemma 2: There exists $\delta_0 > 0$, that does not depend on γ, such that $S_{tot}(-\gamma) - S_{tot}(0) > \delta_0$.

Proof: Note that the curves $h_{FP}(S)$ and $h_{LK}(S)$ are monotone increasing. Let $S_{FP}(h)$ and $S_{LK}(h)$ denote their inverses, respectively. The assumption that each cell is excitable for fixed levels of input implies that there exists $\delta_0 > 0$ such that $S_{FP}(h) - S_{LK}(h) > \delta_0$ for each h for which both curves are defined.

Now $(h(\xi), S_{tot}(\xi))$ reaches a maximum value of S_{tot} at $\xi = -\gamma$ and then must cross the fixed point curve at some $\xi_0 \in (-\gamma, 0)$ before it can jump up. It follows that

$$S_{tot}(-\gamma) > S_{tot}(\xi_0) \ = \ S_{FP}(h(\xi_0)). \tag{13}$$

Moreover, $h'(\xi) < 0$ for $\xi \in (\xi_0, 0)$, and hence $h(\xi_0) > h(0)$. Since $S_{LK}(h)$ is monotone increasing, it follows that

$$S_{LK}(h(\xi_0)) > S_{LK}(h(0)) \ = \ S_{tot}(0). \tag{14}$$

The last equality holds because the jump-up is at $\xi = 0$. From (13), (14), and the definition of δ_0, we conclude that

$$S_{tot}(-\gamma) - S_{tot}(0) \ > \ S_{FP}(h(\xi_0)) - S_{LK}(h(\xi_0)) \ > \ \delta_0$$

as claimed.

To derive *a priori* bounds on the wave speed, we obtain from (12) and Lemma 1 the upper bound

$$c \ = \ a\left\{\tau_R \ln\frac{h(0)}{h_{RK}(0)}\right\}^{-1} \ < \ \left\{\tau_R \ln\frac{h_{LK}(0)}{h_{RK}(0)}\right\}^{-1}.$$

In order to obtain a lower bound, we can calculate that if $a < 1 - \gamma$, then

$$\begin{aligned} S_{tot}(-\gamma) &= \frac{1}{2(1-\gamma)} \left(\frac{c}{\beta}(1 - e^{\frac{\beta}{c}(\gamma+a-1)}) + a \right) \\ &< \frac{1}{2(1-\gamma)} \left(\frac{c}{\beta} + a \right) \; = \; \frac{c}{2(1-\gamma)} \left(\frac{1}{\beta} + \tau_R \ln \frac{h_J}{h_{RK}(0)} \right) \\ &< \frac{c}{2(1-\gamma)} \left(\frac{1}{\beta} + \tau_R \ln \frac{1}{h_{RK}(0)} \right). \end{aligned}$$

Together with Lemma 2, this implies that

$$c \; > \; 2\delta_0(1-\gamma) \left(\frac{1}{\beta} + \tau_R \ln \frac{1}{h_{RK}(0)} \right)^{-1}.$$

If $a \geq 1 - \gamma$, then a lower bound for c follows from (12).

Next, we find a lower bound on the gap size. First we assume that $\gamma < \min\{a, (1-a)\}$, then using Lemma 2, we find that

$$\begin{aligned} \delta_0 < S_{tot}(-\gamma) - S_{tot}(0) &= \frac{1}{2(1-\gamma)} \left\{ \frac{c}{\beta} \left(e^{\frac{\beta}{c}(a-1)} - e^{\frac{\beta}{c}(\gamma+a-1)} \right) + \gamma \right\} \\ &< \frac{\gamma}{2(1-\gamma)} \end{aligned}$$

and hence $\gamma > 2\delta_0/(1+2\delta_0)$. A similar analysis holds if either $\gamma > a$ or $\gamma > 1 - a$, with help from the bounds on c.

13.4. Transitions between Irregular and Clustered Activity

Here we consider activity pattern transitions in an excitatory-inhibitory network, models for cells in the basal ganglia that may collectively shift from irregular firing to synchronous bursting during the development of Parkinson's disease. Reviewing results of Best *et al.* [2], we use geometric singular perturbation methods to construct a one-dimensional map that predicts when these cell types may interact to produce irregular, chaotic firing. We then show how to geometrically construct clustered solutions, and we determine parameter changes that can cause the network to transition between these modes of activity.

13.4.1. *The model*

The model involves two cell types. Excitatory (E) cells arise as models for subthalamic nucleus neurons [15] and satisfy differential equations of the form

$$\begin{aligned}
C_m v_E' &= -I_L - I_K - I_{Na} - I_T - I_{Ca} - I_{AHP} - I_{I\to E} \\
[Ca]' &= c(-I_{Ca} - I_T - k_{Ca}[Ca]) \\
X' &= \phi_X (X_\infty(v) - X)/\tau_X(v).
\end{aligned} \tag{15}$$

Here, X can be n, h or r and the currents are $I_L = g_L(v - v_L)$, $I_K = g_K n^4 (v - v_K), I_{Na} = g_{Na} m_\infty^3(v) h(v - v_{Na})$, $I_T = g_T a_\infty^3(v) b_\infty^2(r)(v - v_{Ca}), I_{Ca} = g_{Ca} s_\infty^2(v)(v - v_{Ca})$, $I_{AHP} = g_{AHP}(v - v_K)([Ca]/([Ca] + k_1))$.

Inhibitory (I) cells arise as models for neurons in the external segment of the globus pallidus; these cells satisfy equations similar in form to those for the excitatory cells:

$$C_m v_I' = -I_L - I_K - I_{Na} - I_T - I_{Ca} - I_{AHP} - I_{E\to I} - I_{I\to I} + I_{app}. \tag{16}$$

The ionic currents are modeled with the same formulas and equations given above for the excitatory cells except that the low-threshold calcium current I_T takes a simpler form; parameter values may differ. I_{app} is a constant and represents input to the globus pallidus from the striatum. For details and parameter values for models of both cell types, see Terman *et al* [15].

The synaptic current $I_{A\to B}$ from structure A to a cell i in structure B is given as

$$I_{A\to B} = g_{A\to B}(v_B^i - E_{A\to B}) \sum_j W_{ij} s_A^j.$$

The sum is over cells in A with the synaptic weight given by W_{ij}, and each synaptic variable s_A^j satisfies a first order differential equation of the form

$$s_A' = \alpha(1 - s_A) H_\infty(v_A - \theta_A) - \beta s_A. \tag{17}$$

H_∞ is a smooth approximation of the Heaviside step function.

Figure 13.10 illustrates the network architecture. There is synaptic coupling between the excitatory and inhibitory cell layers as well as between inhibitory cells. Additionally, inhibitory cells receive a constant level of inhibition. The network is *regularly structured* in that each cell of a given type has the same number, type, and spatial distribution of connections; spatially periodic boundary conditions are imposed.

All of our analysis for this model will be done using a fast/slow reduction: we identify processes that evolve on a timescale slower than the other processes and then reduce the full system to equations for just the slow variables. In particular, there will be a single slow variable for an inhibitory cell: the intracellular calcium concentration, $[Ca]_I$ for which we usually just

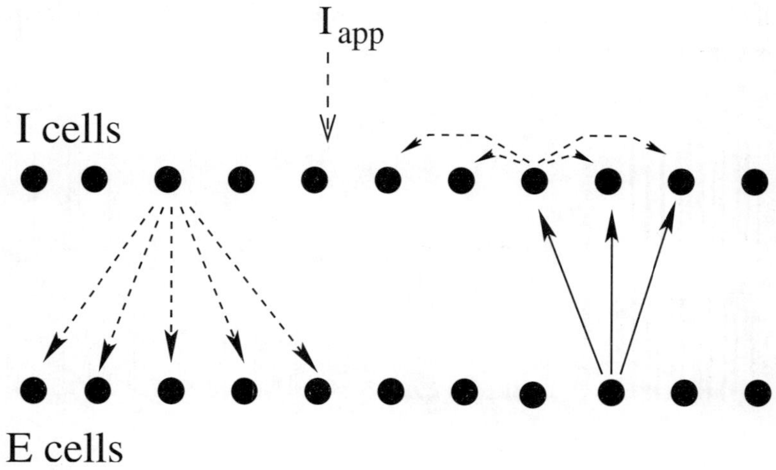

Fig. 13.10. Network architecture. The I cells send synaptic inhibition both to E cells and to other I cells. E cells send excitation to the I cells. The I cells receive an additional constant level of inhibitory input.

write Ca_I. The intrinsic properties of an excitatory cell also give rise to a slow variable: r is the inactivation variable for the slow, depolarizing current I_T that gives these cells the ability to rebound after hyperpolarization. Within the context of the network, we need to associate to each excitatory cell an additional slow variable that reflects the total amount of synaptic inhibition the cell is receiving at a given time:

$$S_{tot} = \sum_j W_{ij} s_I^j.$$

This analysis is often only strictly rigorous in the limit as the rates of the slow processes become zero. Numerical simulations demonstrate that our fast/slow dissections are well-justified in that they accurately predict the qualitative behavior of the system observed when the rates of the slow processes are positive.

13.4.2. *Two distinct activity patterns*

Isolated excitatory cells fire at just a few Hz. However, these cells can exhibit higher frequency firing either in a sustained manner when given sufficient excitatory input or as rebound bursts following release from hyperpolarizing current. The inhibitory cells can fire rapid periodic spikes with sufficient applied current. They also display bursts of activity when subjected to a small constant hyperpolarizing current, as well as an afterhyperpolarization following sustained firing.

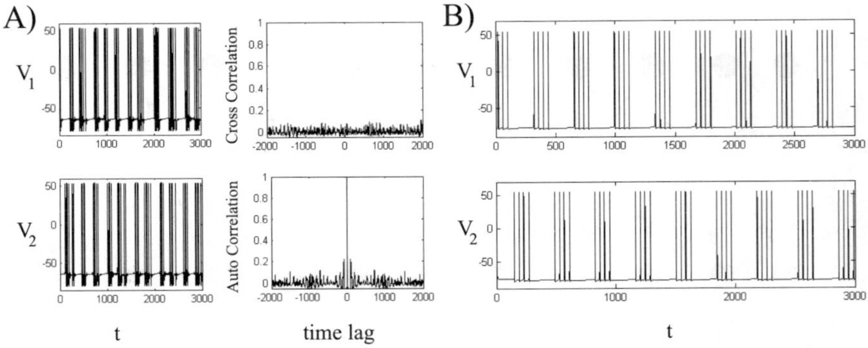

Fig. 13.11. Firing patterns in a network of ten I cells and ten E cells. Here, each E cell sends excitation to the nearest I cell, while each I cell contacts the three closest E cells as well as its two nearest-neighbor I cells; similar activity occurs in networks with different sizes and connection patterns. A) Voltage traces, cross-correlation and autocorrelation for two I cells firing irregularly. B) Voltage traces for two I cells firing in clusters.

We will focus on two types of firing patterns that may be observed when these two classes of cells are connected into a network. We will say that the network activity is *irregular* if the firing of each I cell lacks periodicity as indicated by a single peak in the autocorrelation and if I cells are also unsynchronized as indicated by flat cross-correlation. Figure 13.11(A) illustrates irregular activity generated by the network.

An example of a simple *clustered* rhythm is shown in Fig. 13.11(B). Here the network breaks up into two clusters; cells within each cluster are synchronized with each other while the two clusters fire out of phase. More complicated clustering can also occur involving a larger number of clusters or dynamic cluster membership. The analysis that follows will help clarify how interactions between network architecture and intrinsic and synaptic properties of cells may lead a network to organize itself into clusters.

13.4.3. *Geometric analysis of irregular activity*

How can irregular firing patterns arise in this regularly-structured network? We will see that irregular firing can arise as an interaction between intrinsic properties of the two cell types. Our analysis in this section does not rely on details of the E cells; we only use the fact that an E cell fires intrinsically at a few Hz. On the other hand, we need to know the bifurcation structure for the fast subsystem of a model I cell to understand how the cell responds to this excitatory input. We then show how parameters in the slow equation determine whether the I-cell/E-cell interaction is periodic or irregular.

We begin by considering a single I cell governed by system (16). Numerical simulations indicate that the calcium concentration within an I cell changes more slowly than the other dependent quantities, so we will treat Ca_I as the slow variable in our fast/slow reduction. Regarding Ca_I as a bifurcation parameter and v_I, n_I, h_I and r_I as fast variables, we have the fast subsystem for a single I cell. Its bifurcation diagram is shown in Fig. 13.12(A). Note that for each value of Ca_I there is a unique fixed point; these fixed points are stable for $Ca_I > C_{HB}$ and unstable at $Ca_I < C_{HB}$. There is a subcritical Hopf bifurcation when $Ca_I = C_{HB}$. A branch of unstable periodic orbits bifurcates from the Hopf point and then "turns around" at a saddle-node of limit cycles when $Ca_I = C_{SN}$; there exist stable limit cycles for $Ca_I < C_{SN}$. Note that for $C_{HB} < Ca_I < C_{SN}$, the fast system is bistable: there exist both a stable fixed point and a stable limit cycle.

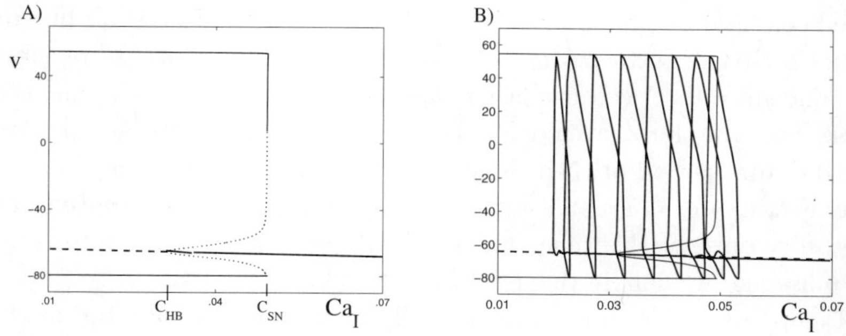

Fig. 13.12. A) Fast/slow analysis of an I cell. Each I cell is an elliptic burster. The projection of a bursting solution onto this diagram is shown in B).

We now include slow variable dynamics in the case when the I cell bursts. The projection of the bursting trajectory onto the bifurcation diagram is shown in Fig. 13.12(B). This is an example of an elliptic burster [7, 12]. During the cell's silent phase, the trajectory tracks close to the branch of fixed points with the slow variable Ca_I decreasing. Once past the Hopf point, the trajectory jumps up to the branch of stable periodic orbits of the fast subsystem. The orbit then tracks close to this branch, generating action potentials, until it reaches the saddle-node of limit cycles. The trajectory is then forced back to the branch of stable fixed points and this completes one cycle of the bursting orbit.

Note that there is a delay in the silent phase from when the orbit passes the Hopf point to when it jumps up to the active phase. This is known as a "delayed bifurcation". Previous analysis has demonstrated that the length of delay is closely related to the distance between the Hopf point and where the cell jumps down [10].

A very important feature of fast/slow analysis is that one can formally reduce the full system (16) to a single equation for just the slow variable Ca_I. There are actually two cases to consider depending on whether the cell is silent or active. Here we will simplify our qualitative analysis by using the observation that Ca_I changes approximately linearly as it decreases during the silent phase and also as it increases during the active phase: we will assume that the slow dynamics are given as

$$Ca_I' = \begin{cases} -\lambda_S & \text{when the cell is silent} \\ \lambda_A & \text{when the cell is active.} \end{cases} \tag{18}$$

Now we define a *phase response curve* (PRC) for an I cell. While PRCs have been used before, a novel feature here is that the I cells are bursters. We must first define a notion of phase. We define the phase to be simply the time since the I cell has last fallen down from the active to the silent phase. Suppose, for convenience, that the I cell jumps down at time $t = 0$ and the total period of the cell is T_I; that is, it jumps down again at this time. Now fix $t \in [0, T_I]$ and suppose we stimulate the I neuron with a small excitatory pulse at this time. The I cell will jump down at some time after the pulse and we denote this time by $\phi(t)$. This is the PRC.

Figure 13.13(A) shows a numerically generated PRC for the model I cell. Note that there exists $T_S \in (0, T_I)$ such that the PRC increases in an almost linear fashion for $0 < t < T_S$ and is nearly constant for $T_S < t < T$; these features are easily understood using the geometric methods discussed earlier. We assume that if the cell is silent then an impulse will force the cell into the active phase, with the same value of the slow variable. This is a reasonable assumption, as Fig. 13.12(B) shows, because during most of the silent phase, the cell's trajectory is evolving close to a branch of unstable fixed points of the fast subsystem. Finally, we assume that if the cell is active, then the impulse has a negligible effect on the cell's trajectory. Again, this assumption is reasonable because while in the active phase, the cell lies close to a branch of stable fixed points of the fast subsystem. A perturbation will push this trajectory a short distance from the periodic branch and the trajectory will then quickly move back.

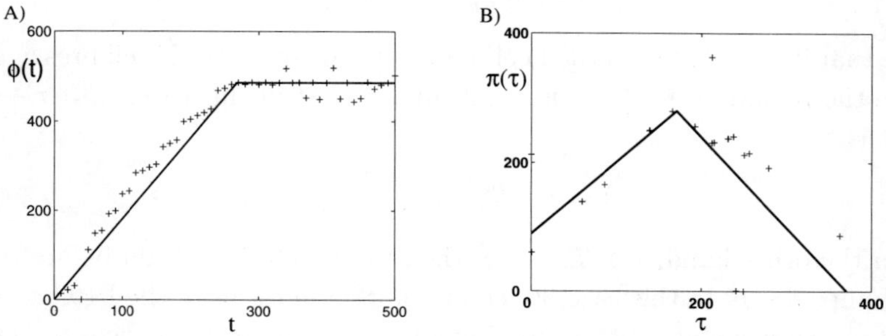

Fig. 13.13. The numerically computed (+) and the analytically computed (solid line) of A) the PRC of a bursting I cell, and B) the one-dimensional map associated with an I cell periodically forced by an E cell.

Choose T_S so that the unperturbed I cell is silent for $0 \leq t < T_S$ and is active for $T_S < t < T_I$. We first consider the case when the I cell's phase t satisfies $0 < t < T_S$. From (18), the cell is a distance $t\lambda_S$ away from C_{SN}, the jump-down value of Ca_I. A perturbation forces the cell to the active phase. The distance to C_{SN} is still $t\lambda_S$; however, according to (18), Ca_I now increases at rate λ_A until it jumps down again. It follows that the time it takes to reach C_{SN} is $(\lambda_S/\lambda_A)t$ and the time when it actually jumps down is

$$\phi(t) = \left(\frac{\lambda_S + \lambda_A}{\lambda_A}\right) t \quad \text{for} \quad 0 < t < T_S. \tag{19}$$

Now suppose the cell is active; that is, $T_S < t < T_I$. Then the perturbation has no effect on the slow dynamics; hence, the cell jumps down when it would if there were no perturbation and

$$\phi(t) = T_I \quad \text{for} \quad T_S < t < T_I. \tag{20}$$

Now consider the subnetwork consisting of just one I cell and one E cell, and imagine that $I \to E$ inhibition is weak enough that we can ignore it. Since the E cell intrinsically fires at a few Hz, it periodically sends excitatory input to the I cell. We will construct a map, closely related to the PRC, that determines the resulting firing pattern of the I cell.

Let T_E be the period of the E cell, assume that the E cell fires at time 0, fix $\tau \in [0, T_E)$ and suppose that the I cell jumps down at time τ. Finally, assume that the next time that the I cell jumps down is at τ_0. We define the map $\pi : [0, T_E) \to [0, T_E)$ as

$$\pi(\tau) = \begin{cases} \tau_0 & \text{if } \tau_0 < T_E \\ \tau_0 - T_E & \text{if } \tau_0 > T_E. \end{cases}$$

Note that if $\tau_0 < T_E$, then the I cell jumps down before the E cell fires again. Since the period of the I cell is T_I, it follows that in this case, $\tau_0 = \tau + T_I$. That is,

$$\pi(\tau) = \tau + T_I \quad \text{if } \tau < T_E - T_I. \tag{21}$$

If, on the other hand, $\tau > T_E - T_I$, then the E cell fires again before the I cell jumps down. In this case, we compute $\pi(\tau)$ in terms of the PRC ϕ. The I cell jumps down at τ before receiving the E input at T_E, hence, the I cell is at phase $T_E - \tau$ when it receives the E input. According to the definition of the PRC, it follows that the I cell next jumps down at $\tau + \phi(T_E - \tau)$. Hence,

$$\pi(\tau) = \tau + \phi(T_E - \tau) - T_E \quad \text{if } \tau > T_E - T_I. \tag{22}$$

Finally, we use the explicit formula for ϕ given earlier and conclude that

$$\pi(\tau) = \begin{cases} \tau + T_I & \text{if } \tau < T_E - T_I \\ \tau + T_I - T_E & \text{if } T_E - T_I < \tau < T_E - T_S \\ (\lambda_S/\lambda_A)(T_E - \tau) & \text{if } T_E - T_S < \tau < T_E. \end{cases}$$

Figure 13.13(B) shows a graph of this function along with simulation results.

We can use the map $\pi(\tau)$ to predict when periodic forcing of an I cell will result in an irregular firing pattern: if iterating the one-dimensional map $\pi(\tau)$ leads to a chaotic attractor, we expect the I cell to fire irregularly. So when does $\pi(\tau)$ have a chaotic attractor? When $\lambda_S/\lambda_A > 1$, this map would be piecewise expanding if not for the intervals where $\pi' = 1$. Consider instead the map $\pi^m(\tau)$ where $m - 1$ is the smallest positive integer such that $\pi^{m-1}(0) = (m-1)(T_I - T_E) > T_E - T_S$; this is the smallest iterate of $\pi(\tau)$ such that every orbit visits an interval on which $\pi(\tau)$ is expanding. For the maps $\pi(\tau)$ and $\pi^m(\tau)$, Lyapunov exponents exist for all but countably many points and are positive. We restrict our attention to the subinterval $[\pi^2(T_E - T_S), \pi(T_E - T_S)]$, since all orbits enter this interval and remain there. For the map $\pi^m(\tau)$, this interval decomposes into a finite number of subintervals on which $|(\pi^m)'| \geq \lambda_S/\lambda_A > 1$; moreover, if J_i and J_j are any two of these subintervals, there exists an integer k such that $(\pi^m)^k(J_i) \cap J_j$ is nonempty. It follows that $\pi^m(\tau)$ (and therefore also $\pi(\tau)$) has a chaotic attractor [1]. In particular, the positive Lyapunov exponents imply that periodic orbits cannot be attracting for the map $\pi(\tau)$ when $\lambda_S > \lambda_A$.

This analysis suggests that the I cell will have irregular dynamics whenever $\lambda_S > \lambda_A$; however, since we constructed $\pi(\tau)$ as an approximation, we should also consider the behavior of nearby maps. If we take a C^3 approximation to $\pi(\tau)$ for which the derivative at the fixed point is still $-\lambda_S/\lambda_A$, we may expect to observe the behavior typical of an S-unimodal map: an attracting periodic orbit for values of λ_S/λ_A slightly greater than 1 with a period-doubling cascade to a chaotic attractor for steeper slopes [8, 19]. This is precisely what one sees when varying parameters in the equation for Ca_I to increase λ_S/λ_A past 1.

The picture just described holds for a single E cell periodically forcing a single I cell, in a parameter regime where the I cell can burst spontaneously. In other words, $g_{I \to E}$ is small so that synaptic input from the I cell to the E cell is too weak to have significant effect on the firing rate of the E cell, and I_{app} is not so strongly hyperpolarizing that I cells need excitation to fire. As Fig. 13.11(A) shows, in this parameter regime these irregular dynamics may be also observed in the full network.

13.4.4. *Geometric analysis of clustered activity*

Clusters arise because the ability of E cells to rebound endows $I \to E$ inhibition with dual action, silencing a cell now while assuring the cell will rebound later. Several factors combine to govern the timing of a rebound within the network; following Wang and Rinzel [20], we will speak of the outcome in terms of the 'escape' or the 'release' of the silent cluster. That is, the active cluster may release the silent cluster from inhibition by ceasing to fire. A silent cluster escapes from ongoing inhibition when it begins firing and the resulting inhibition suppresses the previously active cluster. A given network may exhibit multiple mechanisms for either escape or release depending on intrinsic and synaptic parameters. Moreover, there is often no clear distinction between escape and release.

We will give examples of these mechanisms below, but to explain them it is necessary to know when an E cell will fire: we need a geometric understanding of the condition for a single E cell with inhibitory input to fire a rebound burst. Recall that r is the inactivation variable for the current underlying the rebound and S_{tot} is a measure of the synaptic inhibition an E cell is receiving; these are the slow variables for the E cell. We consider system (15) with

$$I_{I\to E} = g_{I\to E}(v_E - E_{I\to E})S_{tot};$$

thus there are six dependent variables: $v_E, [Ca], n, h, r, S_{tot}$. Viewing r and S_{tot} as bifurcation parameters gives a four-dimensional fast subsystem, and we need to identify the regions in (S_{tot}, r) phase-space where this fast subsystem exhibits steady behavior or oscillations.

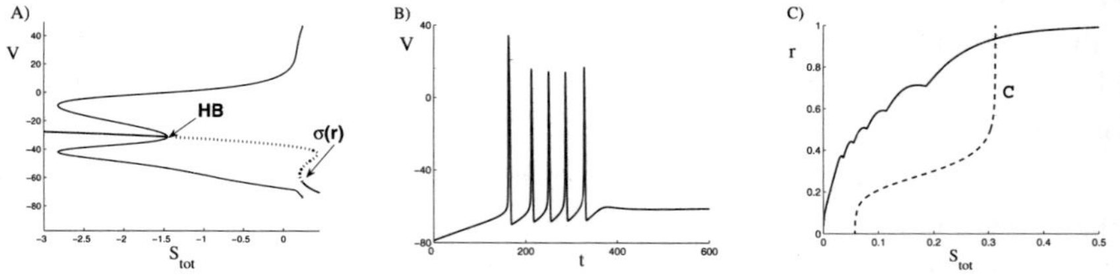

Fig. 13.14. A) Fast/slow analysis of an E cell. There are Hopf bifurcations at points labeled HB and $\sigma(r)$. B) A rebound burst of an E cell after release from sustained inhibition. C) The projection of the solution shown in B) onto the (S_{tot}, r) phase-space. Spiking begins when the trajectory crosses the curve $\mathcal{C}$.

The first step is to fix r and treat S_{tot} as a single bifurcation parameter. The bifurcation diagram is shown in Fig. 13.14(A). Note that there is a z-shaped curve of fixed points. Along the lower branch, there is a Hopf bifurcation at $\sigma(r)$, and fixed points with $S_{tot} > \sigma(r)$ are stable with respect to the fast subsystem. There is also a subcritical Hopf bifurcation HB along the upper branch of the curve of fixed points; from here bifurcates a branch of periodic orbits. This branch extends to the right beyond $\sigma(r)$ before turning around and terminating at a homoclinic orbit with $S_{tot} \approx \sigma(r)$.

This bifurcation structure persists for each r, $0 \leq r \leq 1$. The two-parameter bifurcation diagram is shown in Fig. 13.14(C). The fast subsystem exhibits sustained oscillations for $S_{tot} < \sigma(r)$ and a stable resting state for $S_{tot} > \sigma(r)$.

We now treat r and S_{tot} as dynamic variables in the full E-cell model and consider how the cell responds to an inhibitory input. Fig. 13.14(B) shows a rebound burst from an E cell given a constant level of synaptic inhibitory input and then released from inhibition. In the following analysis, we derive simplified equations for the slow variables that explain the general character of the cell's response.

We will reduce the full model to equations for just the slow variables r and S_{tot}. To simplify the analysis, we will assume that both $r_\infty(v)$ and

$\tau_r(v)$ are piecewise constant; that is, during the active phase, $r_\infty(v) = 0$ and $\tau_r(v) = \tau_A$, while in the silent phase $r_\infty(v) = 1$ and $\tau_r(v) = \tau_S$.

Since r and S_{tot} are slow variables, we will write $\phi_r = \varepsilon$, $\beta = \varepsilon\kappa$, and $\tau = \varepsilon t$. Now suppose that the E cell receives a constant level of inhibitory input for $0 \leq \tau \leq T_0$. During this time, the slow variables satisfy

$$S_{tot} = 1 \tag{23}$$

$$r' = (1 - r)/\tau_S \tag{24}$$

where differentiation is with respect to τ. The cell is released from inhibition at $\tau = T_0$. For $\tau > T_0$, S_{tot} decays according to the equation $S'_{tot} = -\kappa S_{tot}$. As long as $S_{tot} > \sigma(r)$, r satisfies (23). The trajectory must eventually cross the curve $\mathcal{C} \equiv \{S_{tot} = \sigma(r)\}$, after which r decays according to the equation

$$r' = -r/\tau_A. \tag{25}$$

The projection of the rebound burst in Fig. 13.14(B) onto the (S_{tot}, r) slow phase-plane is shown in Fig. 13.14(C). The E cell rebounds and begins to fire action potentials when (S_{tot}, r) crosses the curve $\mathcal{C}$. At $\mathcal{C}$, the spike frequency is positive because the stable periodic orbit is away from the homoclinic orbit; the frequency decreases as (S_{tot}, r) evolves through the firing region. The rebound is a graded response: a longer inhibitory input allows r to increase to a higher level and leads to a more powerful burst. Eventually $(S_{tot}, r) \to (0, 0)$ and the E cell approaches its low, intrinsic firing rate.

We now use geometric methods to analyze the clustered solutions for the network shown in Fig. 13.10. We will focus on mechanisms by which two distinct clusters may switch between one being active and the other silent. For simplicity, we consider the network shown in Fig. 13.15(A) in which each cluster contains just one pair of cells — *Cluster 1* consists of E_1 and I_1 while *Cluster 2* consists of E_2 and I_2.

We will describe two mechanisms that can be responsible for clustered rhythms. In the first example, the switch between one cluster being active and the other silent depends solely on properties of the E cells; here, the I cells simply respond to E input. In the second example, the switch depends on the I cells.

The closed curve in Fig. 13.15(B) is the projection onto (S_{tot}, r) phase-space of an E-cell trajectory for a clustered solution, our first example. Cells E_1 and E_2 have the same projected trajectory in this plane, but they are

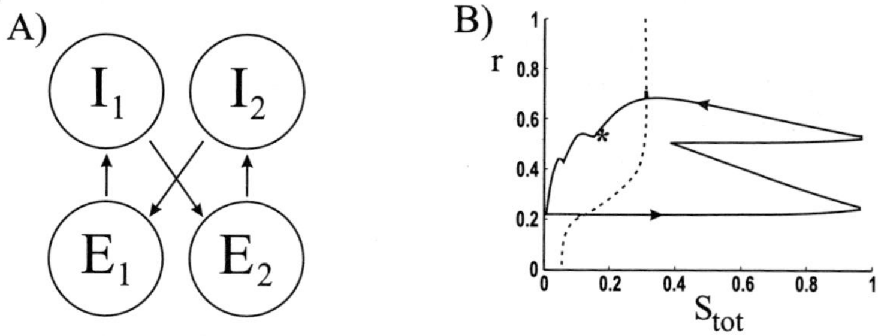

Fig. 13.15. A) The simple E-I network used in the analysis. B) The projection of a clustered solution onto the (S_{tot}, r) phase-space.

out of phase. We follow the solution beginning at a time when E_1 is just about to fire a spike; at this time, (S^1_{tot}, r_1) is at the point marked $*$ in the figure and (S^2_{tot}, r_2) is at the lower left corner of the closed curve. The slow variables corresponding to both E cells lie in the firing region $S_{tot} < \sigma(r)$ with $r_2 < r_1$. When E_1 fires its action potential, it induces I_1 to fire which, in turn, sends inhibition to E_2 causing (S^2_{tot}, r_2) to shoot nearly horizontally out of the firing region.

While Cluster 1 is active, the slow variables (S^1_{tot}, r_1) lie in the firing region and E_1 is able to spike and induce I_1 to fire. As Cluster 1 continues to fire, the slow variable r_1 decreases (see (25)), resulting in a decrease of the spike frequency of E_1. Moreover, continuing inhibition to Cluster 2 allows r_2 to increase, allowing E_2 to more easily rebound (see (23)).

Once r_2 is high enough and E_1 firing is slow enough, E_2 is able to rebound from an I_1 spike. At this time, the positions of (S^1_{tot}, r_1) and (S^2_{tot}, r_2) have switched with respect to their initial positions. In the example shown in Fig. 13.15(B), there are just two spikes per burst.

We note that this mechanism for clustering involves both escape and release. In order for Cluster 2 to begin firing, r_2 must be sufficiently high so that E_2 can 'escape'; that is, rebound from inhibition. However, escape is not possible until the frequency of E_1 is slow enough; that is, Cluster 1 also 'releases' the silent cluster.

We now consider a different mechanism, illustrated in Fig. 13.16, in which the switch between silent and active clusters depends on the slow current I_{AHP} in the I cells. With each I spike, the calcium level Ca_I increases; this enhances I_{AHP}, which tends to hyperpolarize the cell. This in turn makes the I cell less sensitive to excitation from the active E cell. It

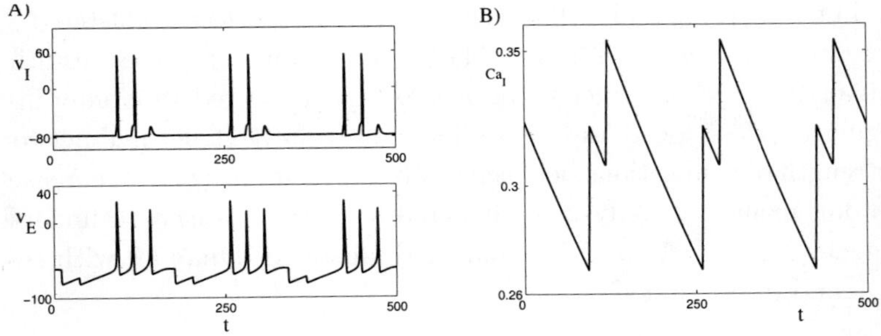

Fig. 13.16. Clustered activity in the simple E-I network. Firing in the active cluster terminates when calcium builds up in the I cell so that it can no longer respond to excitatory input. A) Membrane potential of the I cell (top) and E cell (bottom). B) I cell calcium concentration.

is possible that if Ca_I is sufficiently large then the I cell will no longer be able to respond to E-cell excitation and this terminates the cluster's active phase. Once the I cell stops firing, the silent cluster is able to rebound from inhibition and this cluster 'takes over'. Figure 13.16(A) illustrates this phenomenon: note that an E cell fires three spikes in a burst but the I cell responds to only the first two spikes.

In this section, we have assumed that I_{app} was chosen sufficiently hyperpolarizing so that the I cell can fire only in response to E input. For higher values of I_{app}, isolated I cells fire continuously or in bursts. Each I spike may induce an E cell to fire, by the same mechanism described above. In this case, the network behavior may simply reflect the intrinsic I dynamics. More complicated behavior is certainly possible. For example, the E cell may not respond on every I cycle or E $\rightarrow$ I excitation may disrupt I firing.

13.4.5. *Transitions and dependence on parameters*

Figure 13.17 shows *principle component analysis* (PCA) of network activity for different values of I_{app} and $g_{I\rightarrow E}$ for a regularly-structured network without direct connections between inhibitory neurons. Over this range of parameter values, the network dynamics may be irregular, perfectly clustered, or *nearly clustered*; near-clustering occurs in this network when there are two groups of cells that take turns firing, but the cells within a group are not precisely synchronized. In order to account for the small time differences in firing within near-clusters, we average the time series data over a moving window before performing standard PCA computation. As indicated in the figure, network dynamics tend to be irregular when I_{app} is large but $g_{I\to E}$ is small, while cells tend to be perfectly clustered when I_{app} is small and $g_{I\to E}$ is large. The set of parameter values resulting in irregular dynamics is larger if the network is connected randomly instead of regularly [15]; it decreases in size for the regularly-structured network as the strength of connections between inhibitory neurons ($g_{I\to I}$) increases [2]. From our geometric analysis of clustered activity, it is easy to understand this general distribution of irregular and clustered dynamics with respect to I_{app} and $g_{I\to E}$ values.

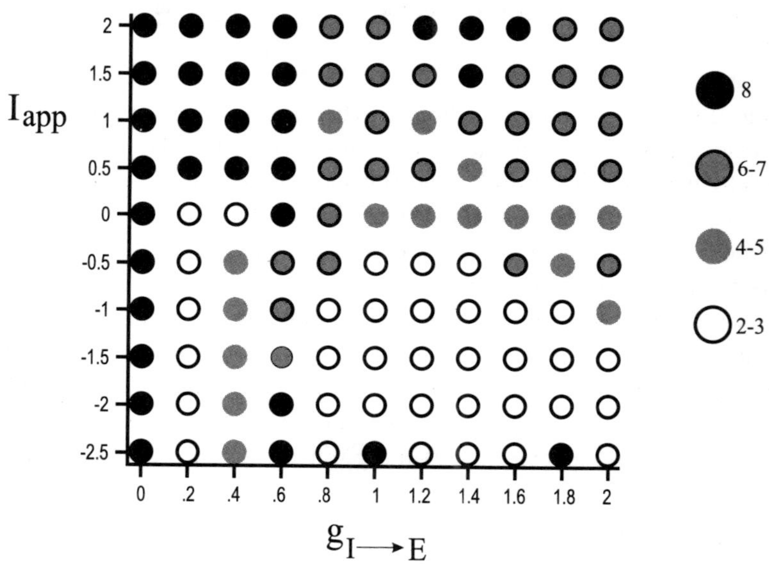

Fig. 13.17. Dependence of clustering on the strength of inhibition to I cells (I_{app}) and $I \to E$ inhibition for a network of ten I cells (each inhibiting the three nearest E cells) and ten E cells (each contacting the closest I cell). Voltage time series of I cells were averaged over 5 msec time windows before PCA. The legend shows the number of components required to explain 80% of the variance for the time series.

Consider the regularly-structured network with high $g_{I\to E}$ and low I_{app}; this corresponds to the lower right portion of Fig. 13.17. Recall that for low values of I_{app}, the I cells can fire only in response to E input. Since $g_{I\to E}$ is high, these I response spikes send strong inhibition to E cells, increasing their r values and thereby supporting their ability to rebound.

In this region of parameter space, these effects dominate network dynamics, and the full network breaks into two clusters with transitions as described in the previous section for I-driven clusters: when inhibitory cells in the active cluster can no longer respond to the excitatory cells, they release silent excitatory cells from inhibition. Figure 13.11(B) illustrates a clustered solution from this parameter regime.

Moving to the left in Fig. 13.17, corresponding to decreasing $g_{I \to E}$, the synchronizing influence of inhibition becomes less powerful. Cells may still organize into clusters, but at a much slower rate, and E cells increasingly display their intrinsic firing patterns. When clustering occurs, transitions are determined by E cell escape and release mechanisms as described above.

When $g_{I \to E} < 0.8$, increasing I_{app} to nonnegative values disrupts the ability of the network to separate into distinct groups of cells. At these parameter values, isolated I cells exhibit bursting behavior for nonnegative levels of I_{app}. Within the network, the I cells sometimes fire bursts without prompting from an E cell; additionally, I cells respond to E-cell input. The number of spikes in the I cell response may depend sensitively on recent cell interactions as expressed by the function $\pi(\tau)$ described in section 13.4.3; the result is irregular network activity as shown in Fig. 13.11(A).

Spontaneous activity of I cells does not necessarily prevent clustering, though it may disallow synchronization within a cluster. Consider again the parameter region represented in the lower right portion of Fig. 13.17 where clustering is strong and precisely synchronized. As I_{app} increases, I cells are more able to respond to E-cell spikes; bursts lengthen. In fact, bursts no longer terminate when an I-cell fails to respond to an E-cell spike; rather an active I cell falls silent only after excitation from an E-cell ends. The mechanism for transitions must then be the mechanism that silences an active E cell: the arrival of inhibition from a spontaneously active I cell. This mechanism prevents synchronization of the E cells within a cluster: the spontaneously active I cell sends inhibition to a set of E cells that includes both active and silent cells. These particular silent cells are then receiving more inhibition than any other cells in the network; they are unable to join the newly active cluster until a significant portion of it decays, a slow process compared to the recruitment of unaffected cells.

Acknowledgments

This work was supported by the NSF grant DMS-0414057 to DT and NSF Agreement No. 0112050.

References

[1] K. Alligood, T. Sauer, and J. Yorke, *Chaos: An Introduction to Dynamical Systems*, Springer-Verlag, New York, (1997).

[2] J. Best, C. Park, D. Terman, and C. J. Wilson, Transitions between irregular and rhythmic firing patterns in a model for the indirect pathway of the basal ganglia, *In Preparation.*

[3] T. R. Chay and J. Rinzel, Bursting, beating, and chaos in an excitable membrane model, *Biophys. J.* **47**, 357–366, (1985).

[4] E. J . Doedel, A. R. Chapneys, T. F. Fairgrieve, Y. A. Kuznetsov, B. Sandstede, and X. Wang, AUTO97: continuation and bifurcation software for ODEs (with HOMCONT), *Concordia University Technical Report* (1997).

[5] N. Fenichel, Persistence and smoothness of invariant manifolds for flows, *Indiana Univ. Math. J.* **21**, 193–226, (1971).

[6] D. Golomb, X. J. Wang, and J. Rinzel, Propagation of spindle waves in a thalamic slice model, *J. Neurophysiol.* **75**, 750–769, (1996).

[7] E. M. Izhikevich, Neural excitability, spiking, and bursting, *International J. of Bifurcation and Chaos* **10**, 1171– 1266, (2000).

[8] O. S. Kozlovski, Getting rid of the negative Schwarzian derivative condition, *Annals of Mathematics* **152**, 743–762, (2000).

[9] E. Lee and D. Terman, Uniqueness and stability of periodic bursting solutions, *J.D.E.* **158**, 48–78, (1999).

[10] A. I. Neishtadt, Persistence of stability loss for dynamical bifurcations. 2, *Differential Equations* **24**, 171–176, (1988).

[11] J. Rinzel, D. Terman, X. J. Wang, and B. Ermentrout, Propagating activity patterns in large-scale inhibitory neuronal networks, *Science* **279**, 1351–1355, (1998).

[12] J. Rinzel, A formal classification of bursting mechanisms in excitable systems, *Pro. Inter. Congress of Math.*, Ed. A. M. Gleason, American Mathematial Society, p. 1578–1594, (1987).

[13] J. Rubin and D. Terman, Geometric singular perturbation analysis of neuronal dynamics, *Handbook of Dynamical Systems II: Towards Applications*, Ed. B. Fiedler, Elsevier, Amsterdam, p. 93–146, (2002).

[14] J. Rubin and D. Terman, Analysis of clustered firing patterns in synaptically coupled networks of oscillators, *J. Math. Biology* **41**, 513–545, (2000).

[15] D. Terman, J. Rubin, A. C. Yew, and C. Wilson, Activity patterns in a model for the subthalamopallidal network of the basal ganglia,

J. Neuroscience **22**, 2963–2976, (2002).

[16] D. Terman, G. B. Ermentrout, and A. C. Yew, Propagating activity patterns in thalamic neuronal networks, *SIAM J. Applied Math.* **61**, 1578–1604, (2001).

[17] D. Terman, Chaotic spikes arising from a model of bursting in excitable membranes, *SIAM J. Appl. Math.* **51**, 1418–1450, (1991).

[18] D. Terman, The transition from bursting to continuous spiking in excitable membrane models, *J. Nonlinear Sci.* **2**, 135–182, (1992).

[19] H. Thunberg, Periodicity versus chaos in one-dimensional dynamics, *SIAM Review* **43**, 3–30, (2001).

[20] X. J. Wang and J. Rinzel, Alternating and synchronous rhythms in reciprocally inhibitory model neurons, *Neural Computation* **4**, 84–97, (1992).

CHAPTER 14

ELLIPTIC BURSTERS, DEPOLARIZATION BLOCK, AND WAVES

Bard Ermentrout

Department of Mathematics, University of Pittsburgh, Pittsburgh, PA 15260, USA
e-mail: bard@euler.math.pitt.edu

Joyeeta Dutta-Moscato

Department of Neuroscience, University of Pittsburgh, Pittsburgh, PA 15260, USA

David Pinto

Department of Neurobiology & Anatomy, University of Rochester, Box 603 601 Elmwood Ave., Rochester, NY 14642, USA
e-mail: David_Pinto@URMC.Rochester.edu

Cortical slices bathed in low magnesium with reduced inhibition are able to sustain propagating waves of spikes. Intracellular recordings suggest that a possible mechanism for termination of waves is depolarization block of the sodium channels. In some instances, repeated waves occur with a frequency of 10-15 Hz. In other instances, the waves splinter into locally active regions. We describe a bursting model based on the interplay between slow synaptic depolarization and block. We show that waves can oscillate and break-up depending on parameters. A simplified normal form permits some insight into the underlying dynamics.

14.1. Introduction

The propagation of activity in biological neural networks is of fundamental importance since activity is information. One highly reduced experimental model is the cortical slice in which a piece of brain is kept alive in a dish while pharmacologically and electrically manipulated. The aim of this preparation is to get at some of the local circuitry in the tissue. Recent recordings [4] and in the Pinto lab show distinctive behavior in slices where the inhibition is blocked and the tissue is bathed in lowered magnesium. A consequence of the latter is that the NMDA receptors are unblocked. Excitatory neurotransmission affects several receptors: AMPA, responsible for short and fast excitation; and NMDA, responsible for longer-lasting excitation. Thus, in the low magnesium slice, the effects of connections between neurons can last for almost 100 milliseconds instead of the typical AMPA response lasting less than 5 milliseconds. Such a slice is quite excited and the dense recurrent connections between the neurons can lead to sustained activity. However, typically, a stimulus produces a propagating transient response (a traveling pulse) with a finite life-time. Under some conditions, the pulse becomes an oscillation in the firing rate of the neuron with bouts of firing followed by silence. There is never a situation when the neurons fire continuously after a stimulus. Thus, we can ask what terminates the repetitive spiking and if it repeats, what causes the re-excitation? One can imagine several possible mechanisms for the termination of activity: 1) slow build up of some extracellular current, e.g., an adaptation current; 2) synaptic depression where the synaptic currents dwindle after repeated firings; or 3) depolarization block. The latter happens to cells which are depolarized so much that the sodium channels cannot recover and so they fail to produce spikes.

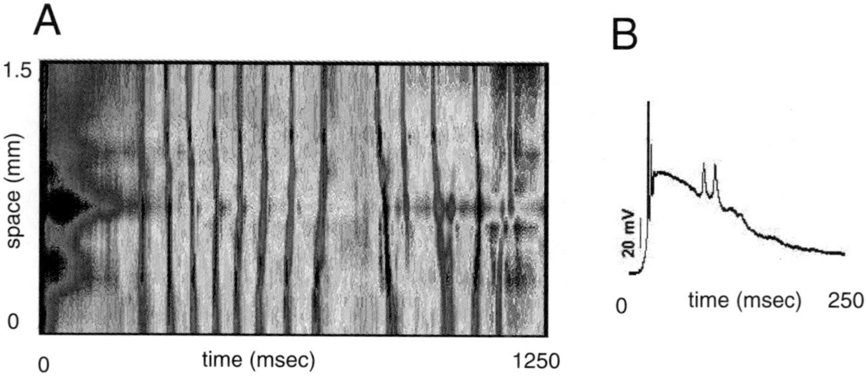

Fig. 14.1. Waves produced in a slice of rat somatosensory cortex. (A) shows the spatio-temporal evolution of the local field potential recorded with a 16 electrode array in a slice bathed in low magnesium. (B) Intracellular recording of a cell in a slice with reduced inhibition showing termination of spikes while the cell remains strongly depolarized.

Figure 14.1 shows two different experiments demonstrating periodic waves in a low magnesium slice (A) and the intracellular potential during a solitary wave in a slice with reduced inhibition (B). The intracellular recording suggests depolarization block. There is a regime of large depolarization which produces a few initial spikes. Then there is a silent region until the potential drops whereby the cell produces two small action potentials. Based on this recording, we will presume that the reason that the waves terminate is depolarization block.

The rest of this chapter is organized as follows. We introduce the model in section 14.2. Next, we analyze the bursting of this and examine the behavior of a one-dimensional coupled array of these cells. We demonstrate some unusual behavior in certain parameter regimes and then explain this with some simplified models.

14.2. Methods

We use a biophysical model of a pyramidal neuron that was first implemented by Golomb and Amitai [2]. The equations are:

$$C\frac{dV}{dt} = -I_L - I_{Nap} - I_{Na} - I_K - I_m - I_{syn} \equiv -I_{ion} - I_{syn} \qquad (1)$$

where $I_L = g_L(V - E_L)$ is a passive leak, $I_{Nap} = g_{NaP}p_\infty(V)(V - E_{Na})$ is a persistent sodium current, $I_{Na} = g_{Na}m_\infty^3(V)h(V - E_{Na})$ is a transient sodium current, $I_K = g_K n^4(V - E_K)$ is the delayed rectifier potassium current, and $I_m = g_m z(V - E_K)$ is a slow potassium current. Parameters for these current are given in Golomb and Amitai [2]. (All simulation files are available from Bard Ermentrout upon request). The synaptic current is excitatory, satisfying $I_{syn}(x) = g_{syn}\sum_{x'} J(x - x')s(x', t)(V - E_{syn})$ where

$$\frac{ds}{dt} = 0.4(1 - s)/(1 + \exp(-(V - V_{th})/5)) - \beta s. \qquad (2)$$

The parameter β sets the decay rate of the synapses and is varied in this chapter. The parameter V_{th} determines the voltage threshold for the activation of a synapse and is also important. All synapses are excitatory so that $E_{syn} = 0$. We do not include a magnesium block term (which affects the slow NMDA excitatory synapses) since the experiments of interest were carried out in low magnesium. All simulations were carried out with XPPAUT using an adaptive time-step integrator.

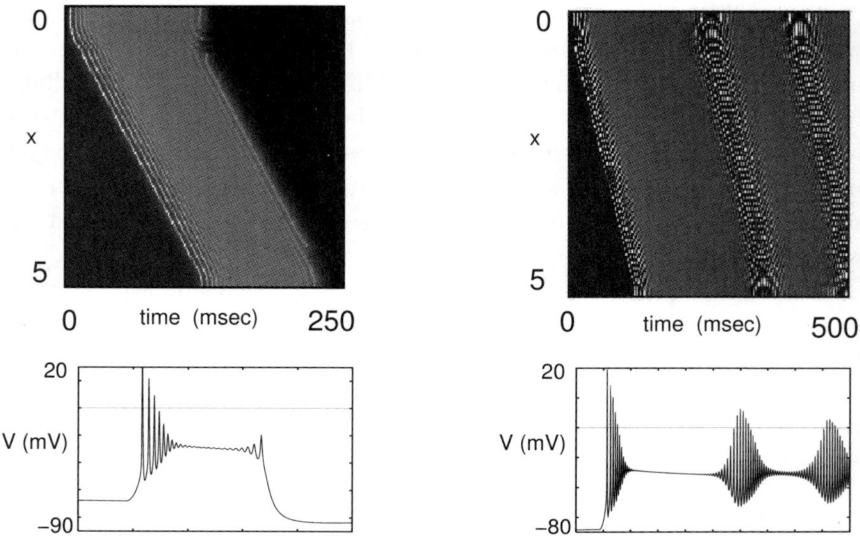

Fig. 14.2. Simulation of 100 cells in a line with a square footprint. Left figure shows a transient wave of excitation propagating across the medium. The potassium conductance, $g_K = 2$ is reduced slightly from the default, $g_K = 3$ to prevent repolarization of the spikes, $\beta = 0.04$, and $V_{th} = 0$ making oscillatory activity more difficult. The right figure is the same except that $g_K = 3$, $\beta = 0.01$ and $V_{th} = -10$.

14.3. Results

Figure 14.2 shows a pair of simulations of a line of 100 cells with a square-wave footprint, $J(x) = H(10 - |x|)/21$,where $H(x)$ is the step function. In each case, the network was started at rest and a group of 5 cells was excited at one end. Depending on the parameters in the model, the network is able to produce either a single broad wave of activity (left panel) or a sustained oscillatory response. The left and right panels in Fig. 14.2 should be compared to Fig. 14.1. Our goal in the rest of this chapter is to explain the simulations in Fig. 14.2 and thus shed some light on the mechanisms underlying the activity in Fig. 14.1.

14.3.1. *The burster*

In order to understand the basic rhythmicity of the present model, we suppose that the synaptic time course is slow relative to the spiking of the individual neuron. Thus, we make the usual slow-fast ansatz [1] in order to dissect the burster. The idea at the single cell level is as follows. If the cell is excited, it turns on the synapse which further depolarizes the cell. This causes the cell to fire faster and release more transmitter. As the level of depolarization increases, it becomes more difficult for the sodium channels to deinactivate so that the spikes become smaller and disappear. This stops synaptic transmission and causes the cell to slowly repolarize towards rest. If the repolarization is sufficiently fast, then the cell will drop to rest. If it is slow enough, then as the synaptic current to the cell diminishes, the cell can begin to spike again. This depolarizes the cell into block and the cycle begins. We now make this intuitive mechanism precise.

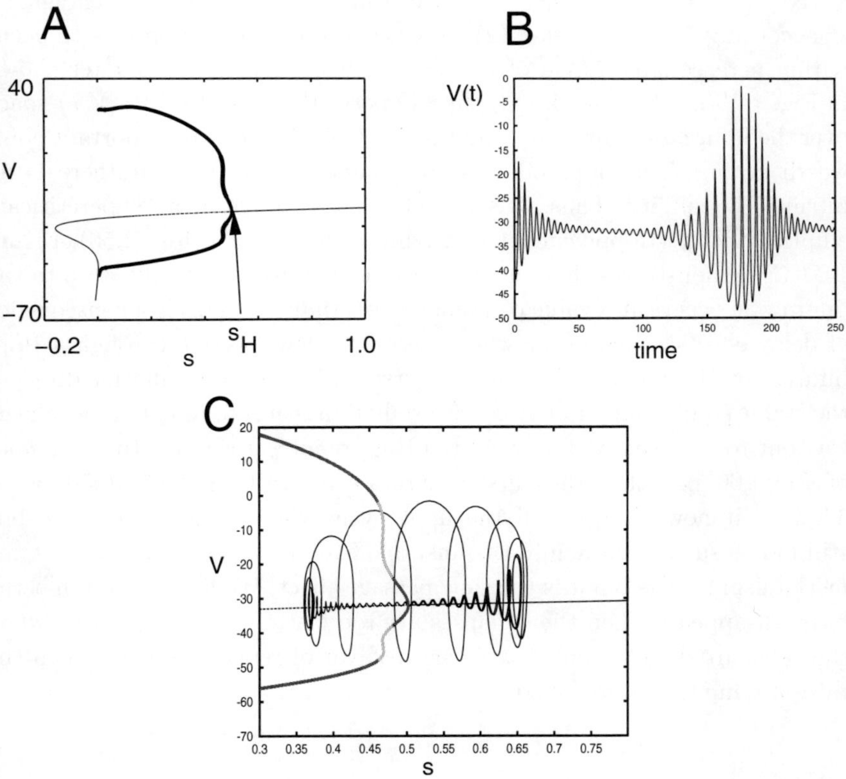

Fig. 14.3. The single elliptic burster. (A) Bifurcation diagram as the synaptic gate, s increases with $g_{syn} = 0.3$ and parameters as in Fig. 14.2(B). Note the block at about $s = 0.5$ as the upper state is restabilized at a Hopf bifurcation (S_H). The large branch of periodic orbits terminates at a saddle node near $s = 0$. (B) Voltage of the single cell burster where s obeys equation (2). (C) Single cell burster in (s, V)-plane overlaid on the bifurcation diagram. Light-gray-unstable periodic orbits; dark gray - stable periodic orbits; dashed line - unstable fixed point; solid line - stable fixed point or trajectory.

We consider equation (1) where I_{syn} is replaced by $I_{syn} = g_{syn}s(V - E_{syn})$ with s constant. Since the synapse is "slow" (or at least, that is our simplifying assumption), we compute the bifurcation diagram for equation (1) with s as a parameter in Fig. 14.3(A). For small values of s, there is a single stable fixed point at a relatively negative potential. As s increases, this fixed point is lost at a saddle-node bifurcation giving rise to large amplitude periodic orbits. Further increases in s depolarize the membrane causing the amplitude of the spikes to decrease until a Hopf bifurcation is reached at $s = s_H$. For larger values of s, the depolarized state is stable and depolarization block occurs.

Next, we consider a self excited cell in which s is itself dependent on V according to the equation (2). If we choose the activation of s to occur within a reasonable range of potentials, then we create a burster shown in Fig. 14.3(B). Figure 14.3(C) superimposes the trajectory in (V, s)-space over the bifurcation diagram from Fig. 14.3(A). There is an important point worth noting. The Hopf bifurcation is supercritical, so that there is no intrinsic bistability. Thus, this model is an example of a "supercritical" elliptic burster (Hoppensteadt and Izhikevich, 1997 [3], Fig. 2.59). Figure 14.3(C) demonstrates that the jump from the unstable steady state to the limit cycle occurs at a value of s much lower than s_H. This is a consequence of delay effects which occur when there is a slow passage through a Hopf bifurcation [1]. There is also a large overshoot before the oscillation drops to the stable equilibrium. (That is, the oscillation seems to remain large all the way out to $s = 0.65$, well beyond the Hopf point.) If we slow the dynamics of s by 100-fold, then the burst occupies a region $0.48 < s < 0.50 \approx s_H$. That is, it now "jumps" off the limit cycle where it is expected to but still moves substantially into the unstable fixed point. This means that the mechanism for the burst is the slow passage effect. We finally note that the burst disappears when the synapses are too fast. The burst persists when the rates are doubled but disappears in favor of repetitive firing when the rates are multiplied four-fold.

14.3.2. *Breaking up is easy to do*

What happens to the oscillatory waves in Fig. 14.2 if the synaptic time course is sped up. Bursts are robust as long as the synapses do not run too fast. Figures 14.4 (A), (B) show an interesting effect if the synaptic rate is doubled. The figure shows the initial formation of oscillatory waves, but these eventually breakup into distinct local regions that look very much

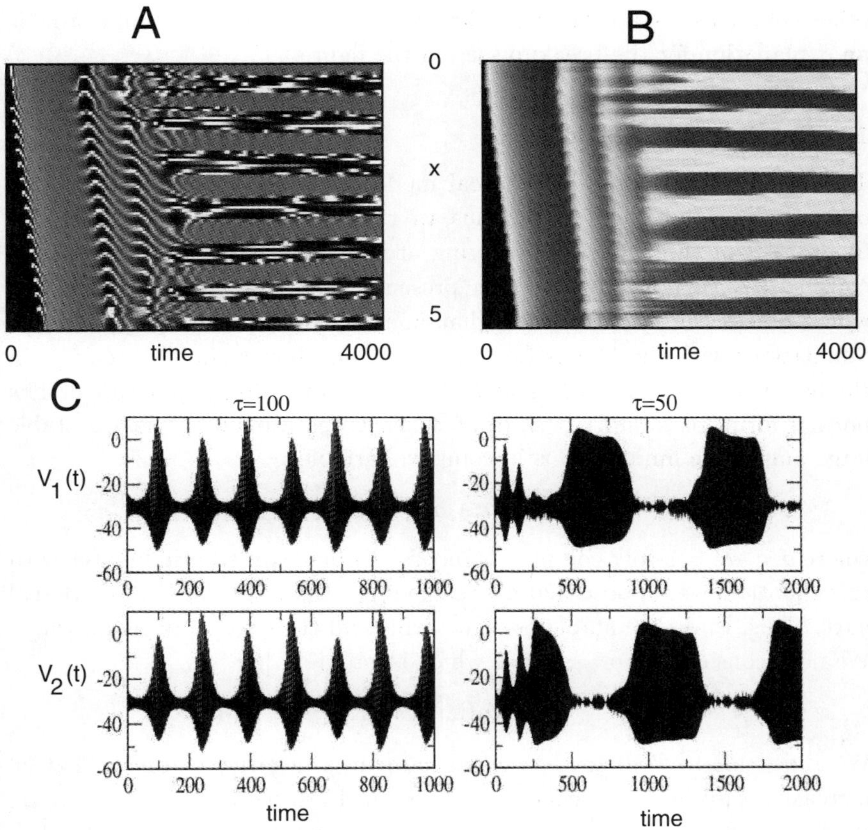

Fig. 14.4. Break-up of the oscillatory waves. A. Spatio-temporal evolution of the potential when the synapses are twice as fast as in Fig. 14.2(B). Synaptic gating variables, $s_j(t)$. C. Behavior of a pair of coupled neurons as a function of τ. Left panel shows that they are almost synchronous with a slight asymmetry in the amplitudes for $\tau = 100$ msec. Right panel shows an extreme asymmetry in the behavior for $\tau = 50$ msec.

like stripes of alternating activity. Figure 14.4(B) shows this more clearly through the synaptic gates, s_j. This is an example of pattern-formation with *no inhibition.* There is only excitatory coupling. However, the coupling is effectively inhibitory. For increasing the presynaptic spiking actually reduces the postsynaptic ability to spike. We illustrate this in Fig. 14.4(C), where we couple just two cells. (Each cell receives half its synaptic input from the other cell, so that they receive identical input.) Even when $\tau = 100$ msec, there is a slight asymmetry. (This disappears when $\tau = 200$ msec.) At $\tau = 50$ msec, there is a strong asymmetry with one cell suppressing the other cell. This instability of synchrony at short values of τ could provide an explanation for the breakup seen in the figure.

14.3.3. *A normal form*

The complexities of the biophysical model preclude any kind of analysis other than careful simulations. Thus, we turn to a caricature of the present model. All of the action is occurring around the Hopf bifurcation so we consider a normal form model. The present system has a supercritical Hopf which makes the bursting somewhat non-robust and difficult to analyze. Simulations with the Morris-Lecar (ML) model show a similar break up in the behavior but in the ML model, the Hopf bifurcation is subcritical. The normal form for a subcritical Hopf which turns around to yield a stable large amplitude limit cycle is in complex variables:

$$z' = z(c + a|z|^2 - |z|^4)$$

where a, c are possibly complex numbers. To make an elliptic burster with this equation, we suppose that c is real and positive and a has a positive real part. Thus, there is a stable periodic orbit and the fixed point is unstable. We next consider a slow synapse which is gated by $|z|$:

$$s' = (|z| - s)/\tau.$$

We allow this to feedback to the oscillator in a negative manner. That is, increasing s pushes the oscillator back to rest. In the coordinates, $z = u+iv$, the burster is three variables; the fast system consists of (u, v) and the slow system consists of s:

$$\begin{aligned} u' &= (c + ar^2 - r^4 - ds)u - v \\ v' &= (c + ar^2 - r^4 - ds)v + u \\ s' &= (r - s)/\tau \\ r &= \sqrt{(}u^2 + v^2). \end{aligned}$$

Since s only depends on the magnitude $r \equiv |z|$ we can separate out the magnitude and s to obtain a two variable burster for the envelope, r of the burst and s. Writing $z = r\exp(i\theta)$, the burster is:

$$r' = r(c - ds + ar^2 - r^4) \quad \text{and} \quad s' = (r - s)/\tau.$$

The phase θ satisfies the trivial equation $\theta' = 1$. We first note that d must be sufficiently large in order for there to be a burster. The r-nullcline for this system is $r = 0$ and $ds = F(r) \equiv c + ar^2 - r^4$. In order for there to be an oscillation, the equilibrium point, $r = s$ and $F(r) - dr = 0$ must be on the middle branch.The maximum of $F(r)$ occurs at a value $F^* = c + a^2/4$ when $r = \sqrt(a/2)$. The minimum value of d will thus be that value for which $dr^* = F^*$; that is $d > d_{min} = (c + a^2/4)/\sqrt(a/2)$.

As with the full biophysical model, we can arrange these in a one-dimensional network which has the complex form:

$$z_t = z(c - d \int J(x-y)s(y)\ dy + a|z|^2 - |z|^4)$$
$$s_t = (|z| - s)/\tau.$$

Figure 14.5(A) shows a simulation of this simple model, plotting $r(x,t)$ As with the cortical model, the network breaks into spatial domains of activity separated by silent domains. Unlike Fig. 14.4, however, the spatial domains are more irregular.

14.3.4. *Elliptic dentistry*

Figure 14.5(B) shows the profile of $r(x)$ from the simulation in Fig. 14.5(A). Note the appearance of many tooth-like structures; none of them particularly broad. These are stationary with respect to the (r,s) system, so that the existence of these reduces to an analysis of $s(x) = |z|(x) \equiv r(x)$ where

$$0 = r(x)[F(r(x)) - d \int_\Omega J(x-y)r(y)\ dy].$$

Here Ω is the domain of the network; it is not very important. Consider a single stationary peak on the interval $a < x < b$ contained in Ω. We show that as long as $d > d_{crit}$, there is a maximal width that such a peak can take. Such a pulse must satisfy:

$$F(r(x)) = d \int_a^b J(x-y)r(y)\ dy \equiv dW(x)$$

for $a < x < b$. The function F is parabola-shaped, so that for each value of $dW \in (c, F^*)$, there will be two roots to $F(r) = dW$. We conjecture that only those values of $r > r^*$ correspond to stable solutions. (This is typical in many bistable systems with cubic nonlinearities; the "middle branch" is generally unstable.) Since J is positive and integrates to 1 over the domain Ω, we see that as the width of the pulse gets larger, $W(x) > r*$ since $r(x) > r^*$. Thus $dW(x) > dr^*$. However, in order for there to be an elliptic burster for the scalar model, we required that $dr^* > F^*$, thus, we have $dW(x) > F^*$ so there are no roots to $F(r) = dW$. This shows that the width of a pulse is bounded above. We note that the width is not bounded below; pulses can be as thin as possible. (You can never be too thin ...?) A proof of the general existence of these pulses will be provided elsewhere. $W(x)$ is smallest at the edges of the pulse, near $x = a$ and $x = b$ and since $F' < 0$ to the right of r^*, this means that the center of the pulse will be smaller than the edges, giving the "tooth"-like profiles seen in Fig. 14.5(B). Figure 14.5(Cb), (Cc) illustrate what happens if the pulse is too large. It splits into two smaller pulse. Another interesting property is as follows. Suppose a single pulse exists. Now introduce a second pulse a long distance away. As this moves close, it contributes to the integral and thus can cause the original pulse to split. Figure 14.5(D) shows this. There is a wide pulse for $100 \leq x \leq 125$. This pulse is supported by the medium and is shown in the dashed lines in the figure. A new pulse is created between $130 \leq x \leq 140$. Since it is close to the original pulse, it contributes enough to the integral so that $dW(x)$ becomes larger than F^*. The middle of the first pulse collapses as it is split into two. These interactions appear to be sufficient to completely explain Fig. 14.5(A), (B) and thus the original biophysical model.

14.4. Discussion

We have shown that one possible way to stop sustained recurrent activity in a disinhibited network is through depolarization block. Furthermore, by allowing the synapses to be slow enough, we suggest a mechanism underlying the slow oscillations seen in Fig. 14.1. One of the consequences of this mechanism is strong sensitivity to the time course of synaptic activation. This is because the coupling is rendered effectively inhibitory since synaptic inputs from other cells make it *less likely* that the neurons fire action potentials. One of the interesting effects of this is the appearance of spatially segregated patterns of activity. A simplified model based on normal forms and bifurcation theory provides an explanation for the spatial patterns.

There are many other possible mechanisms for the termination of sustained activity during waves. Golomb and Amitai [2] used synaptic depression to terminate their waves. We would not expect the spatial pattern formation seen in the present scenario since excitation from other cells does not suppress the spiking of the individual cell. There may be a possibility of sustained oscillations in this model; it remains to be investigated. Another reasonable mechanism for termination is a slow outward current such as a calcium dependent potassium channel. Preliminary results (Golomb,

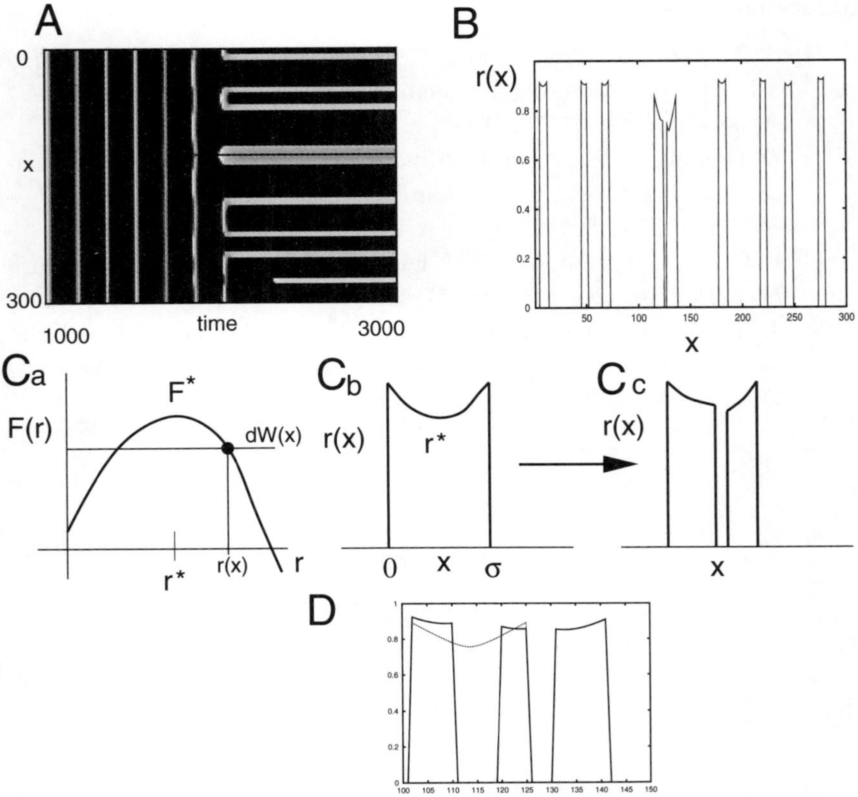

Fig. 14.5. Normal form model. (A) Breakup of the wave into active and "dead" regions – shown is the amplitude r. (B) Spatial profile of (A) at steady state showing regions of excited media separated by "dead" regions. (C) Construction of tooth-like structures. (a) $F(r) = c + ar^2 - r^4$ with maximum, F^* at $r = r^*$ and the solution at a point x satisfying $F(r(x)) = dW(x)$; (b) single tooth at maximal width; (c) breakup into a pair of smaller teeth. (D) Interaction between pulses. Original pulse is dashed. New pulse is introduced to the right which cleaves the original pulse.

Ermentrout, Curtu, unpublished) show that this model can produce slow oscillations. Since the coupling does not effectively inhibit the cells, however, there will not be spatial patterns.

Acknowledgements

Bard Ermentrout acknowledges support in part by NIMH and NSF.

References

[1] S. M. Baer, T. Erneux, and J. Rinzel, The slow passage through a Hopf bifurcation: delay, memory effects and resonance, *SIAM J. Appl. Math.* **49**, 55–71, (1988).

[2] D. Golomb and Y. Amitai, Propagating neuronal discharges in neocortical slices: computational and experimental study, *J Neurophysiol.* **78**, 1199–211, (1997).

[3] F. C. Hoppensteadt and E. M. Izhikevich, Weakly Connected Neural networks, Springer NY, (1997).

[4] J. Y. Wu, L. Guan, and Y. Tsau, Propagating activation during oscillations and evoked responses in neocortical slices, *J. Neurosci.* **19**, 5005–15, (1999).

INDEX